Periodontology Today

Proceedings of the Conference '**Periodontology Today**' held in Zurich May 6–8, 1988, on the Occasion of the 20th Anniversary of the Foundation of the European Research Group for Oral Biology (ERGOB)

Periodontology Today

Editor: *B. Guggenheim, Zurich*

Chairman of the Department for Oral Microbiology and General Immunology, Dental Institute of the University of Zurich

32 figures and 29 tables, 1988

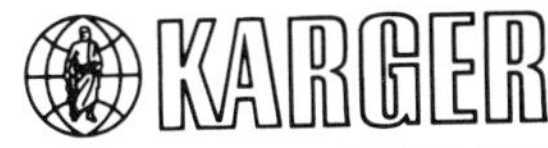

Basel · München · Paris · London · New York · New Delhi · Singapore · Tokyo · Sydney

Periodontology Today

Library of Congress Cataloging-in-Publication Data
Periodontology today.
Includes bibliographies.
1. Periodontics – Congresses. I. Guggenheim, B. II. ERGOB
[DNLM: 1. Periodontics – congresses. WU 240 P4487]
RK361.P467 1988 617.6'32 88-13725
ISBN 3-8055-4843-5

Drug Dosage
The authors and publisher have exerted every effort to ensure that drug selection and dosage set forth in this text are in accord with current recommendations and practice at the time of publication. However, in view of ongoing research, changes in government regulations, and the constant flow of information relating to drug therapy and drug reactions, the reader is urged to check the package insert for each drug for any change in indications and dosage and for added warnings and precautions. This is particularly important when the recommended agent is a new and/or infrequently employed drug.

Printed in Switzerland by Börsig Druck AG, Erlenbach
ISBN 3-8055-4843-5

Contents

Host Defense

Treatment

Summaries of Panel Discussions

Preface

The international conference **Periodontology Today** was organized to commemorate the 20th anniversary of the European Research Group for Oral Biology (ERGOB). This group was founded in 1968 during the Basel congress of the European Organization for Caries Research (ORCA). A group of young, angry, and ambitious researchers were frustrated by the 10-minute-paper-frame offered by established scientific organizations for the exchange of new information.

In consequence, ERGOB was founded with a constitution which seemed to guarantee a permanent revitalization and regeneration process. Since 1968 two meetings have been held annually. The size of the group was limited to a maximum of twelve participants to allow the free exchange of thoughts and the informal discussion of a wide spectrum of topics related to oral biology. These activities were sponsored on a long-term basis by AKZO Consumenten Produkten b. v., The Hague, ELIDA Cosmetic, Zurich, and UNILEVER Research, Port Sunlight. We are most grateful to these companies for their long-lasting generous support which will keep ERGOB afloat also in the future.

In spite of a very successful operation during the past twenty years, ERGOB was not fully immune against a certain wear and the temptation of becoming a part of the scientific establishment. I am, however, convinced that these problems will be solved and ERGOB will keep its avant-garde position distinguishing this organization from other scientific bodies.

Leaving these thoughts which are a part of the self-examination process linked to anniversaries, we would prefer to explain the purpose of this conference and herewith the context of this book. The scope of this meeting was to assess the state of the art in periodontology today. There are a number of reasons for doing it at this point in time:

A great part of the world-wide dental research potential has gradually shifted to the periodontal area. Dental caries prevalence is substantially declining at least in developped countries. Years of basic caries research efforts and especially of preventive and community dentistry are bearing fruit. Further progress will be made, however, although it appears to be rather technical than conceptual. In contrast, periodontology is today a passionately debated issue. There is little consensus in fundamental perceptions of the pathogenesis, etiology and certain epidemiological aspects of periodontal diseases in spite of the fact that therapy and prevention of certain forms have steadily advanced in recent years.

Currently at debate are e.g. most simplistic concepts of the microbial etiology and indiscerning narrow views of the immunopathology of periodontal diseases. None of these concepts are really new. They rather have kept surfacing in various wrappings with a sinus-like function for almost a century. Some of the currently still widely accepted paradigms – like chronic gingivitis progressing inevitably to periodontitis – are not based on the strict experimental doctrine of Claude Bernard but have evolved by empirical thinking. On the other hand, many results of strictly controlled *in vitro* experiments using most advanced technology have provided a flood of new hypotheses on pathomechanisms of these diseases. However, the gap between the integration of the results of most elegant *in vitro* studies and the results of empirical thinking is not as wide as many might believe.

These are the issues which are addressed in this book and were discussed at the conference **Periodontology Today.** The scientific committee has carefully selected speakers known to take a stand for one or the other side on many debated issues in periodontology today. While the overall structure of the resulting main chapters is not different from other publications, the titles within each chapter were formulated in a rather provocative way. This book is therefore not a volume of discovery of new research data but rather a document describing how existing data could be integrated into conceivable concepts. It furthermore contains a summary of the discussions which took place at the conference. They have been edited by the moderators of each session. From an intellectual point of view, it is a pleasure to read how this concentration of the best brains in the field coped with the polarity of views. As limited as the syntheses achieved may be, it was well worthwile arranging the conference and publishing this book.

B. Guggenheim

Periodontology Today. Int. Congr., Zürich 1988, pp. 1–5 (Karger, Basel 1988)

What is a Clinically Healthy Periodontium?

Jan L. Wennström

Department of Periodontology, School of Dentistry, University of Göteborg, Göteborg, Sweden

Introduction

The periodontium is a functional system of tissues supporting the teeth, including gingiva, periodontal ligament, root cementum and alveolar bone. Clinically, a normal periodontium is characterized by a gingiva which (i) has a pale pink color and a firm consistency, (ii) shows a scalloped outline of the soft tissue margin and occupies the entire space below the contact area of neighboring teeth and (iii) does not bleed on gentle probing in the gingival sulcus/pocket area.

In a histological section, the normal gingiva shows absence of infiltrates of inflammatory cells and only few neutrophilic granulocytes and mononuclear cells may be found within the marginal portion of the junctional epithelium (ATTSTRÖM, GRAF-DE BEER and SCHROEDER 1975, LINDHE and RYLANDER 1975). A gingival sulcus is seldom seen and the most apical cells of the junctional epithelium are located at or close to the cementoenamel junction which coincides with the most coronally located collagen fibers of the periodontal ligament. Furthermore, histologically as well as radiographically, the alveolar bone crest of the normal periodontium is found approximately 1 mm apical to the cementoenamel junction.

A normal periodontium is rarely found in humans, but may be established under experimental conditions. Biopsies obtained from areas with clinically healthy periodontium have revealed that a small infiltrate of inflammatory cells is always present in the coronal portion of the gingiva adjacent to the junctional epithelium (PAGE and SCHROEDER 1976). Should this inflammatory response be considered as a pathologic process indicating periodontal disease, i.e. gingivitis? Or, could the periodontium be classified as healthy despite the presence of such an inflammatory cell infiltrate? If so, where should we then draw the borderline between health and disease?

Clinical evaluation

Since it is not possible to obtain a histopathological diagnosis in each particular area of a dentition, we have to rely upon clinical signs and symptoms of the pathological process in the periodontium when determining the condition of the supporting apparatus. In order to distinguish between a clinically healthy and a clinically diseased periodontium, a proper understanding of the biological mechanisms underlying these signs and symptoms is fundamental. Clinically, periodontal disease is recognized by (1) inflammatory alterations of the gingiva, such as swelling and redness of the gingival margin, (2) bleeding on gentle probing in the gingival sulcus/pocket area and (3) reduced resistance of the periodontal tissues to probing, i.e. increased probing or pocket depth. In addition, tissue recession and reduced alveolar bone height may be evident.

Color and texture alterations

A clinically healthy gingiva is generally described to have a pale pink color. However, the color of the healthy marginal tissue may vary depending on (i) the dimensions of the tissue, (ii) the degree of keratinization of the covering epithelium and (iii) the vascularity of the connective tissue. A healthy dentogingival unit with only a narrow zone of gingiva will often appear reddish, while a gingival unit exhibiting a thick keratin layer, which may be found in patients who are smokers, can mask even pronounced inflammatory alterations in the gingiva. Furthermore, the thinning of the epithelium and the diminished keratinization, which occur with increasing age of the individual (for review see VAN DER VELDEN 1984), as well as various amounts of pigmentation of the gingiva may also influence the color of the marginal tissues.

The color and texture alterations associated with gingival inflammation are caused by alterations of the vasculature of the dentogingival plexus. The number of functioning vascular units increases both as a result of proliferation and of opening of previously inactive vascular units. In addition, the vasculature exhibits an increased permeability which is clinically detectable by an increased gingival fluid flow and a swelling of the gingival margin. The extent to which these vascular alterations are clinically detectable depends on the morphology of the tissues of the dentogingival region (for review see WENNSTRÖM 1982). Hence, a thick gingival tissue covered by a well-keratinized epithelium may not display any visible signs of inflammation despite the presence of an established gingival lesion. Consequently, the mere absence or presence of color and/or texture alterations cannot be considered as reliable criteria for determinations of the periodontal conditions.

Bleeding on probing

Since the symptom "bleeding on probing" to the bottom of the gingival sulcus/pocket is associated with the presence of an inflammatory infiltrate subjacent to the junctional epithelium (for review see GREENSTEIN 1984), the occurrence of such bleeding is an important clinical indicator of disease. "Bleeding on probing" is also considered to be an earlier and more sensitive sign of inflammation than changes in color and texture. Preferably, a standardized probing force should be used since the tendency towards bleeding increases with increasing probing force. If bleeding is not provoked from the apical area of the probeable pocket, the gingiva can, from a clinical point of view, be regarded as healthy. However, the lack of the symptom "bleeding on probing" does not necessarily mean an absence of an inflammatory cell infiltrate.

Increased probing depth

The healthy, collagen-rich gingival connective tissue offers a certain resistance to periodontal probing. Hence, in a clinically healthy site, the probing depth, i.e. the distance from the gingival margin to the bottom of the probeable gingival pocket, will seldom exceed 3 mm.

It is today well established that a variety of factors may influence the result of a measurement made with a periodontal probe (for review see LISTGARTEN 1980). Of particular interest is the degree of inflammatory cell infiltration in the soft tissue and accompanying loss of collagen. Destruction of collagen within the inflammatory lesion of the gingiva results in reduced resistance of the periodontal tissues to probing. The increased probing depth measured at an inflamed gingival site may to a various degree also be due to edematous swelling of the gingiva. A probing depth exceeding 4-5 mm may therefore not be considered as compatible with periodontal health. Support for this opinion was generated from the studies by BADERSTEN and collaborators (for review see BADERSTEN 1984) on the effect of nonsurgical periodontal therapy. They reported that, whereas the attachment level was maintained during a 2-year follow-up period in sites which following treatment showed a probing depth of <6 mm, further loss of probing attachment was observed in sites with remaining probing depths of 6 mm or more.

Tissue recession and reduced height of the alveolar bone

Although soft tissue recession is a common feature in periodontal disease (LINDHE and NYMAN 1980), such a finding can not be used to discriminate between a clinically healthy and a clinically diseased periodontium. In fact, the main causative factor in the development of tissue recessions is toothbrushing trauma and, recessions caused by faulty toothbrushing are usually associated with a healthy gingiva.

A reduced height of the alveolar bone is a sign of a defective periodontium rather than a sign of disease. However, repeated assessments of the alveolar bone height over a certain period of time may be a useful parameter in the differentiation between a clinically healthy and a diseased periodontium. In this context, computer-assisted subtraction of serial radiographs offers a tool by which the accuracy and reliability with respect to detection of small changes in the alveolar bone crest can be improved (for review see GRÖNDAHL 1987).

In summary; the absence of visible signs of inflammation (redness and swelling) in the gingiva does not necessarily indicate periodontal health. With respect to probing assessments, "bleeding on probing" and probing depths of 6 mm or more should not be regarded as signs compatible with a clinically healthy periodontium. Furthermore, tissue recessions and reduced height of the alveolar bone can be found in conjunction with clinically healthy supporting tissues. However, longitudinal bone loss is a sign of disease. It is also evident that more sensitive clinical methods than the ones used today are needed in order to improve the diagnostic accuracy.

Clinical considerations

As discussed above, histological studies have revealed that, in a clinically healthy gingiva, a small inflammatory cell infiltrate always will be found. Consequently, from a histopathological point of view, the clinically healthy gingiva could be considered to represent a stage of gingivitis. Clinically, however, gingivitis will be possible to diagnose first when the inflammatory lesion occupies a larger portion of the gingival connective tissue. Should the borderline between periodontal health and disease be the appearance of clinical signs of inflammation (redness, swelling, bleeding, etc.)?

Gingivitis can be considered as a host defence reaction against the bacterial challenge in the dentogingival area. Such a gingivitis lesion may be maintained for years without any major clinical changes. But how often will gingivitis lesions convert into destructive periodontal disease? Recent epidemiological data indicate that, although the prevalence of gingivitis in the population is high, only around 10% of the individuals may develop advanced periodontal disease (HUGOSON and JORDAN 1982, LÖE ET AL. 1987). Moreover, results from recent longitudinal studies of patients with untreated periodontal disease (GOODSON ET AL. 1982, LINDHE, HAFFAJEE and SOCRANSKY 1983, GOODSON, HAFFAJEE and SOCRANSKY 1984) showed that the frequency of sites developing clinically significant loss of probing attachment during a 1 year period was only 2-6%. These data indicate that the gingiva may be a very effective defence barrier against most bacterial plaques, i.e. the gingiva is capable to serve as protection for the underlying connective tissue attachment. Hence, recognizing the low figures for development of destructive periodontal disease in the studies referred to, the question is whether the mere presence of clinical signs of gingival inflammation should be regarded as incompatible with periodontal health. Maybe the borderline between periodontal health and disease should be an evidence of <u>destructive</u> periodontal disease, i.e. loss of connective tissue attachment and/or alveolar bone?

<u>References</u>

ATTSTRÖM, R.; GRAF-DE BEER, M., AND SCHROEDER, H.E.: Clinical and histological characterization of normal gingiva in dogs. J. Periodont. Res. <u>10</u>: 115-127 (1975).

BADERSTEN, A.: Nonsurgical periodontal therapy. Thesis. University of Lund, Malmö, Sweden (1984).

GOODSON, J.M.; HAFFAJEE, A.D., and SOCRANSKY, S.S.: The relationship between attachment level loss and alveolar bone loss. J. Clin. Periodontol. <u>11</u>: 348-359 (1984).

GOODSON, J.M.; TANNER, A.C.R.; HAFFAJEE, A.D.; SORNBERGER, G.C., and SOCRANSKY, S.S.: Patterns of progression and regression of advanced destructive periodontal disease. J. Clin. Periodontol. <u>9</u>: 472-481 (1982).

GREENSTEIN, G.: The role of bleeding upon probing in the diagnosis of periodontal disease. J. Periodontol. <u>55</u>: 684-688 (1984).

GRÖNDAHL, K.: Computer-assisted subtraction radiography in periodontal diagnosis. Thesis. University of Göteborg, Göteborg, Sweden (1987).

HUGOSON, A., and JORDAN, T.: Frequency distribution of individuals aged 20-70 years according to severity of periodontal disease. Community Dent. Oral Epidemiol. <u>10</u>: 187-192 (1982).

LINDHE, J.; HAFFAJEE, A.D., and SOCRANSKY, S.S.: Progression of periodontal disease in adult subjects in the absence of periodontal therapy. J. Clin. Periodontol. <u>10</u>: 433-442 (1983).

LINDHE, J., and NYMAN, S.: Alterations of the position of the marginal soft tissue following periodontal surgery. J. Clin. Periodontol. <u>7</u>: 525-530 (1980).

LINDHE, J., and RYLANDER, H.: Experimental gingivitis in young dogs. Scand. J. Dent. Res. <u>83</u>: 314-326 (1975).

LISTGARTEN, M.A.: Periodontal probing: What does it mean? J. Clin. Periodontol. <u>7</u>: 165-176 (1980).

LÖE, H., ANERUD, A.; BOYSEN, H., and MORRISON, E.: Natural history of periodontal disease in man. Rapid, moderate and no loss of attachment in Sri Lankan laborers 14 to 46 years of age. J. Clin. Periodontol. 13: 431-440 (1986).

PAGE, R.C., and SCHROEDER, H.E.: Pathogenesis of chronic inflammatory periodontal disease. A summary of current work. Lab. Invest. 33: 235-249 (1976).

VAN DER VELDEN, U.: Effect of age on the periodontium. J. Clin. Periodontol. 11: 281-294 (1984).

WENNSTRÖM, J.L.: Keratinized and attached gingiva - regenerative potential and significance for periodontal health. Thesis. University of Göteborg, Göteborg, Sweden (1982).

Jan L. Wennström, Department of Periodontology, School of Dentistry, Faculty of Odontology, University of Göteborg, Box 33070, S-400 33 Göteborg, Sweden.

Periodontology Today. Int. Congr., Zürich 1988, pp. 6–14 (Karger, Basel 1988)

Does the Developmental Origin of Cementum, Periodontal Ligament and Bone Predetermine their Behaviour in Adults?

Antony H. Melcher

Faculty of Dentistry, University of Toronto, Toronto, Ontario, Canada

I suspect that the answer to the question that has been posed by the organizing committee may be difficult to find unless one attempts to focus the question. It could be argued that the developmental origin of a tissue depends on the origin of the cells that synthesize it and that, equally, the behaviour of the tissues in the adult depends on the phenotypes expressed by the cells that are associated with it. Consequently, I intend to restrict this discussion to the lineage of the cells that synthesize cementum, periodontal ligament and bone during development and in the adult, to the phenotypes that they express, and to aspects of their regulation. For convenience of presentation, it could be useful to divide the topic into three categories:

a) The lineage of the cells, their phenotypic expression and aspects of their regulation during development.

b) The lineage of the cells, their phenotypic expression and aspects of their regulation in the adult.

c) Do events during development predetermine events in the adult?

a. The Lineage of the Cells, Their Phenotypic Expression and Aspects of Their Regulation During Development

There now appears to be quite good evidence that the layer of the dental follicle that invests the tooth germ contains cells that differentiate to express the phenotype for cementoblasts, periodontal ligament fibroblasts and, perhaps, alveolar bone. Further, there are indirect lines of evidence that suggest that these cells take origin from the dental papilla. HOFFMAN (1960) has shown that cells of tooth germs transplanted subcutaneously to host animals can give rise to the three connective tissues of the alveolar part of the periodontium, but has interpreted his data to suggest that the periodontal ligament and bone were synthesized by host cells that had been induced so to do by those of the transplanted organ. TEN CATE et al. (1971) and TEN CATE and MILLS (1972) subsequently provided evidence obtained from similar transplants that had first been labelled in vitro with ^{3}H Thymidine, and from the ultrastructure of the transplanted germs and their products, that the cementum, periodontal ligament and some of the alveolar bone were synthesized, at least in part, by cells taking origin from the transplants, specifically from the investing layer of the dental papilla.

By enzymatically dissecting the dental epithelium from the dental papilla and the investing layer of the dental follicle, and then by dissecting the investing layer from the dental papilla, YOSHIKAWA and KOLLAR (1981) and PALMER and LUMSDEN (1987) have provided confirmatory evidence that the cells of the investing layer of the dental follicle give rise, at least in part, to cementum, periodontal ligament and bone, and indirect evidence that these cementoblasts, fibroblasts and osteoblasts take origin form the dental papilla. In these experiments, the dental epithelium, dental papilla and investing layer from mouse first mandibular molar were recombined in different combinations and growth together in the anterior chamber of the eye of host mice. When all three were recombined, they produced, with reasonable regularity, teeth together with cementum, periodontal ligament and some bone, provided that the donor embryos were aged 16 days i.u. However, while the former authors found that each of the investing layer and dental papilla could express teeth and their supporting structures equally well when combined with dental epithelium, Palmer and Lumsden found the presence of the investing layer to be essential for osteogenesis, and, that further, while the other two tissues were expressed in the absence of the investing layer, the success rate was low. Palmer and Lumsden claim that their results are attributable to a superior technique for dissection. While this may be so, a difference between the two sets of experiments may also lie in the method by which the tissues were recombined: Yoshikawa and Kollar recombined their tissues and maintained them in vitro for 24 hours before transplantation in vivo whereas Palmer and Lumsden transplanted them singly and recombined them in the anterior chamber of the eye. I think successful recombination is more likely to be guaranteed by the former method, and could explain the difference between their results.

Both groups of experiments showed donor age to be important in the phenotypes expressed. Yoshikawa and Kollar found that the investing layer rapidly loses its inducing capacity after 16 days i.u. and Palmer and Lumsden found the pulp of newborn mice to be inactive. These results are possibly explained by the differention of the cells of these two tissues with age to express other phenotypes. HERITIER (1982) has shown that the cells of dental follicle left in the crypt after removal of first and second molars of 9 day p.p.

mice still have the capacity to synthesize cementum. These cells may be different from those of the investing layer: the former reside in the tissue that is left behind after removal of the developing teeth, while the cells of the investing layer presumably are removed with the developing teeth. Indeed, the former could be expected to have been excluded from the transplants in the experiments described in the preceding paragraph, although they may have contributed as contaminants. One source of difficulty in Heritier's work is that he inverted and replaced the dissected teeth into their crypts after removing the reduced enamel epithelium from their crowns. It is evident from his description that the epithelium was not always removed in its entirety, so one must suspect that cells from the investing layer could also have been replaced. It is not clear whether these cells could have made any contribution to cementogenesis.

Questions concerning the capacity of the cells of the investing layer and the rest of the dental follicle of mice to express the phenotype for the three tissues of the alveolar part of the periodontium after 16 days i.u. remain to be asked. The recombination experiments described above required the recombined tissues to develop teeth and their supporting structures; if teeth were not developed, nor were supporting structures. However, they do not appear to answer the question of whether papilla, investing layer and follicle cells from donors older than 16 days i.u. can express the phenotype for cementum, periodontal ligament and bone if presented with the needed substrate, presumably root dentine, and the appropriate, but possibly unknown, regulators. In other words, while the cells of these tissues may lose the capacity to induce and express the phenotype that result in the development of a tooth and its supporting structures, they may not, in appropriate circumstances, lose the capacity to induce and express for the latter. I think that elucidating this question is crucial. In this connection, a kinetic study of erupting mouse molar undertaken by PERERA and TONGE (1981) suggests that the developing periodontal ligament in the vicinity of the developing root diaphragm may provide a font of cells which migrate cervically, possibly providing the secretory fibroblasts, cementoblasts and osteoblasts of the periodontal ligament, and so implicating the tissues associated with the forming root-end as a continuing source of these cells.

The capacity of cells of forming and formed roots to express the phenotypes for cementum, periodontal ligament and bone has also been addressed by BARRETT and READE (1981). Third molar teeth in the form of unmineralized germs, teeth with partly-formed roots and fully-erupted teeth with developed roots were taken from mice of varying age and transplanted beneath the renal capsule of recipient mice. Cells from the incompletely-formed teeth, but not from the fully-formed teeth synthesized the three tissues. Although the paper does not contain any data on rates of success, the observations are consistent with the view that cells from functioning periodontal ligament may not have the capacity to synthesize bone and cementum (see below).

While the experiments described above have done much to elucidate the source of the cells that are responsible for the development of the tissues of the alveolar part of the periodontium, our knowledge is still rudimentary. There is some indirect evidence that the cells in question originate in the dental papilla. Presumably, appropriate ancestral cells in this tissue divide, after which their progeny migrate, perhaps via the investing layer of the dental follicle where, for a limited time, they retain their capacity to interact with other cells and produce teeth. What is not clear, I believe, is the identity and location of the population(s) of ancestral cells that give rise to progeny that become the cementoblasts, periodontal ligament fibroblasts and osteoblasts of the developing periodontium. The experiments undertaken by TEN CATE et al. (1971) and TEN CATE and MILLS (1972) indicate that the cells labelled by ^{3}H Thymidine could have taken origin from either the dental papilla or the dental follicle, and those of PALMER and LUMSDEN (1987) and YOSHIKAWA and KOLLAR (1981) confirm this. But, we do not know whether there is a single population of ancestral cells that gives rise to progeny that can differentiate to express the phenotypes of either cementoblasts, fibroblasts or osteoblasts, or whether each of these cells is derived from its own population of ancestral cells. The former possibility seems to be the more likely as it appears that this may be the case for cells of the skeletal system (GRIGORIADIS et al., 1986). If this holds to be true, then one still needs to know where these stem cells are located, to where their progeny migrate, where and how frequently their progeny divide, and if and where their potential to express the phenotype for cementoblast, fibroblast and osteoblast becomes restricted.

TEN CATE et al. (1971) and FREEMAN and TEN CATE (1971) have pointed out the possibility that the cells of the developing periodontal ligament may take origin from more than a single source, and that connective tissue cells associated with blood vessels that migrate into the forming periodontal ligament may also contribute. Unfortunately, to the best of my knowledge, nothing is known about the origin of the blood vessels of the periodontal ligament, the extent to which cells that may be associated with them, or cells of the dental follicle peripheral to the investing layer, or cells associated with the bone of the crypt, contribute cementoblasts, fibroblasts and osteoblasts to the developing periodontium. We also have no information on the regulators that direct the cells that take origin in the tooth germ to migrate to the sites where they will differentiate to express the phenotype for cementum, periodontal ligament or alveolar bone, nor on what are the regulators that influence this differentiation so that each of the tissues is synthesized in the appropriate site. Finally, one could ask what are the regulators that maintain the distance between the bone of the crypt and the developing tooth, the site where ultimately cementum and periodontal ligament will be synthesized?

b) The Lineage of the Cells, Their Phenotypic Expression and Aspects of Their Regulation in the Adult

There is some evidence that the ancestral cells in the functioning periodontal ligament are located paravascularly (MELCHER, 1970; GOULD et al., 1980; McCULLOCH and MELCHER, 1983a; McCULLOCH, 1985). There is also evidence that cells in this tissue, including their progeny, have the capacity to migrate through the tissue under physiological conditions, therapeutic tooth movement and in response to wound healing (GARANT and CHO, 1979; GOULD et al., 1980; ROBERTS and CHASE, 1981; McCULLOCH and MELCHER, 1983b; DAVIDSON and McCULLOCH, 1986). Newly-born cells and their progeny have been shown to migrate to the surfaces of cementum and alveolar bone where they presumably express the phenotypes for cementoblasts, fibroblasts or osteoblasts (McCULLOCH and MELCHER, 1983b). To the best of my knowledge, there is no direct evidence that the cells that are born paravascularly, or their progeny, are the same cells that migrate to these surfaces to express bone or cementum. Evidence has also been provided to show that cells born in the vascular channels that traverse the alveolar bone of mice migrate, and that they may do so in the direction of the periodontal ligament, raising the possibility that they contribute to the populations of cells in the periodontal ligament, particularly the osteoblasts and cementoblasts (McCULLOCH et al., 1987). This interpretation is supported by the simultaneous finding that the periodontal ligament contiguous with the vascular channels contains a greater concentration of cells that can be labelled with ^{3}H Thymidine than does the rest of the ligament. Consistent with these findings, cells obtained from foetal bone apparently have the capacity to synthesize *in vitro* tissue having the ultrastructural characteristics of bone or cellular cementum, and acellular and afibrillar cementum (MELCHER et al., 1986). Consequently, while it is evident that new cells in the periodontal ligament take origin from paravascular precursors located in the ligament and, possibly, in vascular channels in the alveolar bone, I do not think that we know precisely what is the lineage of the cementoblasts, fibroblasts and osteoblasts in the periodontal ligament, what is, or are, the location(s) of their progenitors, nor whether they stem from a single, two or three different ancestral cells.

It has been suggested that cells of periodontal ligament can provide cementoblasts, fibroblasts and osteoblasts for regeneration of the alveolar part of the periodontium during wound healing (MELCHER, 1976). It has also been claimed that it is these cells that are responsible for the regeneration of the alveolar part of the periodontium that is achieved when the wound is protected from the overlying gingival connective tissue and epithelium by a barrier (NYMAN et al., 1982; GOTTLOW et al., 1984; MAGNUSSON et al., 1985; GOTTLOW et al., 1986). However, to the best of my knowledge, no one has yet shown directly that cells from periodontal ligament have the capacity to express the phenotype for cementum or bone in the absence of cells originating from bone (RICHARDS and KOLLAR, 1986; MELCHER et al., Submitted for publication). Indeed, the wound healing experiments in which a barrier has been employed have not excluded the possibility that bone cells could have migrated into the wound; in fact, the manner in which the barrier is placed makes it highly unlikely that this could have been the case (NYMAN et al., 1982; GOTTLOW et al., 1986). Consequently, I now believe that all of the evidence that currently is available points to the possibility that cells taking origin from bone at least contribute to the osteoblasts and cementoblasts in the periodontium. Questions that need to be answered include those pertaining to the origin of these cells, and to the nature and identity of the regulators that govern their birth and their orderly migration and appropriate expression of phenotype under physiological conditions and in wound healing.

Mammalian teeth of limited eruption drift through the bone of the jaws physiologically, requiring remodelling of the tissues of the periodontium (KRAW and ENLOW, 1967; VIGNERY and BARON, 1980). Despite this, the width of the periodontal ligament is normally maintained throughout life, and bone does not colonise it. However, if the periodontal ligament is extirpated, ankylosis supervenes (HAMMER, 1955; LÖE and WAERHAUGH, 1961; MELCHER, 1970), suggesting that the regulators responsible for the maintenance of the width of the periodontal ligament are present in the ligament (MELCHER, 1969; LINE et al., 1974; MELCHER, 1976). We have recently found that cells obtained from human periodontal ligament and rat skin depress significantly the capacity of rat bone marrow cells to synthesize mineralized bone-like tissue *in vitro* and that this is achieved, at least in part, by an agonist produced by these cells (MELCHER and CHEONG, In Preparation). We are now endeavouring to isolate and purify this substance. It could be postulated that periodontal ligament fibroblasts control the extent of osteogenesis in physiological remodelling of the periodontium and in wound healing through this and, possibly, other mechanisms.

c) Do Events During Development Predetermine Events in the Adult?

PALMER and LUMSDEN (1987) claim that their work supports

the view that "The tooth-related ligament appears to contain the cementoblast precursors and the bone-related ligament osteoblast precursors". This certainly would suggest that events during development predetermine events in the adult. While, I do not think that at the present time we can be certain that this is not the case, I submit that it is not proven. Although there is evidence that at appropriate times relatively early in development, cells having the capacity to express the phenotypes for cementum, fibrous connective tissue and bone take origin from a common tissue or tissues, there is no evidence of which I am aware that this is their only source of origin. Do cells arising from sites associated with developing blood vessels, the peripheral part of the dental follice and from the bone of the crypt also contribute? There is also no direct evidence, of which I am aware, to support the belief that cells of periodontal ligament from fully erupted teeth have the capacity for osteogenesis or cementogenesis, nor that experiments showing regeneration of cementum, periodontal ligament and bone in the healing of wounds of periodontium, have demonstrated unequivocally that cells originating from bone were excluded from the wound. It does seem to be distinctly possible that at least some of the cells of the developing and developed periodontium take origin from paravascular precursors in the developing and developed periodontal ligament. To this extent, events in development may cast their shadow before them but, in both the developing and developed organ, the contribution made by these cells needs to be elucidated fully.

It is not clear how the domain separating the tooth germ and the bone of the crypt or that separating cementum and alveolar bone are maintained. We may be on the threshold of obtaining some understanding of this phenomenon in the functioning organ. If sufficient progress can be made, it should be of interest to determine whether the same regulatory mechanisms operate during development.

In conclusion, I do not think that we have sufficient knowledge of either cell lineage or regulatory mechanisms in the developing or developed tooth to answer the question that has been posed. However, a clearer understanding of cellular events in the developing and developed periodontium, and, particularly, of whether or not the cementoblasts, fibroblasts and osteoblasts in the developing and developed periodontium take origin from a single stem cell, should eventually provide the answer.

References

BARRETT, A.P., and READE, P.C. The relationship between degree of development of tooth isografts and the subsequent formation of bone and periodontal ligament. J. Periodont. Res. 16: 456-465 (1981)

DAVIDSON, D., and McCULLOCH C.A.G. Proliferative behaviour of periodontal ligament cell populations. J. Periodont. Res. 21: 414-428 (1986)

FREEMAN, E., and TEN CATE, A.R. Development of the periodontium: An electron microscopic study. J. Periodontol. 42: 387-395 (1971)

GARANT, P.R., and CHO M.I. Autoradiographic evidence of the coordination of the genesis of Sharpey's fibres with new bone formation in the periodontium of the mouse. J. Periodont. Res. 14: 95-104 (1979)

GOTTLOW, J.; NYMAN, S.; KARRING, T., and LINDHE, J. New attachment formation as the result of controlled regeneration. J. Clin. Periodontol. 11: 494-503 (1984)

GOTTLOW, J.; NYMAN, S.; LINDHE, J.; KARRING, T., and WENNSTROM, J. New attachment formation in the human periodontium by guided tissue regeneration. J. Clin. Periodontol. 13: 604-616 (1986)

GOULD, T.R.L.; MELCHER, A.H., and BRUNETTE, D.M. Migration and division of progenitor cell populations in periodontal ligament after wounding. J. Periodont. Res. 15: 20-42 (1980)

GRIGORIADIS, A.E.; AUBIN, J.E., and HEERSCHE, J.N.M. Glucocorticoid induces the differentiation of progenitor cells present in a clonally-derived rat calvaria cell population. 9th International Conference on Calcium Regulating Hormones and Bone Metabolism. Nice, France, Abstract #478 (1986)

HAMMER, H. Replantation and implantation of teeth. Int. Dent. J. 5: 439-457 (1955)

HERITIER, M. Experimental induction of cementogenesis on the enamel of transplanted mouse tooth germs. Archs. Oral Biol. 27: 87-97 (1982)

HOFFMAN, R.L. Formation of periodontal tissues around subcutaneously transplanted hamster molars. J. Dent. Res. 39: 781-798 (1960)

KRAW, A.G. and ENLOW, D.M. Continuous attachment of the periodontal membrane. Am. J. Anat. 120: 133-148 (1967)

LÖE, H., and WAERHAUG, J. Experimental replantation of teeth in dogs and monkeys. Archs. Oral Biol. 3: 176-184 (1961)

LINE, S.E.; POLSON, A.M., and ZANDER, H.A. (1974) Relationship between periodontal injury, selective cell repopulation and ankylosis. J. Periodontol. 45: 725-730 (1974)

MAGNUSSON, I.; NYMAN, S.; KARRING, T., and EGELBERG, J. Connective tissue attachment formation following exclusion of gingival connective tissue and epithelium during healing. J. Periodont. Res. 20: 201-208 (1985)

McCulloch CAG (1985) Progenitor cell populations in the periodontal ligament of mice. Anat Rec 211:258-262.

McCULLOCH, C.A.G., and MELCHER A.H. Cell density and cell generation in the periodontal ligament of mice. Am. J. Anat. 167: 43-58 (1983a)

McCULLOCH, C.A.G., and MELCHER, A.H. Cell migration in the

periodontal ligament of mice. J. Periodont. Res. 18: 339-352 (1983b)

MCCULLOCH, C.A.G.; NEMETH, E.; LOWENBERG, B., and MELCHER, A.H. Paravascular cells in endosteal spaces of alveolar bone contribute to periodontal ligament cell populations. Anat. Rec. 219: 233-242 (1987)

MELCHER, A.H. Repair of wounds in the periodontium of the rat. Influence of periodontal ligament on osteogenesis. Archs. Oral Biol. 15: 1183-1204 (1970)

MELCHER, A.H. On the repair potential of periodontal tissues. J. Periodontol. 47: 256-260 (1976)

MELCHER, A.H.; CHEONG, T.; COX, J.; NEMETH, E., and SHIGA, A. Synthesis of cementum-like tissue in vitro by cells cultured from bone: A light and electron microscopic study. J. Periodont. Res. 21: 592-612 (1986)

NYMAN, S.; GOTTLOW, J.; KARRING, T., and LINDHE, J. The regenerative potential of the periodontal ligament. An experimental study in the monkey. J. Clin. Periodontol. 9: 257-265 (1982)

PALMER, R.M., and LUMSDEN, A.G.S. Development of periodontal ligament and alveolar bone in homografted recombinations of enamel organs and papillary, pulpal and follicular mesenchyme in the mouse. Archs. Oral Biol. 32: 281-289 (1987)

PERERA, K.A.S., and TONGE, C.H. Fibroblast cell population kinetics in the mouse molar periodontal ligament and tooth eruption. J. Anat. 133: 281-300 (1981)

RICHARDS, D., and KOLLAR, E. Human pulp and periodontal ligament fibroblast-like cells do not form mineralized matrix in in vivo diffusion chambers. J. Dent. Res. 65: 212 (1986) Abstract

ROBERTS, W.E., and CHASE, D.C. Kinetics of cell proliferation and migration associated with orthodontically-induced osteogenesis. J. Dent. Res. 60: 174-181 (1981)

TEN CATE, A.R.; MILLS, C., and SOLOMON, G. The development of the periodontium. A transplantation and autoradiographic study. Anat. Rec. 170: 365-379 (1971)

TEN CATE, A.R., and MILLS, C. The development of the periodontium: The origin of alveolar bone. Anat. Rec. 173: 69-77 (1972)

VIGNERY, A. and BARON, R. Dynamic histomorphometry of alveolar bone remodelling in the adult rat. Anat. Rec. 196: 191-200 (1980)

YOSHIKAWA, D.K., and KOLLAR, E.J. Recombination experiments on the odontogenic roles of mouse dental papilla and dental sac tissues in ocular grafts. Archs. Oral Biol. 26: 303-307 (1981)

Dr. A.H. Melcher, University of Toronto, Faculty of Dentisty,
School of Graduate Studies, 124, Edward St., Totonto, Ontario M56 1G6, Canada

Periodontology Today. Int. Congr., Zürich 1988, pp. 15–23 (Karger, Basel 1988)

Continuous Tooth Eruption in the Light of Adult Growth

Geerte R. J. Mazeland

Department of Orthodontics, Academic Center for Dentistry, Amsterdam, The Netherlands

Introduction

According to Gottlieb and Orban (1936) continuous eruption of the dentition is normal in human adults, leading to a loss of attachment and support for the teeth and, eventually, to loss of the teeth. The observations of Waerhaug (1952), Manson (1963), Loë (1967) and many others made it difficult to accept the idea of physiological apical movement of the gingival attachment with continual occlusal movement of the dento-alveolar complex. Continuous eruption does not necessarily lead to bone loss and to ultimate loss of the teeth in subjects with a healthy periodontal condition.

An increase in ginvival width in adults has been reported by Ainamo and Talari (1976). It has been postulated by these authors that the increase in gingival width is associated with an increase in face height. They found no differences, among different adult age groups, in the location of the mucogingival junction in relation to the lower border of the mandible or of the nasal floor (Ainamo et al 1981). This suggests a relationship between the increase in gingival width and continuous eruptive movements of the teeth and of their investing tissues. In a longitudinal investigation over five years in young adult males, Mazeland (1980a) found a slight increase in the width of the gingiva at the upper incisors but no increase could be shown in the width at the lower incisors. Ainamo and Talari (1976) postulated that the increase in gingival width in adults is associated with increase in face height; the vertical growth is thought to occur within the area of the alveolar processes. Mazeland (1980b) found a relationship between the width of the gingiva and the height of the lower face in young adults and also confirmed that gingival width at anterior teeth is primarily related to the height of the alveolar process.On the basis of these results it seems likely that continuous eruption of teeth in human adults takes place and is accompanied by an increase in height of the gingiva and the alveolar process.

Development of the mucogingival complex and the alveolar process

In the human embryo the first morphologic changes in the ectoderm of the primitive oral cavity occur near the end of the fourth week, when the basal cell layers differentiate into cuboidal cells and columnar cells. The cuboidal cells are located in the oral epithelium of the future lips, cheeks and soft palate. The columnar cells are observed in the epithelium of the furure gum ridge, hard palate and epidermis (Coslet and Cohen 1967). In the 8th week, the dense fibrous periosteum of the developing mandibular and maxillary alveolar bone is continuous with the dense collagenous connective tissue of the gum ridge. In the anterior portion of the mouth the lip furrow band, an epithelial mass of cells, separates the gum ridge and the lip primordia (Coslet and Cohen 1968). In the 12th to 14th week the vestibular trough develops in the anterior portion of the mouth. The topography of the epithelial tissues of the trough reflects the anatomy of the adult. The alveolar portion of the bottom of the vestibular trough is covered with epithelial tissue derived from the labial portion. These morphologic relationships appear to result from a difference in growth rates between the gum ridge and the developing alveolar bone on the one hand and the future lip on the other (Coslet and Cohen 1969). In the 16th to 19th week of fetal life keratinization of the epithelium begins. At 20 weeks keratin is present on the gingival portion of the vestibule and absent on the labial portion (McFall and Kraus 1963,1965). At 30 weeks a remarkable distribution of keratinized areas is observed: keratin is present on the buccal and palatal regions of the alveolar ridge, but not on the crest of the ridge. The distribution remains thus at birth (Bowman and Latham 1968).

At birth the primary teeth, of which the crowns are half calcified, lie in a thin shelter of bone covering the apical, buccal and lingual surfaces. There is no bone over the coronal surfaces. The primary teeth begin to erupt at 6-8 months post partum.The jaws grow rapidly in a vertical direction by appositional bone growth at the alveolar crests. This apposition of bone continues even after the crowns of the deciduous teeth are in occlusion and root formation is complete. Thus, the deciduous dentition continues to move occlusally (Brodie 1948).

In the primary dentition the gingiva varies in width from one tooth to another and from one child to another. The greatest gingival width is found at the maxillary and mandibular incisors. In both jaws the width of the gingiva decreases towards the molar region. The narrowest zone is observed in the area of the first decidous molars Bowers 1963, Ainamo and Loë 1966, Rose and App 1973, Maynard and Ochsenbein 1975, Mieler et al 1985, Tenenbaum and Tenebaum 1986).

Concurrent with the exfoliation of the primary incisors and the eruption of the permanant ones, the alveolar processes are reduced in height (Helman 1932, Nanda 1955, Falck and

Fränkel 1973); the gingival sulcus shows a temporary deepening (Manson 1963,Rose and App 1973); and the gingiva narrows (Rose and App 1973, Maynard and Ochsenbein 1975, Mieler et al 1985, Tenenbaum and Tenenbaum 1986). Later, with the continuing eruption of the permanent teeth, the alveolar processes regain height (Helman 1932, Nanada 1955, Falck and Fränkel 1973, Riolo et al 1974). This increase continues even after the teeh have come into occlusion (Björk 1963). In the maxilla, the growth in height of the alveolar process on its occlusal surface is accompanied by a resorption, at the nasal surface and floor of the sinus. This causes a reduction which amounts to about one third of the appositional increase (Björk and Skieller 1976). There is a difference in growth rates with regard to chronological age in boys and girls. In the adolescent and adult, males have higher alveolar processes than females (Riolo et al 1974).

The gingival height also increases with age during childhood, puberty and adolescence (Vincent,Machen and Levin 1976, Mieler et al 1985, Tenenbaum and Tenenbaum 1986). In the mature dentition the gingiva is wider than in the primary dentition, but the pattern of variation is similar (Bowers 1963, Ainamo and Löe 1966). However, in a three years longitudinal study in children from 9-13 years of age an increase in width of the attached gingiva was reported, but very little change in width of the keratinized gingiva (Bimstein et al 1986).

Muscle attachments and crowding produce local anatomical variation in the vertical dimension of the gingiva. However, even when all of the mandibular incisors are properly aligned, there may still be a very narrow zone of gingival tissue (Maynard and Ochsenbein 1975, Boyd 1978). Gingival width at anterior teeth was found to be related to alveolar process height and lower anterior face height in young adults (Mazeland 1980b).

Adult growth

Growth does not cease entirely at the end of the adolescence, head and face measurements seem to increase steadily from 20 to 60 years of age. Cross-sectional anthropometric studies report a variety of findings. During the third decade of life Baer (1956) found a decelerating increase in facial and nasal height in males, but no increase at all in females. An increase with advancing age, up to age 50, in Finnish woman was reported by Tallgren (1957). Severe attrition of the teeth caused a reduction of face height in a small group of the same sample. According to Israel (1973) craniofacial growth in later life is a magnification process: an overall enlargment takes place by surface remodelling, and the symphysis increases in thickness by apposition. Cross-sectional studies are of little value in determining whether and to what extent morphologic changes occur, as factors of selective survival and secular trend influence the results to an unknown degree (Tanner 1962). In a five years cephalometric study from 21 to 26 years Sarnäs and Solow (1980) Found an increase in lower face height of about

1.5 mm; upper and lower dentoalveolar height increased by about 0.5 mm, in the upper jaw due to eruption of the incisors, in the lower jaw almost exclusively due to an increase in clinical crown height. In a longitudinal study over 9 years, Büchi (1950)found a steady increase of head measurements in Swiss males of different age groups up to age 60. In a 10 years longitudinal study from age 24 to 34 Forsberg (1979) reported an incraese in lower face height of 0.56mm in men and 0.67mm in woman. His findings indicated that the major part of the changes of the bony profile were due to posterior rotation and an adjustment (uprighting) of the upper incisors to the new jaw position.

Cross-sectional studies on gingival width also show a variety of findings. According to Bowers (1963) gingival width shows little change in the adult dentition; a steady increase up to age 60 was found by Ainamo et al (1981); an increase between age 35 and 45 by Wally et al (1983); an increase up to age 29, followed by a decrease until 64 by Mieler et al (1985). In a longitudinal study over five years in male subjects 20 to 25 years of age Mazeland (1980a) found a small increase in gingival width at the upper incisors; at the lower incisors no increase could be shown.

Discussion

The association of continuous eruption of the teeth in adults and increase in lower face height is based on skull studies, in which tooth attrition is compensated for by an increase in alveolar process height. Considering tooth attrition a function of age, it is assumed that without attrition of the teeth, facial height would increase with advancing age (Hellman 1927, Herzberg and Holic 1943, Murphy 1959, Manson 1963). However, whether absence of tooth attrition results in an increase in lower face height cannot be concluded from these studies. In a study of skulls of known sex and age the outcome pointed to a decrease in face height, and it was concluded that people get smaller as they get older (de Froe 1936).

Longitudinal aspects of growth can be assessed in detail only by longitudinal investigations. Longitudinal studies report a slight increase in lower face height; a very small increase in upper alveolar process height; and a very small increase in upper anterior gingival width during the third decade of life. In young adults, especially in males, late maturation of some of the subjects can influence the outcome for the total group, and what is called adult growth, is possibly delayed adolescent growth in a few subjects. In adults where chondrocranial growth, condylar growth and sutural growth is supposed to have ceased (Björk 1966), four possible sites of growth can be associated with an increase in lower face height (figure 1):

1 appositional increase on the lower border of the symphysis (Israel 1973)

2 appostional increase at the crest of the upper anterior alveolar process (Forsberg 1979, Sarnäs and Solow 1980, Ainamo et al 1981)

3 appositional increase at the crest of the lower anterior alveolar process (Ainamo et al 1981)

4 a slight posterior rotation of the mandible with eruption in the molar region and a compensatory adaption of the incisors to a more lingual inclination (Forsberg 1976); or an increase in the distance supradentale-infradentale (SD-ID).

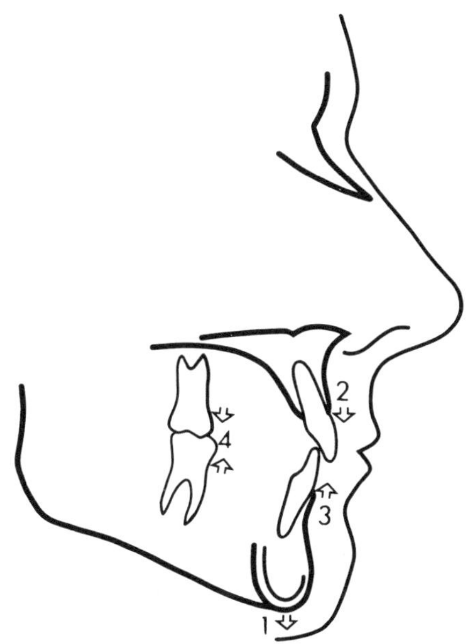

Fig. 1 Possible sites and directions of growth in adults.

Changes in lower face height in adults are very small. The results of the studies of gingival width may point to analogous changes of the human adult dentition. Extrusion and uprighting of front teeth are both associated with an increase in gingival width (Batenhorst et al 1974, Boyd 1978, dorfman 1978). An increase in gingival width in adults may result form uprighting of the teeth. Mieler et al (1985) found that the age group 20-29 years showed the widest zone of attached gingiva; that older age groups showed smaller values may be due to recessions, caused by traumatic tooth brushing combined with the effects of secular tren, the older age groups never having reached the same vertical measurements as their minors in age. The results of the studies of Forsberg(1979) and of Sarnäs and Solow (1980) coincide well with the longitudinal study of gingival width in the same age group (Mazeland 1980a), where a small increase was measured at the upper incisors, but no alterations were found at the lower anterior region.

When methodological errors in clinical and cephalometric measurements are taken into account, the changes in the vertical dimensions of the lower face, asociated with continuous tooth eruption are almost impossible to quantify. In clinical research or epidemiologicl surveys, when more than one examiner is involved, the examiners should be calibrated, as a systematic error is likely to exist (Mazeland 1978). In longitudinal studies duplicate measurements should be taken on each occasion to reduce the method error as much as possible.

In view of the fact that these requirements have not been met in the clinical studies of eruptive movements of teeth, any conclusions must be regarded with caution. There is still no conclusive evidence for continuous tooth eruption and simultanuous increase in height of the gingiva and the alveolar process in man.

References

AINAMO,A.; AINAMO,J.and POIKKEUS,R.:Continuous widening of the band of attached gingiva from 23 to 65 years of age. J. Periodontol. Res.16: 595-599,1981

AINAMO,J and LÖE,H.: Anatomical characteristics of gingiva. A clinical and microscopic study of the free and attached gingiva. J. Periodontol. 37: 5-13, 1966

AINAMO,J. and TALARI, A.: Eruptive movements of teeth in human adults. Colston papers no. 26, pp 97-107 Butterworth, London, 1976

BEAR, M.J.: Dimensinal changes in the human head and face in the third decade of life. Am J. of Physical Anthropology, 14: 557-575, 1956

BATENHORST,K.F., BOWERS, G.M. and WILLIAMS, J.E.Jr.: Tissue changes resulting from facial tipping and extrusion of incisors in monkeys J. Periodontol.,45: 660-668, 1974

BIMSTEIN, E.and EIDELMAN,E.: Dimensional differences in the attached gingiva and gingival sulcus in the mixed dentition J. Dentistry Children 50: 264-267, 1983

BIMSTEIN, E., MACHTEI,E. and EIDELMAN, E.: Dimensional differences in the attached and keratinized gingiva and gingival sulcus in the early permanent dentition: a longitudinal study J. Pedodontics 10: 247-253

BJÖRK, A.: Variations in the growth pattern of the human mandible: Longitudinal radiographic study by the implant method J. Dent. Res.., 42: 400-411, 1963

BJÖRK,A. : Sutural growth of the upper face studied by the implant method Acta Odont. Scand., 24: 109-127

BJÖRK, A. and SKIELLER, V.: Postnatal growth and development of the maxillary complex. Craniofacial Growth Series.6:

pp. 61-99, Ann Arbor, Michigan, Center fo Human Growth and development, 1976

BOWERS, G.M.: A study of the width of attached gingiva J. Periodontol.: 34: 201-2o9, 1963

BOWMAN, A.J. and LATHAM, R.A.: The differential development and structure of keratinizing mucosa of the upper denture bearing area. Dent. Practit., 18: 349-352, 1968

BOYD, R. L. , : Mucogingival considerations and their relationship to orthodontics J. Periodontol., 49: 67-76, 1978

BRODIE, A.G.: The growth of the alveolar bone and the eruption of the teeth. Oral Surg., Oral Med., Oral Path.,1: 342-345, 1948

BÜCHI, E.C.: Änderungen der Körperform beim erwachsenen Menschen Anthropologische Forschungen, Anthr. Gesellsch. Wien, Horn, 1950

COSLET, J.G. and COHEN, D.W.: The basal cell layer of the developing oral mucosa in the human fetus J. Periodontol. Res., 2: 297-316. 1967

COSLET, J.G. and COHEN, D.W.: The basal cell layer of the developing oral mucosa in the human fetus part II J. Periodontol. Res., 3: 194-211, 1968

COSLET, J.G. and COHEN, D.W.: Observations on the development of the vestibular trough in the human fetus J. Periodontol. Res.40: 320-330, 1969

DORFMAN, H.S. Evaluation of mucogingival changes resulting from mandibular incisor tooth movement J. Dent. Res. special issue B, p. 22, 1977

FALCK, F and FRÄNKEL, R.: Die labiale Alveolenwand unter dem Einfluss des durchbrechenden Schneidezahns Fortschr. der Kieferorthop., 34: 37-47, 1973

FORSBERG, C.M.: Growth changes in the adult face. Thesis, Stockholm, 1976

FORSBERG, C.M.: Facial morphology and ageing: a longitudinal investigation of young adults Eur. J. Orthodont.1:15-23, 1979

de FROE, A.: Meetbare variabelen van den meschelijken schedel en hun onderlinge correlaties in verband met leeftijd en geslacht Academisch proefschrift, Universiteit van Amsterdam

GOTTLIEB, B. and ORBAN, B.: Zahnfleischentzûndungen und Zahnlockerungen, 2te Auflage, pp. 31-61, 66,67, Berlin, Berlinische Verlagsanstalt, 1936

HELLMAN,M.: A preliminary study in the development as it affects the human face Dental Cosmos, 69: 250-269,1927

HELLMAN, M.: An introduction to the growth of the human face from infancy to adulthood Int. J. Orthod. 18:777-798,1932

HERZBERG,F. and HOLIC,R.: An anthropologic study of face height Am. J. Orthod. 29: 90-100, 1943

ISRAEL, H.: Recent knowledge concerning craniofacial aging Angle Orthod. 43: 176-184, 1973

LÖE, H.:The structure and physiology of the dentogingival junction, in: Miles, A.E.W.,Structural and chemical of teeth pp.415-455,Academic Press, New York, 1967

MANSON, J.D.:Passive eruption Dent. Pract. 14: 2-9, 1963
MAYNARD,J.G. and OCHSENBEIN,C.: Mucogingival problems, prevalence and therapy in children J. Periodontol. 46: 534-552,1975
MAZELAND, G.R.J.:Jaws and Gums. The mucogingival complex in relation to alveolar process height and lower anterior face height in man. Academisch Proefschrift, Universiteit van Amsterdam, 1978
MAZELAND,G.R.J.: Longitudinal aspects of gingival width J. Periodontol. Res. 15: 429-433, 1980
MAZELAND, G.R.J.: The mucogingival complex in relation to alveolar process height and lower anterior face height J. Periodontol. Res. 15: 345-352, 1980
McFALL,W.T. and KRAUS,B.S.:Histological studies of human prenatal oral mucous membranes Periodontics 3:20-27,1963
McFALL,W.T.and KRAUS,B.S.:Notations in surface morphology of prenatal oral mucous membranes Periodontics 3:141-146,1965
MIELER,I.KLEIN,M. and STIER,H.: Eine Studie zur Breite der befestigten Gingiva in Abhängigkeit von Alters- und Zahngruppen; Zahn-,Mund-,u.Kieferheilk. 73:243-252, 1985
MURPHY,T.:Compensatory mechanisms in facial height adjustments to functional tooth attrition Austr. Dent.J.4:312-323,1959
NANDA,R.S.:The rates of growth of several facial components measured from serial cephalometric röntgenograms Am. J. Orthod. 41:658-673,1955
RIOLO,M.L.,MOYERS,R.E.,McNAMARA,J.A. and HUNTER,W.S.:An atlas of craniofacial growth.Cephalometric standards from the University School of Growth Study, The University of Michigan, Ann Arbor, Michigan, 1974
ROSE,S.T. and APP,G.R.:A clinical study of the development of the attached gingiva along the facial aspect of the maxillary and mandibular anterior teeth in the deciduous, transitional and permanent dentitions. J.Periodontol. 44:131-139, 1973
SARNÄS, KV.V and SOLOW, B.:Early adult changes in the skeletal and soft-tissue profile Eur.J.Orthod.2: 1-12, 1980
TALLGREN,A.: Changes in adult face height due to aging,wear and loss of teeth and prosthetic treatment ActaOdont. Scand. 15, suppl. 24, 1957
TANNER,J.L.:Growth at adolescence.2nd ed.,pp.1.27, Oxford, Blackwell Scientific Publ., 1962
TENENBAUM,H.andTENENBAUM,M.:A clinical study of the width of the attached gingiva in the deciduous, transitional and permanent dentitions.J.Clin.Periodontol:13:270.275,1986
VINCENT,J.W.,MACHEN,J.B. and LEVIN,M.P.: Assessment of attached gingiva using the tension test and clinical measurements J.Periodontol. 47: 412-414, 1976
WALLY,M.,CURILOVIĆ,Z. and STEINER,M.: Mukogingivalzustand 35- und 45järiger Zürcher. Sweiz.Monatschr. Zahnheilk. 93: 163-173, 1983
WAERHAUG,J.:The gingival pocket. Odontologisk Tiskrift 60, suppl. 1, 1952

WINGARD, C.E. and BOWERS, G.M.: The effects on facial bone from facial tipping of incisors in monkeys. J. Periodontol. 47: 450-454. 1976

Address:

Dr. G. R. J. Mazeland
Academic Center for Dentistry Amsterdam
Department of Orthodontics
De Boelelaan 1115
Postbus 7161
1007 MC Amsterdam
the Netherlands

Periodontology Today. Int. Congr., Zürich 1988, pp. 24–31 (Karger, Basel 1988)

Distribution of Collagen Fibres in the Periodontal Ligament and Their Role in Tooth Support

D. C. A. Picton

University College & Middlesex School of Dentistry, London, UK

Introduction

Collagen is the predominant fibre type in the periodontium forming in the order of fifty per cent of the ligament by dry weight. All levels of the hierarchical organisation of collagen could be relevant to this discussion but fibril and fibre bundles will be considered. The close physical and biochemical association of intervening molecules of ground substance, while not strictly part of the collagen aggrigate, probably have a significant contribution to the mechanisms of tooth support (29).

Distribution of collagen fibres

The location and orientation of the fibres was described by the early dental histologists and has remained substantially unchallenged. Standard texts on the periodontium identify admirably the more or less clearly distinguishable groups of dentoalveolar or principal fibres (37), although relatively minor clusters of collagen fibres can be found with the neurovascular bundles passing in the long axis of the ligament. The principal fibres of a tooth of limited growth appear to be arranged to oppose displacing forces from any direction. The oblique groups of fibres predominate and exist as such before fixation (7). Although the alignement of principal fibres is basically radial the variation is reminiscent of wire spokes of a wheel (42).

The groups of fibres can be readilly identified in a wide range of mammals. Thin walled blood vessels, entering the ligament obliquely are enveloped in the fibre network. BIEN (5) has suggested that tension created in the fibres would constrict these vessels with consequent slowing of blood flow and possibly generating gas bubbles. The incisors of rodents, may have interlacing collagen fibrils in the form of sheets rather than bundles in the middle zone of the ligament (42). The fibre bundles are evident at their insertion into cementum and bone, where they are aligned more steeply than for teeth of limited growth (2). The angulation of the fibres is related to forces acting on the tooth as is shown by angular changes which follow sustained intrusive or extrusive forces (40). A striking difference in the rodent incisor ligament is the restriction of the dentoalveolar fibres to the concave surface, while collagen elsewhere is orientated parallel to the enamel surface.

Electronmicroscopy reveals that the fibre bundles from a highly organised three-dimensional network (43). It is not possible to follow a discrete fibre across the webb from cementum to bone as they interweave and form other cluster fibres (19). Adjustments affecting the position of the tooth probably occur continuously throughout the ligament at a molecular level in view of the high rate of turnover in the tissue elements (44, 39, & 6). The level of activity is also shown by the restoration of structural and functional normality within three weeks of replantation of human teeth(1). The functionally significant waviness of collagen is also manifest under polarized light as crimping of fibrils which are generally in phase (14).

The Tooth in Function

The effect of any force to the crown relates to the geometry and surface area of the root to which the force is transmitted. Thus, for example, intrusive forces would place all but crestal, furcation and apical fibre groups under tension. Almost all forces tend to cause the tooth to tilt and probably rotate to some degree. The axis of tilt depends on the magnitude of the force (25) and changes dynamically as the force increases (33). As all the tissues of the periodontium are viscoelastic time is important in the response to force, while rate of loading and previous loading history also affect the magnitude of displacement (23).

Theories of Tooth Support

Unequivocal evidence on the mechanisms of tooth support is in short supply since, like eruption, most findings are subject to several interpretations while the experimental procedure itself invariably influences tissue elements other than those primarily being studied.

Tooth Support by Tension

Tension is the mechanism which seems to have most structural evidence in its favour. The fibre orientation appears to be designed to resist force from any direction. Further, long-term increase in the number and density of principal fibres correlates with increasing masticatory loads (18). The waviness of the fibres corresponds well with the two phases in the force displacement curves for collagen (16) and for tooth mobility (25). The first phase was explained experimentally as being due to straightening of the fibres by force below 1 Newton, as the root is moved across the ligament, but that tension develops in the fibres thereafter and is conveyed to the socket as the force increases. The marked reduction in mobility of the tooth as the individual matures also corresponds with the increase in fibre density (27).

Although the biomechanical characteristics of fresh periodontal ligament have been studied _in vitro_ (9, 38) and are comparable to those for collagen fibres in tendon, the mechanisms _in vivo_ are probably more complex. Sustained force causes the tooth to creep (26) and histologically clear evidence is given of elongation and realignement of fibres in areas of presumed tension. Extrusive force produced significantly less displacement than intrusive force (32) which is consistent with short apical and furcational fibres being tensed with less displacement of the root than fibres oblique to the line of displacement. Transducers on the socket margins detected displacement in the wake of the tooth when horizontal force above 0.5N was applied to the crown (31), while a thin steel blade cutting the tissue in presumed sites of tension caused a significant increase in mobility (36).

To account for the experimental findings it is necessary to accept that force is transmitted across a three dimensional net rather than to simple ties directly from tooth to bone, and that collagen can transmit tension although it undergoes dimensional change with repeated loadings. Thus PARFITT (28) recorded progressively deeper penetration of incisors into their sockets with a series of loadings. Similarly, vasoconstructors and exsanguination caused a reduction in vertical mobility (41, 47) probably causing increasing collapse of the vessels and elongation of the fibre net as the tooth becomes progressively intruded and less mobile. However, it is difficult to explain on the basis of tension the marked reduction in displacement as the loading rate is increased (17).
At impact rates the ligament seems to be almost rigid with no time for fluid to be displaced while the tooth itself bends under horizontal force.

Biochemical alterations to the fibres also gives indirect support to the tension hypothesis. Thus reduction in the tensile strength of collagen molecules following systemic lathyrogens weakens the periodontal attachment (8) and increases extrusive mobility of rodent incisors (24). Similarly marmosets rendered scorbytic had loose teeth together with loss of compactness and number of collagen fibres (10).

Tooth Support by Compression

The alternative explanation for many of the same observations is that the fibres form a compressive mattress. Thus the gradual decrease in mobility after eruption can be attributed to the increasing fibre content acting as a more dense filling to the mattress. In 1933 SYNGE (46) showed mathematically that the collagen fibres were too wavy to account for the normal tightness of the tooth and that compression in some regions of the ligament would result in a subatmospheric pressure elsewhere. Although KORBER (17) has shown with rapidly applied force that there is too little time for the fibres on the "tension" side to be straightened, on the opposite side compression would develop instantly. Experimentally, the socket margin was distorted as though the ligament was under compression when horizontal loads were applied (31) while intrusive force produced dilation of the socket (34).

Gabel (12) proposed that tissue in zones of compression would be displaced towards areas of lower pressure and would cause the principal fibres to come under tension in a series of catenary cures. Surgical trauma to selected sites, however, cutting the oblique fibres on the mesial and distal aspects of incisors produced no change in horizontal mobility (36). Recently, excision of a complete band of coronal ligament 3-4 mm wide produced little or no increase in intrusion for half the insisors tested in monkeys (33). Thus tangential flow of tissue either around or along the root, seems to be of little importance under these conditions.

If the SYNGE hypothesis (46) is correct the whole periodontium would function as a single entity. However, clinically teeth with alveolar fenestrations, teeth having incompletely formed roots or following apicectomy are not dramatically more mobile under intrusive force than their intact neighbours. Similarly, little change in mobility with intrusive force followed removal of root apices in pig mandibles (13) or in living monkeys (35). Thus compression is not of importance in the apical region, at least under these conditions.

Support by Tension and Compression

Several findings suggest that tension and compression can be generated simultaneously. Thus the alveolar margins were distorted in the same direction as the force on both the presumed tension and compression sides (31). Again, surgical trauma to the approximal ligament caused mobility to increase to the same extent towards or away from the lesion (36).

The dimensions of collagen fibrils which are subjected to tension in rabbit flexor digitorum tendon are larger than in other regions subjected to compression (15, 20). Analysis of the fibre size in the periodontal ligament of rats (4) indicate that the dimensions of the fibres, and the composition of the ground substance are consistent with both tension and compression (21).

Conclusions

While the present discussion has focused on short term loadings histological evidence on long acting forces indicates that both tension and compression develop in the periodontium. From the findings with short acting forces it is apparent that collagen may act as a three dimensional tensional net but may also resist displacement of the tooth as a compressive mat. Compression and tension may develop at different times in the same zone or may operate simultaneously in different sites depending on the direction of force. The loading conditions are important. Indeed the rate of loading may dictate the contribution made by each of the several possible mechanisms.

References

1. ANDERSON, J.O. and HJORTING-HANSEN, E.: Replantation of teeth. Histological study of twenty two replanted anterior teeth in humans. Acta odont. Scand. 24: 287-291 (1966).
2. BEERTSEN, W. and SNYDER, J.: Histologic differences between the periodontal membranes of teeth with continuous and limited eruption. Nederl T. Tandheelk. 76: 542-546 (1969).
3. BERKOVITZ, B.K.B.; MOXHAM, B.J. & SHORE, R.C.: Ultra-structural quantification of the extra cellular matrix of sheep incisor periodontium. J.dent.Res. 64: 687 (1985).
4. BERKOVITZ, B.K.B.; WEAVER, M.E.; SHORE R.C. & MOXHAM, B.J. Fibril diameters in the extracellular matrix of the periodontal connective tissues of the rat. Connect. Tiss. Res. 8: 127-132 (1981).
5. BIEN, S.M.: The pressure gradient in the periodontal membrane. Trans. N.Y. Acad. Sci. 28 (4): 496-506 (1966).
6. BOS, T. van den, and TONINO, G.T.M.: Composition and metabolism of the extra cellular matrix in the periodontal ligament of impeded and unimpeded rat incisor. Archs oral Biol.: 29, 893-897 (1984).
7. BURN-MURDOCH, R.A. & TYLER, D.W.: Physiological evidence that periodontal collagen in rats exists as fibres prior to histological fixation. Archs. oral Biol. 26: 995-999 (1981).
8. CHIBA, M. and OHKAWA, S.: Measurement of the tensile strength of the periodontium in rat mandibular first molar. Archs. oral Biol. 25: 569-572. (1980).
9. DALY, C.H.; WILSON, B.D. and KYDD, W.L.: A mathematical and experimental investigation of tooth mobility. Proc. Amer. Conf. Eng. Med. Biol. 14: 289-290 (1972)
10. DREIZEN, S.; LEVY, B.M. and BERNICK, S.: Studies on the biology of the periodontium of marmosets. J. periodont. Res. 4: 274-280 (1969).
11. EASTOE, J.E. and MELCHER, A.H.: Amino acid composition of whole periodontal ligament from rat incisor. J. dent. Res. 50: 675-680 (1971).
12. GABEL, A.B. A mathematical analysis of the function of the fibres of the periodontal membrane. J. Periodontal 27: 191-196 (1956).

13. GATHERCOLE, L.J.: In-vitro mechanics of intrusive loading in porcine teeth. Archs oral Biol 32: 249-256 (1987).
14. GATHERCOLE, L.J.: Biophysical aspects of the fibres of the periodontal ligament; in Berkovitz: The periodontal ligament in health and disease. pp103-117 Pergamon Press Oxford 1982).
15. GILLARD, G.C.: The proteoglycan content of collagen in tendon. Biochem. J. 163: 145-151 (1977).
16. KELLER, A. and GATHERCOLE, L.J.: Biophysical and mechanical properties of collagen in relation to function; in Poole and Stack, The eruption and occlusion of teeth. Colston Papers, No 27, pp 252-266 (Butterworths, London 1976).
17. KORBER, H.K.: Electronic registration of tooth movements. Int. dent. J. 21: 466-477 (1971).
18. KRONFELD, R.: Histological study of the influence of function of human periodontal membrane. J.Amer.Dent.Assn. 18: 1242-1245 (1931).
19. KVAM, E.: Topography of principal fibres of the periodontal ligament. Scand.J.dent.Res. 81: 553-557 (1973).
20. MERRILEES, M.J. and FLINT, M.H.: Ultra structural study of tension and pressure zones in a rabbit flexor tendon. Amer.J.Anat. 187: 87-106 (1980).
21. MOXHAM, B.J.: Studies on the mechanical properties of the periodontal ligaments; in Lisney and Matthews, Current Topics in Oral Biology; pp.73-81 (Univ.Bristol Press,1985)
22. MOXHAM, B.J. and BERKOVITZ, B.K.B.: A quantitative assessment of the effects of axially directed extrusive loads on displacement of the unimpeded rabbit mandibular incisor. Archs oral Biol. 26: 209-216 (1981).
23. MOXHAM, B.J. and BERKOVITZ, B.K.B.: The effect of external forces on the periodontal ligament - the response to axial loads; in Berkovitz; Moxham and Newman: The periodontal ligament in health and disease: pp.249-270 (Pergmon Press Oxford 1982).
24. MOXHAM, B.J. and BRECOVITZ, B.K.B.: The mobility of lathyritic mandibular incisors in response to axially directed extrusive loads. Archs oral Biol. 29: 773-778 (1984).
25. MÜHLEMANN, H.R.: A method of measuring tooth mobility. J.Oral Surg., Oral Med., Oral Path. 4: 1220-1226 (1951).
26. MÜHLEMANN H.R., SAVDIR, S. and RATEITSCHAK, H.K.: Tooth mobility, its causes and significance, J.Periodontol. 36: 148-152, (1965).
27. MÜHLEMANN H.R. and ZANDER, H.A.: The mechanisms of tooth mobility. J. Periodontol. 25: 128-137 (1954).
28. PARFITT, G.J.: Measurement of the physiological mobility of individual teeth in an axial direction. J.Dent.Res. 39: 608-618.
29. PEARSON, C.H.: The ground substance of the periodontal ligament; in Berkovitz, Moxham and Newman; The periodontal ligament in health and disease; pp.119-149 (Perga-

mon Press, Oxford, 1982).

30. PICTON, D.C.A.: The effect on tooth mobility of trauma to the mesial and distal regions of the periodontal ligament in monkeys. Hel.odont.Acta. 11: 105-112 (1967).

31. PICTON, D.C.A.: Dimensional changes in the periodontal membrane of monkeys due to horizontal thrusts applied to the teeth. Archs oral Biol. 12;1635-1643 (1967),

32. PICTON, D.C.A.: Extrusive mobility of teeth in adult monkeys. Archs oral Biol. 31: 369-372 (1986).

33. PICTON, D.C.A.: The effect on intrusive tooth mobility of surgically removing cervical periodontal ligament in monkeys. Archs oral Biol. (accepted) 1988.

34. PICTON, D.C.A. and DAVIES, W.I.R.: Distortion of the socket with normal tooth mobility; in Anderson, Melcher, Eastoe & Picton; The mechanisms of tooth support. pp.157-161, (John Wrights, Bristol, 1967).

35. PICTON, D.C.A. and PICTON, H.M.: The effect of excision of the root apex on the intrusive mobility of anterior teeth in adult monkeys (M. fascicularis) Archs oral Biol 32: 323-327 (1987).

36. PICTON, D.C.A. and SLATTER, J.M.: The effect on horizontal tooth mobility of experimental trauma to the periodontal ligament in regions of tension or compression. J.Periodont.Res. 7: 35-41 (1972).

37. PROVENZA, D.: Oral histology and Development. Ch.11, pp.326-354. (J.B. Lippencott Co. Philadelphia).

38. RALPH, W.J.: Tensile behaviour of the periodontal ligament. J.Periodont.Res.17: 423-426, (1982).

39. RIPPIN, J.W.: Collagen turnover in the periodontal ligament under normal and altered functional forces.II Adult rat molar. J.Periodot.Res. 13: 149-154 (1978).

40. SIMS, M.R.: Angular changes in collagen cemental attachment during tooth movement. J.Periodont.Res. 15: 638-645 (1980).

41. SLATTER, J.M. and PICTON, D.C.A.: The effect of intrusive tooth mobility of noradrenaline injected locally in monkeys. J.Periodont.Res. 7: 144-150. (1972).

42. SLOAN, P.: Scanning electron microscopy of the collagen fibre architecture of the rabbit incisor periodontium. Archs oral Biol. 23: 567-572, (1978).

43. SLOAN, P.; SHELLES, R.P. and BERKOVITZ, B.K.B.: Effect of specimen preparation in the appearance of the rat periodontal ligament in the scanning electron microscope. Archs oral Biol. 21: 633-634 (1976).

44. SODEK, J.: A comparison of the rates of synthesis and turnover of collagen and non-collagen proteins in adult rat periodontal tissues. Archs oral Biol. 22: 655-665, (1977).

45. SYNGE, J.L.: The equilibrium of a tooth with a general conical root. London Philos. Mag. 15: 969-974 (1933).

46. WILLS, D.J.; PICTON, D.C.A.; and DAVIES, W.I.R.: A study of the fluid systems of the periodontium in macaque monkeys. Archs oral Biol. 21: 175-185, (1976)

Dr. D.C.A. Picton, University College & Middlesex School of Dentistry, Mortimer Market, London WC1E 6JD, UK

Periodontology Today. Int. Congr., Zürich 1988, pp. 32–40 (Karger, Basel 1988)

Origin, Structure and Distribution of Cementum and its Possible Role in Local Periodontal Treatment

Hubert E. Schroeder

Department of Oral Structural Biology, Dental Institute, University of Zurich, Switzerland

Introduction

Very recently, JONES (1981) and SCHROEDER (1986) proposed and adopted a new classification of root cementum, differentiating between four varieties according to the absence or presence of cells and to the source of collagen fibers contained within. This classification distinguishes between acellular afibrillar cementum (AAC), acellular extrinsic fiber cementum (AEFC), cellular, mixed stratified cementum (CMSC), and cellular intrinsic fiber cementum (CIFC). Apart from a mineralized ground substance, AAC contains neither cells nor ex- or intrinsic collagen fibers. In the human, it is found as coronal cementum covering portions of the enamel surface and as an occasional part of AEFC. The latter lacks cells and is composed almost entirely of densely packed bundles of Sharpey's fibers. In the human, it is found primarily on the cervical third of the root, but it may extend further apically. CMSC is a mixture of extrinsic (Sharpey's) and intrinsic fibers, varying in proportion, and contains cells with uneven distribution and density. It is usually a stratified deposit, with layers of AEFC and CIFC being superimposed on one another. In the human, it occurs primarily in the apical third of the roots and in the furcations. CIFC contains cells but its collagen fibers are all intrinsic, i.e., it lacks Sharpey's fibers. In the human, it is found mainly in situations of repair, filling resorption lacunae or recombining root fragments during root fracture healing (SCHROEDER, 1986).

As AEFC and CMSC are the two major varieties covering the root surface, their origin, structure and function will be described on the basis of recent data (OWENS, 1972, 1973, 1976; SCHROEDER, 1986).

Acellular extrinsic fiber cementum (AEFC)

Following the separation of Hertwig's root sheath from the initially formed root dentine, cells of the dental follicle proper gain access to the outer root surface. At this stage of development and up to the time of tooth eruption, the tooth surface is covered by a thin layer of external predentine which is seen to be continuous with pulpal predentine around the apical rim of the growing root. As shown by sequential Tetracyclin labeling (OWENS, 1973), the about 20 to 40 μm thick external predentine undergoes delayed mineralization only after about three quarters of the root have been formed and the tooth has started to erupt. This external predentine is comprised of a dense layer and an outermost fringe of fibers, and serves as an organic base to which follicular and later periodontal ligament fibers become attached. Produced by fibroblasts, these fibers obviously have a rather complicated genesis. As suggested by the fine structural composition of AEFC and the adjacent ligament (SCHROEDER, 1986), the synthesized collagen fibrils must first be bundled in parallel, then orientated perpendicular to the root surface, and, with their terminal ends, intermingled with the still non-mineralized external predentine. Eventually, the external predentine mineralizes together with the terminal portions of the densely stacked bundles of collagen fibrils of the ligament and, thereby, the first layer of AEFC is formed. In an erupting human tooth, this may happen first in the apical region and spread coronally (OWENS, 1976).

As seen on fractured root surfaces and on the inorganic external surface of newly-formed AEFC, this cementum variety consist almost exclusively of densely packed, well orientated bundles of collagen fibrils, the fibers of Sharpey. These fibers run uninterrupted into the periodontal ligament, forming its principal fibers. Thus, all AEFC-fibers are extrinsic. Additional layers of AEFC arise from the conversion of a layer of the radially ordered periodontal ligament fibers into cementoid and its eventual mineralization. Therefore, AEFC becomes thicker with age. There are about 30,000 fibers inserting into 1 mm^2 of AEFC-surface, each fiber being about 4 μm in diameter. All fibers are fibroblast-products while the contribution of cementoblasts to AEFC is in doubt. AEFC is densely and homogeneously mineralized and shows mineral-rich incremental lines. Its function is to anchor the tooth via principal fibers of the periodontal ligament to the alveolar bone proper. AEFC is nothing more than calcified periodontal ligament fibers attached to the root surface.

Cellular, mixed stratified cementum

CMSC is a mixed deposit containing layers of pure CIFC and AEFC, with Sharpey's fibers often being discontinued. The CIFC-component undoubtedly is a cementoblast product. It is often the first to develop in the course of root genesis, at least on all surfaces facing a furcation, over root concavities, and around the apex. Cementoblasts are generated from the dental follicle proper and the periodontal ligament derived from it. Early CIFC formation often occurs patchwise and in irregular layers directly on the external predentine or over a thin, first-formed layer of AEFC. These CIFC-layers may later be covered by AEFC, which in turn may again be overlaid by one or several layers of CIFC. Thus, so-called resting lines as seen in routine histological sections may, at least in part, represent thin layers of AEFC coating previously formed or the most superficial layer of CIFC. Sharpey's fibers originating from a deep layer of AEFC may or may not run continuously through the superimposed layers of CIFC. Unfortunately, details of cellular cementum formation and the deposition of CMSC are still unknown.

However, the above stated remarks are in agreement with the microscopic structure of CMSC, as observed in the light- and the scanning electron microscope (SCHROEDER, 1986). CMSC is a rather heterogeneous deposit of varying thickness. Cells, contained within the CIFC-component, the cementocytes, occur with varying distribution and density. Because of this, the cementocyte lacunae (6 to 12 µm in diameter) and their fine canaliculi extending up to 15 µm render CMSC variably porous. Sharpey's fibers are irregularly distributed. Some extend through several cementum layers and, because of their rather hypomineralized cores, form channels of organic material. Others seem to be rather short and related to the next following AEFC-layer only. The intrinsic collagen fibers are the main structural component of all CIFC-layers and these fibers run a spiral course around the root, i.e., parallel to the root surface. The stratification of consecutive or alternating layers of AEFC and CIFC results in a lamellation which, occasionally, may be rather regular but most often is very irregular and scale-like. For all these reasons, CMSC is very inhomogeneously mineralized, porous and rather soft. As the surface of CMSC may or may not, at a particular point in time, be coated with AEFC, CMSC contributes to tooth support to a variable degree. The average number of inserting fibers of Sharpey (about 10- to 20,000/mm^2) is smaller than that of AEFC. The main functional role of CMSC is the adaptational, dynamic reshaping of the root surface as the tooth shifts and drifts in its socket.

Material and Methods

A total of 48 extracted human teeth including maxillary and mandibular central and lateral incisors, canines, and single-rooted first premolars were collected from patients of varying ages. All teeth were fixed in formalin and stored in cacodylate buffer. From each of these teeth, an about 100 to 200 µm thick, central ground section was produced along the tooth axis in the vestibulo-oral direction, using the Exakt-Cutting-Grinding System (Exakt-Apparatebau, Norderstedt, BRD). These axial sections were dehydrated in ethanol and mounted on glass slides with Permount[R]. From all sections, low-power light-micrographs were taken with a Leitz-Aristophot equipment. Enlarged glossy prints were produced at a standardized magnification of x 7.8. Regions along the root surface covered with either AEFC or CMSC were marked on these pictures and their proportional contribution to the total root surface was determined. This was done either by tracing the respective portion of the root surface profiles with the pencil cursor of the MOP-AMO-I system (Kontrol AG, Zürich) or by measuring the distance (in mm), buccally and orally, between the cemento-enamel junction (CEJ) and the root apex along the root axis and determining the height (in mm) of the apical root portion covered with CMSC. In both cases, the contribution of either cementum variety was expressed in percentages of the total root surface profile or total root length. Buccal and oral measurements were pooled and averages (± standard deviation) were calculated for individual teeth and each type of tooth. Furthermore, using data on the actual average length of such teeth (SCHUMACHER and SCHMIDT, 1983), the axial length of AEFC-covered root surfaces, extending from the CEJ apically, was calculated.

Results

As both, the profile- and the length-related measurements yielded analogous data, only the length-related data are presented here. The mean percentage of the root length covered with AEFC ranged from 91±8 (mandibular lateral incisor) to 59±16 (mandibular first premolar); Table I). In the maxillary jaw, the proportion of AEFC-coating was highest in lateral incisors and lowest in central incisors and canines. In the mandibular jaw, the proportion of AEFC-coating was heighest in lateral incisors and lowest in first premolars (Table I). The amount of CMSC-coating was indirectly proportional. In terms of the actual root length, AEFC covered 8.5 to 10.7 mm in maxillary and 8.0 to 12.5 mm in mandibular teeth, when expressed as the apical extension from the CEJ along the root axis (Table II). This extension was larger in lateral incisors and canines than in central incisors and premolars, both in the maxillary annd the mandibular jaw (Table II).

Discussion

The distribution of AEFC and CMSC in single-rooted human teeth and the proportional and actual length of the cervical root surface covered with AEFC was determined in one plane of sectioning and with a limited number of teeth only. Nevertheless, it became clear that, because of their opposite distribution at cervical or apical parts of the root, AEFC and CMSC extended to a variable degree in incisors, canines and premol-

Table I. Mean percentage of total root length covered with acellular or cellular cementum, as measured on vestibular and oral aspects of single-rooted human teeth.

Parameters		Percentage cementum on teeth			
CMSC ($\bar{x}\pm s$, apical)		35±18	17±17	33±13	25±19
AEFC ($\bar{x}\pm s$, cervical)		65±18	83±17	67±13	75±19
N		6	8	3	9
Tooth index	Maxillary	11,21	12,22	13,23	14,24
	Mandibular*	41,31	42,32	43,33	44,34
N		6	3	9	4
AEFC ($\bar{x}\pm s$, cervical)		79±15	91±8	72±14	59±16
CMSC ($\bar{x}\pm s$, apical)		21±15	9±8	28±14	41±16

N = number of teeth
AEFC = acellular extrinsic fiber cementum
CMSC = cellular mixed stratified cementum
* Molars present 30-60% CMSC which also covers all of the furcation

Table II. Actual root length (mm) of single-rooted human teeth and length (mm) of the coronal root portion covered with acellular cementum.

Parameters		Actual root length and AEFC on teeth			
AEFC-covering		8.5	10.7	10.6	10.2
Root length* ($\bar{x}\pm s$)		13.0±1.7	12.9±1.6	15.9±2.4	13.6±1.8
Tooth index	Maxillary	11,21	12,22	13,23	14,24
	Mandibular	41,31	42,32	43,33	44,34
Root length* ($\bar{x}\pm s$)		12.8±1.6	13.7±1.6	15.3±2.0	13.7±1.6
AEFC-covering		10.1	12.5	11.0	8.0

AEFC = acellular extrinsic fiber cementum
* Data from SCHUMACHER and SCHMIDT (1983)

ars. This distribution pattern may play a role in the success of local periodontal treatment.

AEFC is a very dense, homogeneously mineralized, and rather thin deposit, ranging in width from about 50 to 250 µm. Conversely, CMSC is a variably porous, inhomogeneously mineralized deposit of variable thickness, ranging from about 100 to 600 µm or more. Both variations are very much softer than dentine, i.e., 40 versus 70 KHN, but CMSC is much more permeable than AEFC (SCHROEDER, 1986). For these reasons, AEFC and CMSC supposedly react differently when subjected to scaling and root planing. Neither AEFC nor CMSC is completely removed from human teeth undergoing their first scaling and root planing. Extensive instrumentation (i.e., 50 strokes per test surface) of incisors, premolars and molars with freshly sharpened scalers and curettes does not result in the complete removal of root cementum, particularly in the apical region covered with CMSC (O'LEARY and KAFRAWY, 1983). Only rigorous root planing removes all cementum and exposes dentine, at least in a 5 mm wide cervical region (as measured from the CEJ; LASHO, O'LEARY and KAFRAWY, 1983). Thus, long-term treatment with scaling and root planing performed at regular intervals may eventually result in the complete removal of AEFC but not CMSC. In other words, for an unknown period of time, repetitive root instrumentation may deal with either planing AEFC and dentine, or CMSC only.

Scaling and root planing with hand-instruments or rotating burs coated with ultrafine diamond particles, however, does not result in a microscopically smooth root surface. It has been shown repeatedly (JONES, LOZDAN and BOYDE, 1972; PANMEIJER, 1972; EWEN and GWINNETT, 1977), that any kind of root instrumentation changes the character and structure of the root surface. Depending on the type, form and sharpness of the instrument used, depending on the force and direction of strokes, about three different surface features are produced. These are a somewhat blurred but close to normal surface structure, a grooved pattern representing a range of alterations from fine and shallow grooves to large and deep troughs, and a smeared pattern characterized by an inelastic deformation and squeezing or flattening of the root surface. As JONES, LOZDAN and BOYDE (1972) have suggested, the latter type of alteration results from very high pressure applied locally. In addition, the root surface may fracture with splintering of cementum portions. Dull instruments tend to produce troughs and a smeared pattern rather than fine grooves, scratches or open tears and cavitations which are due to freshly resharpened instruments (EWEN and GWINNETT, 1977). Fine diamond burs produce a pattern of variably short and very fine grooves (SCHWARZ et al., 1988). No exact data are available today, however, on the effect of root planing and instrument pressure on CMSC, as in all probability the quoted literature refers to AEFC-coated surfaces only.

Table III. Percentage loss of individual teeth during periodontal long-term treatment (15 to 22 years) of all patients and of a well-responding subgroup of patients, as observed in two clinical studies.

Groups/patients	Loss of teeth during long-term treatment			
Total loss				
H.W.* (600 p.)	5.3	5.5	3.6	6.3
McF.** (100 p.)	8.2	7.9	4.7	10.2
Well-responding p.				
H.W.* (500 p.)	0.8	0.7	0	1.3
McF.** (77 p.)	1.4	0	0	2.1
Tooth index – Maxillary	11,21	12,22	13,23	14,24
Tooth index – Mandibular	41,31	42,32	43,33	44,34
Total loss				
H.W.* (600 p.)	6.3	3.4	0.8	1.6
McF.** (100 p.)	9.0	6.5	0.5	5.8
Well-responding p.				
H.W.* (500 p.)	1.2	0.6	0	0.6
McF.** (77 p.)	0.6	0.6	0	0.7

* Data from HIRSCHFELD and WASSERMAN (1978)
** Data from McFALL (1982)
p. = patients

Nevertheless, the present knowledge on the character and properties of AEFC versus CMSC, and on the damage done to these tissues by scaling and root planing allows to postulate the following: Because of its density, its limited thickness and the underlying core of harder dentine, AEFC is likely to withstand this treatment for a longer period of time, while retaining a relatively dense, smooth and tight surface pattern. On the other hand, CMSC, because of its heterogeneous and porous character, its irregular lamellations and relative thickness, may be subject to coarser artifacts and surface splintering, eventually revealing a grossly irregular and porous surface. In fact, porosity may increase with the exposure of deeper layers of CMSC.

For these reasons, local periodontal long-term treatment of single-rooted teeth may be assumed to meet with favorable conditions and success, provided root instrumentation remains within the realm of AEFC-coated surfaces. Instrumentation of CMSC-covered surfaces may involve a less favorable prognosis. This hypothesis can be tested on the basis of data provided by HIRSCHFELD and WASSERMAN (1978) and by McFALL (1982): In Table III, the reported percentage loss of individual single-rooted teeth during local periodontal long-term treatment is listed for all patients as well as for the major subgroup of well-responding patients, supervised by these authors. In the maxillary jaw, the greatest loss was seen with central incisors and first premolars, while lateral incisors and canines were less often lost. In the mandibular jaw, the lateral incisors and canines were also less often lost than the central incisors and first premolars (Table III). This pattern of tooth loss correlates rather well with the length of the coronal root portion coated with AEFC (Table II). If this correlation were real, the success of local periodontal long-term treatment of single-rooted teeth would, at least in part, be a function of the distribution and character of root cementum varieties.

References

EWEN, S.J. and GWINNETT, A.J.: A scanning electron microscopic study of teeth following periodontal instrumentation. J. Periodontol. 48: 92-97 (1977).

HIRSCHFELD, L. and WASSERMAN, B.: A longterm survey of tooth loss in 600 treated periodontal patients. J. Periodontol. 49: 225-237 (1978).

JONES, S.J.; LOZDAN, J. and BOYDE, A.: Tooth surfaces treated in situ with periodontal instruments. Brit. dent. J. 132: 57-64 (1972).

JONES, S.J.: Cement; in OSBORN, Dental anatomy and embryology; pp. 286-294 (Blackwell Scientific, Oxford/London 1981).

LASHO, D.J.; O'LEARY, T.J. and KAFRAWY, A.H.: A scanning electron microscope study of the effects of various agents on instrumented periodontally involved root surfaces. J. Periodontol. 54: 210-220 (1983).

McFALL, W.T.: Tooth loss in 100 treated patients with periodontal disease. A long-term study. J. Periodontol. 53: 539-549 (1982).

O'LEARY, T.J. and KAFRAWY, A.H.: Total cementum removal: A realistic objective ? J. Periodontol. 54: 221-226 (1983).

OWENS, P.D.A.: Light microscopic observations on the formation of the layers of Hopewell-Smith in human teeth. Archs. oral Biol. 17: 1785-1788 (1972).

OWENS, P.D.A.: Mineralisation in the roots of human deciduous teeth demonstrated by tetracycline labeling. Archs. oral Biol. 18: 889-897 (1973).

OWENS, P.D.A.: The root surface in human teeth. A microradiographic study. J. Anat. 122: 389-401 (1976).

PANMEIJER, C.: Surface characteristics of teeth following periodontal instrumentation. A scanning electron microscope study. J. Periodontol. 43: 628-633 (1972).

SCHROEDER, H.E.: The Periodontium. Handbook of Microscopic Anatomy; Vol. V/5, pp. 26-28, 54-129 (Springer, Heidelberg/New York 1986).

SCHUMACHER, G.H. and SCHMIDT, H.: Anatomie und Biochemie der Zähne; 3. Aufl., p. 438 (Fischer, Stuttgart/New York 1983).

SCHWARZ, J.P.; GUGGENHEIM, B.; RATEITSCHAK, E. and RATEITSCHAK, K.H.: The effectiveness of curettes and diamond burs in open flap root debridement. J. Clin. Periodont. in press (1988)

Author's Address

Hubert E. Schroeder, DMD, Department of Oral Structural Biology, Dental Institute, University of Zurich, Plattenstrasse 11, 8028 Zurich (Switzerland)

Periodontology Today. Int. Congr., Zürich 1988, pp. 41–49 (Karger, Basel 1988)

Factors Influencing the Stability of the Gingival Sulcus

Ian C. Mackenzie

Dows Institute for Dental Research, University of Iowa, College of Dentistry, Iowa City, Ia, USA

As it erupts, a mammalian tooth breaks the continuity of the surface mucosal epithelium, leaving a cuff which surrounds the tooth and forms a "free edge" of epithelium at the cemento-enamel junction. The significance of this unique anatomical arrangement to the pathogenesis of periodontal disease has been discussed extensively in terms of attachment of epithelium to the tooth, its cell turnover and permeability and to gingival fluid flow and other possible self cleansing mechanisms. Apical migration of epithelium is one of the many tissue responses which occur during periodontal disease and was once thought to be a primary event in its pathogenesis. Now the prevailing view is that epithelial downgrowth occurs as a consequence of other destructive tissue changes (16), but the evidence for either view remains equivocal. Regardless of whether it is a primary or secondary phenomenon, epithelial downgrowth is of central importance to the progression of periodontal diseases. Surface epithelia functionally separate the internal environment of the body from the external one and apical migration of epithelium leads to areas of cementum which had previously been situated within the internal environment, being excluded from defensive and regenerative processes occurring there. Thus reattachment of connective tissue to cementum is inhibited and this is probably a major factor in perpetuating small intermittent increases in pocket depth. Normally when the continuity of epithelium is interrupted, by wounding or by foreign bodies such as sutures or implants which pass through it, there is epithelial migration in an attempt to restore continuity. From this point of view it is puzzling why the unusual arrangement of epithelium, tooth and connective tissue that forms the healthy gingival sulcus should normally be stable. It is of importance to understand the mechanisms by which this stability is achieved before the question can be addressed as to what changes occur during periodontal disease to initiate or permit epithelial downgrowth.

Phenotypic Markers of the Gingival Epithelia

Epithelia synthesize a wide range of macromolecules which differ regionally, from one epithelium to another, and between basal and terminally differentiating cells within the same epithelium. Epithelial expression of particular macromolecules changes during their embryonic development and is influenced by pathological involvement, but regionally specific patterns of differentiation are normally consistent in the adult animal. Examination of the pattern of macromolecular expression of an epithelium provides a powerful method of identifying its characteristics. This has been aided by the development of monoclonal antibodies (mAbs) against two classes of macromolecules, blood group antigens (17), and the cytokeratins, the latter of which will be discussed here.

Keratins form the intermediate filaments of epithelial cells and consist of two families of polypeptides, Type II keratins which are relatively large and basic, and Type I keratins which are smaller and more acidic. Differences in electrophoretic mobility have indicated allocation of eight keratins (numbers 1-8) into the basic subgroup, and 10 keratins (numbers 9-19) into the acidic subgroup (12). A particular epithelium expresses only a few of the total possible number of keratins and mAbs with specificity for individual keratin polypeptides permits their immunohistological localization (6,13,14,23). An outcome of such studies has been the formulation of "rules" of keratin expression (23) which may, in a very simplified form, be generally summarized as: (a) the formation of intermediate filaments requires copolymerization of a pair of keratins, one acidic and the other basic, (b) that the basal cells of all stratifying epithelia express keratins 5 and 14, (c) that the keratins expressed by the terminally differentiating cells of stratifying epithelia differ regionally; for example, the differentiating cells of cornifying epithelia produce keratins 1 and 10, but those of non-cornifying epithelia, keratins 4 and 13, and (d) that keratins 7 and 19, and 8 and 18 are usually found in simple epithelia.

Keratin expression in the gingival epithelia. The ultrastructural studies of Schroeder and Listgarten (21) removed much of the previous uncertainty about the structure and arrangement of the gingival epithelia and about the epithelial attachment to the tooth. These investigations also demonstrated unique characteristics of the junctional epithelium which, unlike other epithelia, forms a basal lamina against the non-vital substrate of the enamel and which, although stratified, shows no distinct ultrastructural evidence of cell maturation. The patterns of keratin expression in the oral gingival, oral sulcular and junctional epithelia show further clear differences between them (10,13). Human oral gingival and oral sulcular epithelia both express keratins 5 and 14, markers of stratifying epithelia, but the oral gingival epithelium is similar to palatal epithelium, expressing keratins 1 and 10, and the oral sulcular epithelium similar to lining epithelium, expressing keratins 4 and 13. Junctional epithelium shares with these epithelia the expression of the stratifying markers, keratins 5 and 14, but does not express differentiation markers typical of other oral epithelia. Instead, it expresses keratin 19, which is usually a marker of simple epithelia although it is sometimes detectable in the basal cells of oral epithelia (13). There is a similar pattern in rodents where the oral gingival, oral sulcular and junctional epithelia all express keratins 5 and 14 but differ in their expression of the differentiation markers keratins 10, 13 and 19 (Fig. 1).

Terminal differentiation in junctional epithelium. It was previously reported that mAbs which bind only to the basal cells of stratifying epithelia bind to all strata of junctional epithelia but some recently produced mAbs show preferential staining of basal cells of both oral epithelia and junctional epithelium. Further evidence for differences between basal and suprabasal cells of junctional epithelium were found when rodent epithelia were screened with a large panel of mAbs against various keratins. The suprabasal cells of rat junctional epithelia stain for keratin 19 (Fig. 1) and were also found to show weak but consistent binding of mAbs with specificity for keratin 8. This was an unexpected finding as keratin 8 is usually a marker of the simple epithelial phenotype and human junctional epithelium has been reported not to show such reactivity (13). However, recent examination of a series of human gingival biopsies has indicated that suprabasal staining with mAbs directed against keratin 8 and also keratin 18, is a feature of human junctional epithelium (Fig. 2). There are thus several differences between basal and suprabasal cells in junctional epithelium suggestive of an unusual pattern of terminal differentiation.

Epithelia similar to junctional epithelium. Coexpression of keratins typical of stratifying and of simple epithelia occurs in some epithelia of the respiratory tract (14) but is not normally found in stratifying oral epithelia. Quite complex patterns of coexpression of keratins occur during embryonic development of the epidermis and periderm but information about keratin expression in developing oral and odontogenic epithelia is lacking. However, to consider the junctional phenotype simply as a legacy of its epithelium of origin would not explain its expression in junctional epithelium reformed from oral epithelia. Expression of both simple and stratifying markers is seen in the linings of periapical cysts (2), which are derived from odontogenic epithelia, but mucosal epithelia also show this pattern in two differing experimental systems. When full-thickness mucosa is transplanted to a graft bed of deep connective tissue the epithelium differentiates normally over its own lamina propria but does not migrate out to epithelialize the exposed surface of the graft bed (7,10). There is a small outgrowth of epithelium onto the deep connective tissue which resembles junctional epithelium in a number of ways. It is proliferative, forms a basal lamina, stratifies without the normal pattern of terminal differentiation and shares a passive, non-migratory behavior. Such outgrowths of murine mucosal epithelium similarly express basal markers of stratifying epithelia, lack the differentiation markers of the epithelium of origin, and express simple epithelial keratins suprabasally (Fig. 2). A similar pattern of keratin expression is also seen when epithelial cells isolated from murine mucosal epithelia are plated on collagen gels and allowed to grow and stratify in supplemented culture media (Fig. 2).

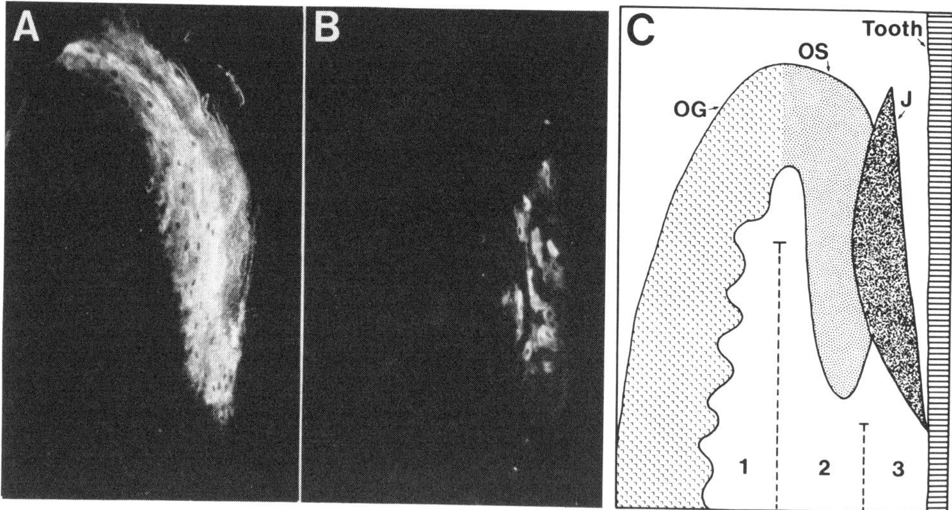

Fig. 1. Rat gingiva stained with antibodies against keratin 13 (A) and against keratin 19 (B) which stain suprabasal cells of the oral sulcular and junctional epithelium respectively. A scheme in which 3 zones of differing connective tissue influences determine the phenotypes of the gingival epithelia is shown in C.

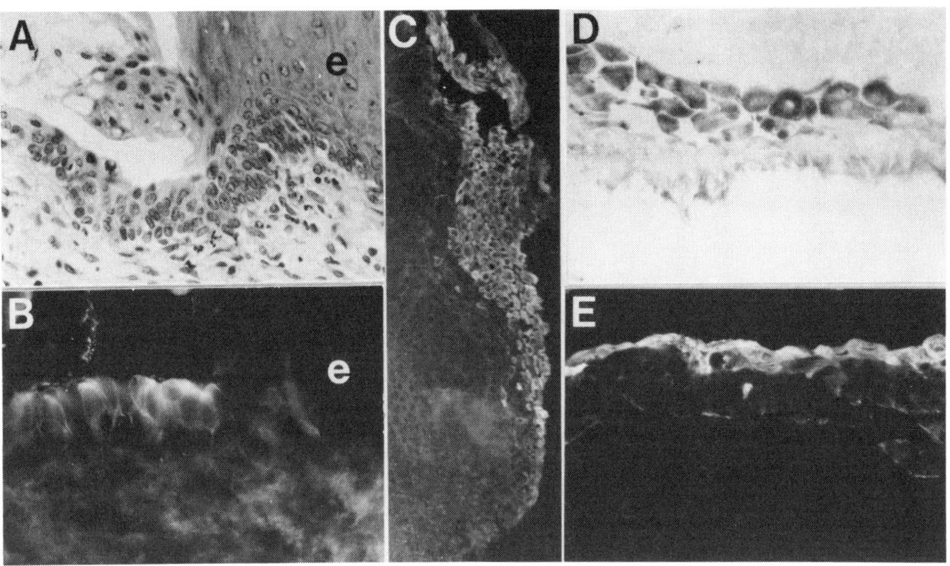

Fig. 2. A: the epithelial outgrowth onto the deep connective tissue adjacent to a transplant of murine palatal mucosa. The outgrowth lacks the normal pattern of differentiation seen in the epithelium (e) overlying the transplanted lamina propria. B-E show reactivity of the suprabasal cells of various epithelia with antibodies against simple epithelial keratins. B: outgrowth epithelium similar to that shown in A. C: human junctional epithelium. D: the epithelial lining of a periapical cyst and E: a stratifying culture of epithelial cells from mouse palate.

Influences of Connective Tissue on Patterns of Epithelial Differentiation

The cells initially forming the junctional epithelium may originate from reduced enamel epithelium (21) but the observation that junctional epithelium can reform from oral epithelium indicates that the factors determining the phenotype of junctional epithelium persist beyond the developmental phase. Epithelial-mesenchymal interactions play an essential role during embryonic development and when components of developing tissues are dissociated and variously recombined, the changes observed can be interpreted as resulting from influences of an instructive or permissive nature (19). Similar interactions between connective tissue and epithelium can be demonstrated in adult tissues. For example, dissociation and cross-recombination of the epithelial and connective tissue components of palatal and buccal mucosa alters the pattern of differentiation of the epithelium which acquires characteristics of the epithelium normally associated with the connective tissue component (22). Similar recombinant experiments indicate that in order for epithelium from an adult animal to survive and differentiate, connective tissue normally associated with epithelium (such as dermis or lamina propria) is necessary: other connective tissues, such as muscle fascia, fail to support epithelial growth (3,9). It thus appears that lamina propria (a) differs regionally in the type of instructive influences it provides and (b) differs from "deep" connective tissues in the permissive influences it exerts on epithelial growth and differentiation.

Connective tissue influences on the junctional epithelial phenotype. The connective tissues of the periodontal ligament and of the lamina propria of the gingiva differ in their developmental histories and possibly in the directive or permissive influences they exert on an epithelium with which they are associated. The phenotypic similarities between junctional epithelium and mucosal epithelia related to deep connective tissues or maintained in tissue culture appear to support the previous suggestion that the junctional phenotype results from the periodontal connective tissue being non-permissive for epithelial growth and differentiation. To these may be added the passive behavior and lack of differentiation of the epithelia of rests of Malassez within the normal periodontium (1,2). A scheme which would provide an explanation of the acquisition and regeneration of gingival epithelial phenotypes in terms of connective tissue differences is shown in Figure 2c. Three zones of differing connective tissue influences are postulated. Zones 1 and 2 are considered to exert directive influences similar, but not identical, to palatal and buccal connective tissues respectively. These zones are also considered to provide permissive influences necessary for full expression of the determined phenotype. Zone 3, corresponding anatomically to the periodontal ligament, is considered to be similar to other deep connective tissues and to be neither directive nor permissive.

Effects of Inflammation on the Junctional Epithelium

If non-permissiveness of periodontal connective tissue is accepted as a working hypothesis, the question arises as to why apical migration of the epithelium occurs at all during periodontal disease. The epithelium adjacent to mucosal transplants fails to epithelialize the adjacent deep connective tissue despite the absence of any physical barrier to its outgrowth. Thus loss of attachment of connective tissue to the tooth would not in itself be sufficient to initiate epithelial downgrowth. Within the experimental transplant system, outgrowth of differentiating epithelium has been produced when the deep connective tissue bed surrounding the transplant is seeded with cells isolated from dermis, an observation supporting the concept of permissive factors derived from such cells. However, it has also been observed that epithelial outgrowth occurs when the graft bed is permitted to become infected by exposing it to the external environment. This suggests that factors associated with inflammation can substitute for permissive factors produced by dermal cells or can perhaps act to favor selective outgrowth of fibroblasts of the permissive phenotype from the transplanted lamina propria. A direct role of inflammation in stimulating epithelial growth and differentiation is suggested by the behavior of the rests of Malassez in periapical granulomas (3,4). In their quiescent state in normal periodontal ligament, these rests strongly express only keratins 5 and 19. However, under the influence of inflammation they become activated to a proliferative state and express additional keratins characteristic of both stratifying and simple epithelia (Fig. 2).

The molecular basis of the type of epithelial-mesenchymal interactions discussed here has not yet been elucidated. There is, however, an increasing body of related information about the roles of various cytokines and growth factors in influencing cell proliferation, movement and differentiation in adult and developing tissues. In particular, soluble mediators produced during immunological reactions have been demonstrated to have effects on non-immune cells (5). For example, interleukin-1 (IL-1) causes an increase in epithelial proliferation (18) and type IV collagen synthesis (11) and its effects on fibroblasts include altered proliferation (20) and collagen and prostaglandin E2 (PGE2) synthesis with fibroblast substrains differing in their PGE2 synthetic responses to IL-1 (4). Furthermore, lymphoid cells isolated from gingival tissues of subjects with gingivitis and periodontitis show increased production of lymphokines in response to plaque and various specific oral bacteria (15). Such evidence supports the concept that the presence of inflammation can alter the periodontal connective tissue environment making it either directly or indirectly permissive to the apical migration of epithelium. The use of mAbs to detect early changes in epithelial differentiation should permit these effects to be tested experimentally in order to analyze their role in periodontal diseases.

Acknowledgments. The collaboration of Drs. Erik Dabelsteen, Zhirong Gao, Ania Korszun, Birgit Lane and Irene Leigh in various aspects of these studies is gratefully acknowledged, as is the assistance of Julie Anolik, Cindy Asmussen, Albert Doden and Gillian Rittman.

References

1. GAO, Z.; MACKENZIE, I.C.; WILLIAMS, D.M., and CRUCHLEY, A.T.: Immuocytochemical examination of immune cells in periapical granulomata and odontogenic cysts. J. Oral Pathol. in press.
2. GAO, Z.; MACKENZIE, I.C.; WILLIAMS, D.M.; CRUCHLEY, A.T.; LEIGH, I., AND LANE, B.: Patterns of keratin-expression in rests of Malassez and periapical lesions. J. Oral Pathol. in press.
3. HILL, M.W. and MACKENZIE, I.C.: The influence of differing connective tissue substrates on the maintenance of adult stratified squamous epithelia. Cell Tissue Res. 237: 473-478 (1984).
4. KORN, J.M.: Substrain heterogeniety in prostaglandin E2 synthesis of human dermal fibroblasts. Arthritis Rheum. 28(3): 315-322 (1985).
5. KORSZUN, A.K.; WILTON, J.M., and JOHNSON, N.W.: The in vivo effects of lymphokines on mitotic activity and keratinization in guinea pig epidermis. J. Invest. Dermatol. 76: 433 (1981).
6. LANE, E.B., BARTEK, J., PURKIS, P.E., and LEIGH, I.M.: Keratin antigens in differentiating systems. Ann. NY Acad. Sci. 455: 241 (1985).
7. MACKENZIE, I.C. and HILL, M.W.: Maintenance of regionally specific patterns of cell proliferation and differentiation in transplanted skin and oral mucosa. Cell Tissue Res. 219: 597-607 (1981).
8. MACKENZIE, I.C.: The role of epithelial-mesenchymal interactions in epithelial migration and differentiation. J. Periodont. Res. 19: 397-401 (1984).
9. MACKENZIE, I.C.; RITTMAN, G.A., and ASMUSSEN, C.: Use of athymic mice to examine the role of epithelial-mesenchymal interactions in epithelial maintenance; in Immune-Deficient Animals in Biomedical Research; pp. 141-148 (Karger, Basel, Copenhagen 1987).
10. MACKENZIE, I.C.: Nature and mechanisms of regeneration of the junctional epithelial phenotype. J. Periodont. Res. 221: 243-245 (1987).
11. MATSUSHIMA, K.; BANO, M.; KIDWELL, W.R., and OPPENHEIM, J.: Interleukin 1 increases collagen type IV production by murine mammary epithelial cells. J. Immunol. 134: 904-909 (1985).
12. MOLL, R.; FRANKE, W.W.; SCHILLE, D.L.; GEIGER, B., and KREPLER, R.: The catalog of human cytokeratins. Cell 31: 11 (1982).
13. MORGAN, P.R.; JOHNSON, N.W.; LEIGH, I.M., and LANE, E.G.: Structure of gingival epithelium as revealed by monoclonal antibodies to keratins; in LEHNER and CIMASONI: Borderland between caries and periodontal disease III (Medecine et Hygiene, Geneva 1986).

14. NAGLE, R.B.; MOLL, R.; WEIDAUER, H.; NEMETSCHEK, H., and FRANKE, W.W.: Different patterns of cytokeratin expression in the normal epithelia of the upper respiratory tract. Differentiation 30: 130-140 (1985).
15. O'NEILL, P.A. and WOODSON, D.L.: Lymphokine production by human gingival lymphocytes. J. Periodont. Res. 21: 338-350 (1986).
16. PAGE, R.C. and SCHROEDER, H.E.: Periodontitis in man and other animals. A comparative review; (Karger, Basel, 1982).
17. REIBEL, J.; DABELSTEEN, E.; HAKOMORI, S.; YOUNG, W.W., and MACKENZIE, I.C.: The distribution of blood group antigens in rodent epithelia. Cell Tissue Res. 237: 111-116 (1984).
18. RISTOW, M.-J.: A major factor contributing to epidermal proliferation in inflammatory skin diseases appears to be interleukin 1 or a related protein. Proc. Natl. Acad. Sci. USA 84: 1940-1944 (1987).
19. SAXEN, L.: Directive versus permissive induction: a working hypothesis; in LASH and BURGER: Cell and tissue interactions, vol. 32; (Raven Press, New York 1977).
20. SCHMIDT, J.A.; MIZEL, S.B.; COHEN, D., and GREEN, I.: Interleukin 1, a potential regulator of fibroblast proliferation. J. Immunol. 128: 2177-2182 (1982).
21. SCHROEDER, H.E. and LISTGARTEN, M.A.: Monographs in developmental biology; (Karger, Basel 1971).
22. SCHWEIZER, J. and MACKENZIE, I.C.: The keratin polypeptide patterns in heterotypically-recombined epithelia of skin and mucosa of the adult mouse. Differentiation 26: 144-153 (1984).
23. TSENG, S.C.G.; JARVINEN, M.J.; NELSON, W.G.; HUNG, J.W.; WOODCOCK-MITCHELL, J., and SUN, T.: Correlation of specific keratins with different types of epithelial differentiation: monoclonal antibody studies. Cell 30: 361 (1982).
24. VAN MUIJEN, G.N.P.; WARNAAR, S.O., and PONEC, M.: Differentiation related changes of cytokeratin expression in cultured keratinocytes and in fetal, newborn and adult epidermis. Exp. Cell Res. (1987).
25. WAHL, S.M.; WAHL, L.M., and MCCARTHY, J.B.: Lymphocyte-mediated activation of fibroblast proliferation and collagen production. J. Immunol. 121: 942 (1978).

Dr. I.C. Mackenzie, Dows Institute of Dental Research, University of Iowa, College of Dentistry, Iowa City, Ia. 52242, USA

Periodontology Today. Int. Congr., Zürich 1988, pp. 50–58 (Karger, Basel 1988)

What are the Problems in Defining Periodontal Diseases?

Jukka Ainamo

Department of Periodontology, University of Helsinki, Finland

Introduction

Descriptive epidemiological research deals with recording of signs of disease. In medical research, the individual forms the unit of examination whereas in dentistry, it is common practice to make separate recordings for teeth or tooth surfaces, or for gingival or periodontal units.

According to the Concise Oxford Dictionary, the definition of disease is "unhealthy condition of body or mind, or some part thereof". Signs of disease no doubt are more difficult to define for phychological disturbances than for periodontal diseases. However, also the part of a periodontal diagnosis which relates to observation of signs of current or past disease has its own inherent problems.

A substantial number of index systems have been developed and utilized for the evaluation of periodontal conditions (AINAMO, 1983). The index systems are based on visual inspection, use of a periodontal probe, or examination of x-rays.

Visual Examination

The least problematic indicator of periodontal pathology that can be assessed by visual inspection is the occurrence of supragingival calculus. Visual examination has been used also to define gingivitis and periodontal disease.

Supragingival Calculus

The light-coloured and porous supragingival calculus deposit has obtained its minerals from the saliva and is formed in the areas of the openings of the major salivary ducts. Although not a disease in itself, supragingival calculus contributes to inflammation in the contact area between the mineralized deposit and the gingival tissue. In epidemiological surveys, assessment of supragingival calculus is one of the least complicated issues. Only in case of very small amounts, the question may arise whether calculus is present or not.

Appearence of the Gingiva

In its earliest stage, gingival inflammation has been described as a deviation from normal in the colour, shape, surface structure and firmness of the tissue forming the gingival margin (LÖE and SILNESS, 1963; LÖE, 1967). These clinical signs are the criteria of score 1 in the Gingival Index which has been extensively used in clinical trials since the 1960's and 1970's. If the signs of pathology are quite clear, such criteria can be successfully used. A typical example would be when the gingival margin is of a clearly darker shade of red colour than the adjacent, healthy area of the keratinized gingiva. The problem with all these criteria is the delicate borderline between health and the first sign of pathology. A minor change in colour can best be observed in longitudinal studies where the same subject is being followed for a limited period of time. In cross-sectional epidemiological studies the individual and intraoral variation in the appearance of healthy gingival tissue may well be greater than the minute visual differences between health and disease.

Periodontitis

Past pocket formation with breakdown of tooth attachment was assessed by visual examination alone in the Periodontal Index (PI) of Russell (1956) and in the WHO Periodontal Status Index (WHO, 1977). According to Russell, the "mouth mirror and explorer are supplemented occasionally by a straight Jacquette scaler or the chip blower for demonstration of a periodontal pocket". Although a lot of valuable data was collected by Russell and coworkers, the lack of periodontal probing may have been one of the reasons why other groups of investigators experienced great difficulty in uniform recording according to the Periodontal Index (DAVIES et al., 1969). The WHO Periodontal Status Index, recommending identification of pocketing by means of pressing suspected areas with the finger, was found to be less objective and a less quantitative method for evaluating periodontal status than the Periodontal Index (CUTRESS et al., 1978).

Use of the Periodontal Probe

The periodontal probe is used for measurement, in millimeters, of pocket depth or amount of lost attachment. Other measurements made with the probe are the identification of subgingival calculus and bleeding tendency after probing of the gingival or periodontal pocket.

Probing Force

The main general problem in the use of a periodontal

probe relates to applying of a standard force during probing. Use of excessive force at insertion of the probe into a pocket is known to result in an overestimate of both pocket depth, loss of attachment and gingival bleeding, and may also reduce the examiner's ability to detect small amounts of subgingival calculus such as the thin strand of mineralized plaque at the orifice of the gingival crevice, described with score 1 of the Retention index (LÖE, 1967). On the other hand, a too timid probing may lead to corresponding underestimates. During recent years many attempts have been made both to develop pressure sensitive probes and other gadgets for use in examiner calibration, and to reach agreement with regard to recommended pressure in different situations.

In clinical research, especially in studies in which attachment levels are assessed before and after treatment, a particular problem has been how to evaluate the effect of an initial overestimate of the probing depth of the inflamed pocket as compared to a subsequent underestimate of the healed situation. At evaluation of the healed pocket there may be indications to use a relatively substantial force in order to accurately measure the length of a healthy junctional epithelium and the amount of attachment gained. For such purposes, forces corresponding to 50 or 70 g have been utilized.

In the determination of treatment needs there is no reason to use more force than is required to reach the apical extent of the infected and inflamed area of the gingival or periodontal pocket. During the development of the Community Periodontal Index of Treatment Needs (CPITN) (AINAMO et al., 1982; CUTRESS et al., 1987; WHO, 1987), it was soon realized that detailed directives for the pressure to be used at probing would be necessary for improving the comparability of results from different parts of the world. The original recommendation was to use a force corresponding to 20-25g (AINAMO et al., 1982). This recommendation has subsequently been reduced to 20g or less, based on the clinical experience that in most cases almost no pressure is required to reach the apical border of a pathological pocket (CUTRESS et al., 1987). When assessing treatment needs, it is not meaningful to penetrate between the root surface and a healthy junctional epithelium.

Subgingival Calculus

The dark-coloured and hard subgingival calculus deposit has obtained its minerals from the sulcular fluid and is thus a sign of past gingival inflammation. If located close to the gingival margin, subgingival calculus can sometimes be identified by visual examination. By definition, however, it is in most cases covered by gingival tissue and can be found only by means of meticulous probing. There is reasonable evidence to indicate that the ball-tipped probe (WHO, 1978; JEFFCOAt et al., 1986) is more sensitive than straight periodontal probes in the identification of small quantitites of subgingival calculus, especially in deep pockets. Nevertheless, scoring of subgingival calculus in epidemiological surveys has been found to have definite shortcomings, mainly evidenced by substantial differences between comparable populations when these have been examined by different teams of examiner.

Bleeding after Probing

Bleeding after gentle probing of the gingival or periodontal pocket is understood as a sign of a plaque-induced inflammatory reaction in the soft tissue wall of the pocket. In the Gingival Index the presence of visual signs of gingivitis is required in order to test the gingival unit for bleeding after gentle probing (LÖE, 1967). In the Sulcular Bleeding Index by MÜHLEMANN and SON (1974) a reversed sequence of severity scores was suggested with bleeding after probing being the first sign and bleeding combined with visual colour change, or with colour change and swelling, forming the criteria of more severe gingivitis.

In the Gingival Index (LÖE, 1967), bleeding after probing of the orifice of the gingival sulcus is the criterion of score 2, whereas spontaneous bleeding, for example after a blast of air, is given score 3. During the last 10 years presence or absence of bleeding after probing has in epidemiological research to a great extent replaced previously used multi-graded index systems for assessment of gingivitis. Bleeding from the gingival or periodontal pocket is one of the few available signs of current disease.

Pocket depth

In principle, the pocket depth is measured, with a graduated pocket probe, as the distance, in millimeters, from the gingival margin to the bottom of the pocket. If this distance is in excess of 3mm and gentle probing results in bleeding, the depth of the pocket usually is recorded as a sign of periodontal disease. Correspondingly, a pocket of 3mm or less, with bleeding, represents a gingival pocket. Recently, the ISO has adopted the definitions "healthy gingiva" when there are no clinical signs of disease and "intact gingiva" when signs of neither disease nor recession are present. In epidemiological research, common practice would be to record gingivitis or gingival health, regardless of whether the bottom of the pocket is located on cementum or at the apical border of the enamel. For additional clarity, ATTSTRÖM and LINDHE (1983) use the terms gingivitis with or without loss of connective tissue attachment.

Both gingival and periodontal pockets may have a component of false pocketing when edema has resulted in a coronal extention of the gingival margin. False pockets may occur also around not yet fully erupted teeth, including the distal surface of the most posterior molar where gingival tissue often reaches up to the level of the occlusal surface. The main problem, however, in the measurement of both gingival and periodontal pockets, and of loss of attachment, relates to the difficulty in defining the apical extent of the pocket.

Loss of Attachment

Loss of connective tissue attachment is also a measure of past periodontal disease experience. The amount of lost attachment is measured in millimeters as the distance from the cementoenamel junction to the bottom of the pocket and was first introduced by RAMFJORD (1959). The problems with this measurement are related not only to the difficulty to determine the location of the bottom of the pocket but also to the identification of the location of the cementoenamel junction. For solving the latter problem, RAMFJORD cuts the probe tip perpendicularly to obtain a sharp edge which "allows easy detection of the cementoenamel junction" (personal communication). Another approach was published by JEFFCOAT et al. (1986) who developed a device in which the traditionally straight tip of the periodontal probe is replaced with a 0.5mm ball tip, identical to that recommended for use with the CPITN (WHO, 1978). To improve the reliability of identification of the cementoenamel junction, CARLOS et al. (1986) suggested restriction of measurements of loss of attachment to mesial and buccal surfaces of the teeth.

Gingival recession caused by trauma from toothbrushing is usually included in the measurement of lost connective tissue attachment. Measurement of gingival recession has not been reported to present major problems in itself. The problem involved relates to the fact that especially in young adult age groups the recession caused by excessive toothbrushing, if included in the measurements, gives a false picture of attachment loss due to periodontal disease.

Use of X-rays

The use of x-rays in epidemiological surveys was applied already by MARSHALL DAY (1949) in an extensive comparative study of periodontal conditions in India and the United States. RUSSELL (1956) reported a 21% increase in the PI score from 1.20 to 1.45 after having supplemented his clinical observations from 200 patients with radiographs.

In industrialized countries with an extensive public health service for children and adolescents, the use of x-ray supplementation has been recommended whenever a pocket depth of 4mm or more has been recorded (AINAMO et al., 1984). On the other hand, already available bite-wing radiographs have been utilized for screening teenagers for juvenile periodontitis. In one such study, the bite-wing radiographs of 8000 teenagers were screened, resulting in the clinical examination of 28 of the subjects, and subsequent identification of 8 subjects showing both clinical and radiographic evidence of localized juvenile periodontitis (SAXÉN, 1980).

Reporting of Population Studies

Definitions are needed also for uniform reporting of epidemiological surveys in dentistry. For example, prevalence should indicate the proportion of the population affected but is used in cariology to indicate the average number of teeth with caries experience. During the development of the PI, RUSSELL directly applied the DMF principle to periodontal diseases. Thus, "the score for an individual patient is the arithmetic average of the scores for the teeth in his mouth" and "the population score is the arithmetic average of the individual scores for the persons examined" (RUSSELL, 1956). With the development of treatment need indices in the 1970's (JOHANSEN et al., 1973; AINAMO et al., 1982) the need became apparent to base reporting on age-specific prevalence data instead of population averages.

Severity of Periodontal Disease

Severity of periodontal disease has with the CPITN been illogically used to indicate the average number of sites (sextants) affected with various periodontal disease indicators when, as quite correctly pointed out by CARLOS et al. (1986), severity should indicate the periodontal disease status of the worst affected tooth or site of the individual mouth examined. For example, a 6mm pocket is a more severe clinical sign of disease than a 3mm pocket. With the CPITN, another conceptual flaw in logic was subsequently introduced by starting to define 4 or 5mm pockets as shallow (WHO, 1987) instead of moderate (AINAMO et al., 1982). Such terminology leaves no category for 3mm or less deep gingival pockets and adds to the confusion of severity as a basic concept.

Prevalence of Periodontal Disease

The word prevalence should serve to indicate, per age group, the proportion of the population affected with a given degree of severity of periodontal disease as their highest score, and is given in per cent of the population examined. The "population" usually includes only those subjects who have remaining natural teeth but can, by indication of the corresponding proportions of edentulous subjects, be calculated also for the entire age cohort.

Extent of Periodontal Disease

Extent is another concept introduced by CARLOS et al. (1986). "Extent" more appropriately than "severity" refers to the number of teeth affected with a disease indicator of a given severity. Dividing the data collected into teeth or sites with shallow, moderate and deep pockets, and by expressing the average number of such units per subject, a rather clear picture can be drawn of both past disease experience (CARLOS et al., 1986), and of current treatment needs and manpower requirements (CUTRESS et al., 1987). Additional detail information can with the CPITN be obtained from cross-tabulations showing what proportion of subjects per age group has what number of units affected with a disease indicator of a given severity (AINAMO et al., 1987).

Validity and Reproducibility of Recordings

Validity of an epidemiological recording answers to the question on how well the finding reflects the true disease situation. Due to their relatively even distribution within the dentition, valid scorings can be made for gingivitis and dental calculus even by using examination of selected index teeth only (RAMFJORD, 1959). Such partial examination has in most cases been combined with full recording, i.e., all observations made are also recorded. On the other hand, a number of recent studies have confirmed the impression that advanced periodontal disease predominantly occurs at only one site or sextant per individual (see AINAMO et al., 1987). A valid screening for advanced periodontal disease thus requires full mouth examination although, as with the PTNS (JOHANSEN et al., 1973) and CPITN (AINAMO et al., 1982), partial recording is sufficient for identification of all subjects affected.

Reproducibility of recordings indicates with what accuracy the recordings can be repeated by the same or by a group of examiners. Reproducibility of recordings is essential for comparison of results from different studies. In epidemiological studies, unless the relevant parameter can be measured in millimeters, it has been suggested (WHO, 1978, 1987) that dichotomous scoring offers better reproducibility than systems which have a multi-graded scale for increasing severity of a phenomenon, like for example the GI of LÖE (1967), the SBI of MÜHLEMANN and SON (1971) and many others. There is general agreement that multi-graded indices are difficult to subject to correct mathematical analysis. In addition, the inbetween scores do not alone give meaningful information.

In their Extent and Severity Index, CARLOS et al. (1986) recommend, explicitly for the purpose of improving the reproducibility, examination and recording of buccomesial and buccal tooth surfaces only. As loss of attachment due to gingival recession frequently occurs already at young age, the results obtained with the ESI on loss of tooth attachment are difficult to interpret. Also, in view of current knowledge of the site specificity of advanced periodontal breakdown, the underestimate of the prevalence of deep pocketing should be clearly realized when applying any partial examination system. According to the above definitions, the reproducibility of the recordings with the ESI would seem to have been improved at the expense of the validity of the results.

Discussion and Conclusions

Indices used in epidemiological surveys of periodontal diseases focus mainly on signs of past disease experience. The most typical exmaple is the loss of tooth attachment which represents the sum total of all periods and all types of periodontal breakdown during the lifetime of the examinee, including the loss of attachment caused by excessive oral hygiene measures. All measurements can be criticised for lack of accuracy. Serious researchers such as SHEIHAM (1978) and many others have questioned the importance of periodontal screening as long as enough knowledge is not available on whether the disease will lead to loss of teeth or not. The only direct indicator of current disease is the bleeding after gentle probing and even that is known to be an unreliable sign of disease progression. On the other hand, dentistry is a health service profession. From a health services point of view it would seem "important" to outline and try to reduce the amounts of gingival bleeding, suppuration from periodontal pockets, bad taste in the mouth and fear of bad breath which certainly, for patient comfort, are important in many countries. In addition, achievement of a general improvement in periodontal health at young age, of which there already exists some evidence, would seem like the most logical and promising approch to the prevention of loss of tooth attachment in the future. As with any other disease, medical or dental, there are no absolute predictors for identification of groups at high risk for disease progression in the future. Until such predictors have been made available, periodontal epidemiology should continue to record the signs of past or present disease.

References

AINAMO, J.: Epidemiology of periodontal disese; in LINDHE, Textbook of clinical periodontology; 1st ed., pp. 67-84 (Munksgaard, Copenhagen 1983).

AINAMO, J.; BARMES, D.; BEAGRIE, G.; CUTRESS, T.; MARTIN, J. and SARDO-INFIRRI, J.: Development of the World Health Organization (WHO) Community Periodontal Index of Treatment Needs (CPITN). Int. dent. J. 32: 281-291 (1982).

AINAMO, J.; NORDBLAD, A. and KALLIO, P.: Use of the CPITN in populations under 20 years of age. Int. dent. J. 34: 285-291 (1984).

AINAMO, J.; TERVONEN, T.; NORDBLAD, A. and KALLIO, P.: Use of CPITN cross-tabulations - a research perspective. Int. dent. J. 37: 173-178 (1987).

ATTSTRÖM, R. and LINDHE, J.: Pathogenesis of plaque associated periodontal disease; in LINDHE, Textbook of clinical periodontology; p. 155 (Munksgaard, Copenhagen 1983).

CARLOS, J.P.; WOLFE, M.D. and KINGMAN, A.: The extent and

severity index: a simple method for use in epidemiologic studies of periodontal disease. J. clin. Periodont. 13: 500-505 (1986).

CUTRESS, T.W.; AINAMO, J. and SARDO-INFIRRI, J.: The community periodontal index treatment needs (CPITN) procedure for population groups and individuals. Int. dent. J. 37: in press (1987).

CUTRESS, T.W.; HUNTER, P.B.V.; BECK, D.J. and de SOUZA, P.: A comparison of WHO Periodontal Status Index with the Periodontal and Oral Hygiene Indices. Community Dent. oral Epidemiol. 6: 245-252 (1978).

DAVIES, G.N.; KRUGER, B.J. and HOMAN, B.T.: An epidemiological training course. Aust. dent. J. 12: 17-28 (1967).

JEFFCOAT, M.K.; JEFFCOAT, R.L.; JENS, S.C. and CAPTAIN, K.: A new periodontal probe with automated cemento-enamel junction detection. J. clin. Periodont. 13: 276-280 (1986).

JOHANSEN, J.R.; GJERMO, P. and BELLINI, H.T.: A system to classify the need for periodontal treatment. Acta odont. Scand. 31: 297-305 (1973).

LÖE, H.: The gingival Index, the Plaque Index and the Retention Index systems. J. Periodont. 38: 610-616 (1967).

LÖE, H. and SILNESS, J.: Periodontal disease in pregnancy. I. Prevalence and severity. Acta odont. Scand. 21: 533-551 (1963).

MARSHALL DAY, C.D. and SCHOURIE, K.L.: A roentgenographic survey of periodontal disease in India. J. Amer. dent. Ass. 39: 572-588 (1949).

MÜHLEMANN, H.R. and SON, S.: Gingival sulcus bleeding - a leading sign in initial gingivitis. Helv. odont. Acta 15: 107-113 (1971).

RAMFJORD, S.P.: Indices for prevalence and incidence of periodontal disease. J. Periodont. 30: 51-59 (1959).

RUSSELL, A.L.: A system of classification and scoring for prevalence surveys of periodontal disease. J. dent. Res. 35: 350-359 (1956).

SHEIHAM, A.: Screening for periodontal disease. J. clin. Periodont. 5: 237-245 (1978).

WHO: Oral health surveys. Basic methods; 2nd ed., pp. 33-37 (World Health Organization, Geneva 1977).

WHO: Epidemiology, etiology, and prevention of periodontal diseases. Tehn. Rep. Ser. 621 (World Health Organization, Geneva 1978).

WHO: Oral Health surveys. Basic methods; 3rd ed., pp. 31-33 (World Health Organization, Geneva 1987).

Jukka Ainamo, Dr.Odont., Department of Periodontology, University of Helsinki, Mannerheimintie 172, SF-00280 Helsinki, Finland

Periodontology Today. Int. Congr., Zürich 1988, pp. 59–67 (Karger, Basel 1988)

Why Do Epidemiologic Data Have No Diagnostic Value?

M. A. Listgarten

Department of Periodontics, University of Pennsylvania, Philadelphia, Pa., USA

Epidemiology

Epidemiology is the science that deals with the distribution, cause and control of disease. The epidemiologist is concerned with aspects of disease that affect the population at large, rather than individuals. Epidemiology has played a key role in identifying the prevalence of various diseases, i.e. the proportion of a population affected by a disease, and its incidence, i.e. the rate at which new cases of the disease appear in a population. This information has led to the identification of environmental factors or factors intrinsic to the population studied that are associated with the etiology and development of a disease. A classic example related to periodontics is the association of calculus and dental plaque with inflammatory periodontal diseases.[10]

Epidemiology has been of extreme value in the identification of microorganisms associated with various infectious diseases. In many cases these findings were instrumental in the identification of the key pathogen and the subsequent control of the disease. A recent example of such a sequence of events occurred in 1976 with Legionnaire's disease. Epidemiologic investigations led to the eventual isolation and identification of the etiologic agent, a new genus of microorganism, appropriately named *Legionella pneumophila*. With the identification of the etiologic agent and the ability to examine the antibiotic spectrum to which *Legionella* is sensitive, a cure, in the form of erythromycin administration, was rapidly developed to a frequently fatal infection.[4]

Sources of error

Because the association of a microorganism with a particular infection often precedes the identification of the microorganism as the etiologic agent of the disease, it is tempting to equate microorganisms or other factors associated with a disease as etiologic agents of the disease. In order to demonstrate that a suspected pathogen is, in fact, causing a disease, additional clinical and laboratory studies are needed.

The omission of adequate hypothesis testing may lead to erroneous conclusions about the role of certain factors in the pathogenesis of a disease. For many years the association of calculus with periodontal disease led to the notion that calculus was a direct cause of the disease. This notion was reinforced by the widespread observation that calculus removal resulted in an immediate clinical improvement. The exact role of calculus was clarified after additional experiments demonstrated that it is relatively inert, that sterilized calculus does not act as a significant irritant when implanted subcutaneously, and that its presence in germfree animals does not contribute to the development of periodontal disease.[26] Calculus is harmful only indirectly because it promotes the retention of pathogenic organisms able to initiate and promote periodontal disease. While calculus may also interfere with regeneration of a new connective tissue attachment to denuded root surfaces, it is of interest to note that a new epithelial attachment to clean calculus has been reported under certain experimental conditions.[15]

A strong association between poor oral hygiene and gingivitis, as measured by a variety of epidemiological indices[3,11] has been reported in a number of epidemiologic surveys throughout the world.[1,22] These reports provide a basis for what LOESCHE[17] has described as the <u>non-specific plaque theory</u>, that is the concept that dental plaque is quantitatively rather than qualitatively related to the severity of periodontal disease. Indeed, there is a direct relationship between amount of dental plaque and severity of gingivitis, and when the quantity of plaque is controlled there is a decrease in the severity of gingivitis.[11]

The somewhat arbitrary weighting of scores to measure severity of gingivitis and periodontitis in epidemiologic surveys have suggested a linear evolution or conversion from gingivitis to periodontitis, with plaque mass as the main etiologic agent. However, subsequent research demonstrated that the epidemiological data could be misleading and that under certain clinical conditions plaque quantity did not relate to severity of disease and that the quality or microbial composition of plaque was of greater importance.[6,27] A good example is juvenile periodontitis, a condition in which the presence of <u>Actinobacillus</u> in the sulcus or pocket appears to be of greater significance than the mass of plaque on the affected tooth. Obviously, monitoring Actinobacillus may be diagnostically more relevant for patients with juvenile periodontitis than monitoring plaque mass.[9,25,28,30]

Direct attempts at testing the hypothesis that gingivitis will convert to periodontitis have revealed that the number of conversions is very small and that only a small proportion of sites with gingivitis will convert. Indeed, in a longitudinal study of 61 subjects with gingivitis monitored over a 3-year period, the incidence of conversions to periodontitis was so low as to be undetectable. Although some conversions were detected, their number did not differ significantly from the number of probing depth increases that were expected on the basis of the estimated measurement error inherent in the measurement technique.[16]

Data collected from primitive populations also support the hypothesis that gingivitis does not inevitably lead to periodontitis, even if it is not properly attended to. Reports by AFRICA et al.[2] and REDDY et al.[24] indicate that while gingivitis and poor oral hygiene are very prevalent in certain South African communities, periodontitis and the accompanying loss of attachment has a low prevalence in these populations.

Finally, it should be noted that the recurrence of periodontitis lesions in the periodontally treated dentition does not parallel the more generalized distribution of gingivitis, an observation that casts further doubt on the assertion that periodontitis is simply an end result of gingivitis.[19,23]

Epidemiologic data from the classical longitudinal studies of KNOWLES et al.[8] suggest that conventional maintenance visits are extremely effective in preventing the recurrence of periodontitis in previously treated patients with adult periodontitis. Repeated yearly examinations over an 8-year period indicated relatively stable clinical criteria following the marked clinical improvement reported one year following therapy. The stability was attributed largely to regular maintenance visits which appear to maintain the patients in a relatively healthy periodontal state despite imperfect oral hygiene habits. Similar results have been reported by PIHLSTROM et al.[20]

However, when data from such studies are reexamined with emphasis on the clinical course of individual subjects, it becomes clear that the epidemiologic data can be misleading. Isolated sites in the dentition of susceptible subjects may be deteriorating to a significant degree.[13] However, since most sites in the dentition remain stable, the usual descriptive statistics fail to detect these few sites. Furthermore, since relatively few subjects account for most of the deterioration in the patient population, the epidemiologic data not only fails to detect the existence of deteriorating sites, but also fails to detect the differential susceptibility of individual subjects to periodontal tissue destruction. This error is most likely to occur when data are analyzed, as they often are, on a site by site basis. The clinician who is concerned with individual patients rather than trends in a population needs diagnostic tools to identify in a reliable manner diseased patients and their relative susceptibility to periodontitis.

Most diagnostic techniques in current use in dental practice measure the extent of prior tissue destruction rather than ongoing destructive processes. This unfortunate state of affairs is due to the lack of sufficiently reliable criteria to measure ongoing (active) disease. Nevertheless, the information has been of value to the clinician, since the aim of therapy is not only to control disease, but also to eliminate defects productd by the disease.

Diagnostics

In contrast to epidemiology, which is concerned with studies of diseases in populations, diagnostics is concerned with identification of disease in the individual patient. Specifically, the diagnostician seeks to determine the exact nature of a disease in a subject and to distinguish among closely related disease entities (differential diagnosis). To this end the disease is characterized by clinical signs and symptoms, and assorted laboratory tests. Few signs, symptoms or laboratory test results are pathognomic, i.e. distinctive or characteristic, of a particular disease entity. A laboratory test is used as a diagnostic aid either because it is able to identify with a satisfactory degree of certainty the presence of a given disease, or its absence. Sensitivity refers to the likelihood that a test will be positive when the disease is present. Specificity is the likelihood that a test will be negative when the disease is absent.[5] Generally these two characteristics of a diagnostic test vary inversely with one another. As criteria for interpreting test outcomes are varied to increase sensitivity, the specificity of the test will decrease and the number of false-positive test outcomes will increase. Similarly, increasing the specificity of the test will result in decreased sensitivity and an increased number of false-negative test results. The most useful diagnostic aids are those with good efficiency, i.e. reliability. Such tests combine good sensitivity and specificity, i.e. they can accurately identify both the presence as well as the absence of disease.

By combining the discriminating features of two or more efficient tests that measure different features of the disease the likelihood of making an accurate diagnosis in a given subject at a certain point in time is increased. The theory underlying the decision making process in the diagnosis of disease has been presented in a simple and readable manner by GALEN and GAMBINO.[5]

Currently, severity of periodontitis is usually estimated by prior cumulative loss of periodontal attachment. The latter is assessed most commonly by probing or by radiography. Neither method truly reflects the actual anatomic event, i.e. the loss of attachment of the root surface to alveolar bone.

Drawbacks of evaluation techniques

Measurements of loss of attachment, either by probing or radiography, cannot distinguish between attachment loss due to periodontitis or other causes, such as recessions due to anatomic constraints, or surgically created loss of attachment. Thus assumptions made in epidemiologic studies that equate loss of attachment with loss of the supporting tissues due to periodontitis may not be warranted. Since both techniques measure prior rather than current loss of attachment, neither technique is able to determine in a cross-sectional survey whether the disease process has been temporarily or permanently arrested. Unless longitudinal data are available, it is not possible with current technology to show whether sites are deteriorating or stable.

The most practical method of determining that disease is active remains the demonstration that a significant loss of attachment over time has occurred. Probing is likely to detect loss of attachment at an earlier stage than radiography, i.e. it is a more sensitive test, but the latter is a more specific indicator that bone has been lost.[7,18] It is not known to what extent either probing or radiography truly reflect the actual loss of connective tissue fibers from their insertion into the cementum layer. This is the elusive "gold standard" which, ideally, should serve as a reference for any potential test of disease activity. Since it is impossible to quantify the true attachment level in vivo, reasonable estimates provided by probing or radiography are used. However, no data are available to indicate the fidelity with which either probing or radiography reflect the actual loss of attachment.

It is known that substantial volumes of the alveolar process must be destroyed before the loss is detectable in radiographs. Therefore, radiographs will seldom, if ever, reveal bone loss when no loss has taken place, while bone loss is likely present in many cases where radiographs are unable to detect it. Thus radiographs are not a very sensitive diagnostic tool for bone loss, but may be a relatively specific tool.

Since probing depth is affected by level of fiber insertion into the root, as well as probing force, size of probe and degree of inflammation, variations in probing depth within a certain range may be independent of bone level.[14,29] Thus a significant increase in probing depth is likely to be detected before bone loss actually occurs. The method, therefore, is quite sensitive for bone loss. However, it is not very specific, since absence of bone loss may be accompanied by increases in probing depth due to alterations in the inflammatory status of the gingiva.

By combining probing, a very sensitive test to detect potential cases of alveolar bone loss, and periapical radiographs, a very specific test, as a confirming test, the clinician is able to maximize his efficiency for detecting alveolar bone loss.

Summary

Epidemiology, because of its primary concern with disease characteristics in populations, emphasizes general trends in the dynamics of the disease process. It points out correlations of disease with environmental and other factors. While the information may provide clues as to the etiology of the disease and factors that may modify its progress in large populations, the data cannot be used for diagnostic purposes and the management of individual patients who may not fit the population norm. The development of tests with diagnostic value depends on the utilization of decision-making theory to determine the probability that a test can detect the presence or absence of disease, and its efficiency to do so, i.e. its value in correctly predicting some of the clinical characteristics of the disease. Epidemiology may generate some of the data bases used in developing diagnostic tests; however, the data cannot be directly extrapolated to the management of individual patients.

References

1. ABDELLATIF, H.M. and BURT, B.A.: An epidemiological investigation into the relative importance of age and oral hygiene status as determinants of periodontitis. J. Dent. Res. 66:13-18 (1987).

2. AFRICA, C.W., PARKER, J.R. and REDDY, J.: Bacteriological studies of subgingival plaque in a periodontitis-resistant population. I. Darkfield microscopic studies. J. Periodont. Res. 20:1-7 (1985).
3. BARNES, G.P., PARKER, W.A., LYON, T.C. and FULTZ, R.P.: Indices used to evaluate signs, symptoms, and etiologic factors associated with diseases of the periodontium. J. Periodontol. 57:643-651 (1986).
4. BERKOW, R., ed.: The Merck manual of diagnosis and therapy; ed. 14, pp. 658-660 Merck Sharp & Dohme Research Laboratories, Rahway, NJ, 1982.
5. GALEN, R.S. and GAMBINO, S.R.: Beyond normality: The predictive value and efficiency of medical diagnoses. John Wiley & Sons, New York, 1975.
6. GENCO, R.J., ZAMBON, J.J. and CHRISTERSSON, L.A.: Use and interpretation of microbiological assays in periodontal diseases. Oral Microbiol. Immunol. 1:73-79 (1986).
7. GOODSON, J.M., HAFFAJEE, A.D., and SOCRANSKY, S.S.: The relationship between attachment level loss and alveolar bone loss. J. Clin. Periodontol. 11:348-359 (1984).
8. KNOWLES, J.W., BURGETT, F.G., NISSLE, R.R., SHICK, R.A. MORRISON, E.C. and RAMFJORD, S.P.: Results of periodontal treatment related to pocket depth and attachment level. Eight years. J. Periodontol. 50:225-233 (1979).
9. KORNMAN, K.S. and ROBERTSON, P.B.: Clinical and microbiological evaluation of therapy for juvenile periodontitis. J. Periodontol. 56:443-446 (1985).
10. LINDHE, J.: Textbook of clinical periodontology; pp. 67-84 (Munksgaard, Copenhagen, 1983).
11. LINDHE, J.: Textbook of clinical periodontology; pp. 85-124 (Munksgaard, Copenhagen, 1983).
12. LINDHE, J.: Long-term effect of surgical/nonsurgical treatment of periodontal disease. J. Clin. Periodontol. 11:448-458 (1984).
13. LINDHE, J. and NYMAN, S.: Long-term maintenance of patients treated for advanced periodontal disease. J. Clin. Periodontol. 11:504-514 (1984).
14. LISTGARTEN, M.A.: Periodontal probing: What does it mean? J. Clin. Periodontol. 7:165-176 (1980).
15. LISTGARTEN, M.A. and ELLEGAARD, B.: Electron microscopic evidence of a cellular attachment between junctional epithelium and dental calculus. J. Periodont. Res. 8:143-150 (1973).
16. LISTGARTEN, M.A., SCHIFTER, C.C. and LASTER, L.: 3-year longitudinal study of the periodontal status of an adult population with gingivitis. J. Clin. Periodontol. 12:225-238 (1985).

17. LOESCHE, W.J.: Chemotherapy of dental plaque infections. In: Preventive dentistry: Nature, pathogenicity and clinical control of plaque. Oral Sci. Rev. 9:65-107 (1976).
18. MANN, J., PETTIGREW, J., BEIDEMAN, R., GREEN, P. and SHIP, I.: Investigation of the relationship between clinically detected loss of attachment and radiographic changes in early periodontal disease. J. Clin. Periodontol. 12:247-253 (1985).
19. MORRISON, E.C., RAMFJORD, S.P., BURGETT, F.G., NISSLE, R.R. and SHICK, R.A.: The significance of gingivitis during the maintenance phase of periodontal treatment. J. Periodontol. 53:31-34 (1982).
20. PIHLSTROM, B.L., McHUGH, R.B., OLIPHANT, T.H. and ORTIZ-CAMPOS, C.: Comparison of surgical and nonsurgical treatment of periodontal disease. A review of current studies and additional results after 6 1/2 years. J. Clin. Periodontol. 10:524-541 (1983).
21. RAMFJORD, S.P.: Subgingival curettage versus surgical elimination of periodontal pockets. J. Periodontol. 39:167-175 (1968).
22. RAMFJORD, S.P., EMSLIE, R.D., GREENE, J.C., HELD, A.-J. and WAERHAUG, J.: Epidemiological studies of periodontal diseases. Parodont. Acad. Rev. 2:109-122 (1968).
23. RAMFJORD, S.P., MORRISON, E.C., BURGETT, F.G., NISSLE, R.R., SHICK, R.A., ZANN, G.J. and KNOWLES, J.W.: Oral hygiene and maintenance of periodontal support. J. Periodontol. 53:26-30 (1982).
24. REDDY, J., AFRICA, C.W. and PARKER, J.R.: Darkfield microscopy of subgingival plaque of an urban black population with poor oral hygiene. J. Clin. Periodontol. 13:578-582 (1986).
25. SANDHOLM, L.: Bacteriology in juvenile periodontitis. Finn. Dent. Soc. 81:63-76 (1985).
26. SCHROEDER, H.E.: Formation and inhibition of dental calculus. (Hans Huber Publ., Berne, 1969).
27. SLOTS, J.: Bacterial specificity in adult periodontitis. A summary of recent work. J. Clin. Periodontol. 13:912-917 (1986).
28. TSAI, C.-C. and TAICHMAN, N.S.: Dynamics of infection by leukotoxic strains of Actinobacillus actinomycetemcomitans in juvenile periodontitis. J. Clin. Periodontol. 13:330-331 (1986).
29. VAN DER VELDEN, U.: Periodontal probing. Clinical and histological investigations (Thesis, University of Amsterdam, 1981).

30. **ZAMBON, J.J., CHRISTERSSON, L.A. and GENCO, R.J.: Diagnosis and treatment of localized juvenile periodontitis. J. Amer. Dent. Assoc. 113:295-299 (1986)**

(Supported in part by the National Institute of Dental Research Grants R01-DE06085 and DE-02623, and a grant from the Colgate-Palmolive Co.).

Author's Address

MAX A. LISTGARTEN, D.D.S., Department of Periodontics, School of Dental Medicine, University of Pennsylvania, 4001 Spruce Street, Philadelphia, PA 19104, U.S.A.

Periodontology Today. Int. Congr., Zürich 1988, pp. 68–76 (Karger, Basel 1988)

The Status of Epidemiological Data on Periodontal Diseases

Brian A. Burt

School of Public Health, The University of Michigan, Ann Arbor, Michigan, USA

The science of epidemiology seeks to define the natural history of disease and to discern associations between determinants and disease outcomes. The purpose of this paper is to summarize the evolution of current epidemiological data in periodontal disease, to assess the nature of the data produced, and to suggest areas for further research. Emphasis will be on adult periodontitis.

Epidemiological study of periodontal disease, a generic name for a disease complex, falls into three eras. The first is pre-1950s, when many people were diagnosed as having "pyorrhea", for which extraction was the usual treatment. When added to beliefs prevalent at the time about "focus of infection" (CHILTON 1950), the result was almost universal edentulousness among older people. Supposed causes of "pyorrhea" covered bacterial infection, mechanical irritation, nutritional deficiencies, and manifestations of systemic illness.

The second era began with the Periodontal Index, the PI (RUSSELL 1956), an index which had been extensively validated against the clinical diagnoses of periodontists during its development. With the PI as the major tool, epidemiological studies over the next 20 or so years documented those social and behavioral associations which are now taken as basic knowledge more extensive disease in developing compared to developed countries, greater severity in men than in women, relationships to increasing age, calculus, plaque, deposits, and social class. By the time Waerhaug reviewed the literature at the World Workshop in Periodontics at Ann Arbor (Waerhaug 1966), these relationships could be specified in some detail. The perception of the distribution of periodontal diseases from these studies, which was accepted without much question until fairly recent years, could be summed up as follows:

1. Virtually all persons were susceptible to severe disease if oral hygiene was inadequate
2. Periodontal disease was related to age, gender, social class, race, and extent of calculus and plaque deposits
3. The disease progressed in a linear fashion throughout life from gingivitis to periodontitis to bone loss to tooth loss
4. Periodontal disease was the principal cause of tooth loss in persons aged 35 or older.

The third era, where we seem to be now, began when more precise methods of clinically measuring periodontal diseases, some of which had been introduced earlier in clinical research, were applied in field studies.

Current review of periodontal epidemiology

Some of the social and behavioral relationships with periodontal disease which followed the development of the PI have remained accepted as basic truths. What has changed over the last decade or so is perceptions of (a) the natural history of the disease, and (b) susceptibility, especially susceptibility related to aging.

Natural history of periodontitis

The epidemiological studies of the 1950s-1960s linked oral hygiene levels to PI scores so consistently that these findings were taken as presumptive evidence of cause and effect. The experimental gingivitis studies of LÖE et al (1965) were seen as confirmatory evidence of a bacterial cause from dental plaque, even though this research looked only at gingivitis. Today, however, the evidence is clear that periodontitis is a disease of bacterial etiology (NEWMAN 1985; PAGE 1986). Gram-negative, anaerobic bacteria are the predominant species in deep periodontal pockets (SLOTS 1977), from which it is inferred that the ecological shift from the streptococcal, aerobic, Gram-positive bacteria characteristic of new supragingival plaque to this Gram-negative, anaerobic flora is of etiological significance. Although these anaerobic bacteria are becoming better specified (SLOTS 1986), and although they are used to evaluate therapy and to identify patients at risk (GREENWELL and BISSADA 1984; LISTGARTEN et al 1986), as yet there is no direct evidence to support their etiological role.

Periodontal infections are complex. Over 70 species from plaque around the gingival margin have been positively correlated with gingivitis (MOORE et al 1982), and wide variation has been observed in the composition of flora from moderate periodontal pockets (4-6 mm.) among different people with similar clinical signs (MOORE et al 1984). These studies have also led to the hypothesis that periodontitis results from a sequence of bacterial colonization rather than just an increase in bacterial counts. Research of this type, with very detailed study on a small number of patients, is clinical research rather than classical epidemiology, but if the hypotheses produced are plausible then later epidemiological studies can strengthen them.

Epidemiological and clinical evidence shows that most gingivitis does not progress to periodontitis, but periodontitis has not yet been reported without a preceding gingivitis. If the hypothesis of a bacterial colonization sequence could be supported, then prevention of gingivitis clearly would become the most logical way of preventing periodontitis, and it would also become a public health goal worth achieving. Although the presumptive evidence is strong, however, we cannot be certain at present that preventing gingivitis is a sufficient condition for preventing periodontitis.

Until quite recently, periodontitis was thought to progress in linear fashion throughout life (LÖE et al 1978). By the mid-1980s, however, the concept that adult periodontitis progressed by acute bursts of activity, followed by periods of quiescence, had required some re-examination of the accepted view. Although the "random burst" hypothesis, proposed by the Forsyth group (SOCRANSKY et al 1984) may need some modification, there is other evidence that disease progression fluctuates from year to year in a non-linear fashion (SELIKOWITZ et al 1981). Further epidemiological study of how periodontitis progresses could help specify the nature of the disease. If, for example, periodontitis is an auto-immune disease, epidemiological study could assess how closely it follows the pattern of those other auto-immune diseases characterized by cycles of exacerbation and remission.

Periodontal disease was long assumed to be the major cause of tooth loss in adults, though evidence for this belief was always limited and of questionable quality. Recent data from several countries have shown that periodontal diseases in fact account for few extractions at all ages (BAILIT et al 1987, CAHEN et al 1986, AINAMO et al 1985, KAY and BLINKHORN 1986). By the time the last edentulous person from the "focal infection" era of 1910-50 has passed on, tooth loss from periodontal diseases should be limited to those relatively few teeth that are clearly beyond redemption (WEINTRAUB and BURT 1985).

Susceptibility

Probably the greatest shift away from earlier views comes with susceptibility, where it used to be assumed that virtually everybody was susceptible to serious, generalized periodontitis. Epidemiological evidence now suggests that generalized, destructive periodontitis is unusual among adult populations, even where oral hygiene is poor, gingivitis severe, and professional treatment limited (CUTRESS et al 1982; POWELL 1984; BUCKLEY and CROWLEY 1984; BAELUM et al 1986; LÖE et al 1986; ISMAIL et al 1986). Where oral hygiene is generally better, periodontitis is even more unusual though gingivitis is common (HUGOSON and JORDAN 1980; BECK et al 1984; PILOT and SCHAUB 1985; HALLING and BJORN 1986; HOOVER and TYNAN 1986). The most recent data from a large representative sample is the 1985-86 NIDR Adult Survey in the United States, which found that severe periodontitis (at least one site with loss of attachment of 6 mm. or more) was present in less than 8% of the employed population below 65 years of age (MILLER et al 1987).

Concepts of susceptibility to periodontitis among older persons has undergone particular revision. There is now clear evidence that tooth retention, low periodontal disease scores, and good oral hygiene are closely associated, regardless of age (HUGOSON and JORDAN 1980; BURT et al 1985). While there is evidence from one large-scale survey that severe periodontitis is no more prevalent in older than in younger persons (BECK et al 1984), the recent U.S. national survey found a higher prevalence of severe periodontitis, 34%, among persons over 65 than was seen in the under-65 employed population. The contrasts between these two surveys might reflect sampling variation and cohort effects, though all longitudinal implications from cross-sectional data need to be made with caution. The direct relationship between age and periodontal diseases that cross-sectional studies usually demonstrates may principally reflect the results of long-term plaque accumulations, perhaps exacerbated by poorer plaque tolerance in aging tissues.

There are few longitudinal studies conducted over a long period; those that have been done have come as result of unusual opportunities. Studies in England (SHEIHAM et al 1986) and Ireland (BUCKLEY and CROWLEY 1984) both found that disease progression in factory workers was slow. The Irish study found tooth loss was concentrated in a small number of those examined. Our group in Michigan has just completed field examinations for 195 adults in Tecumseh, Michigan, who were first examined by JAMISON in 1959. Preliminary scanning of the data also suggests that there has been limited disease activity in this group over that 28-year period.

In summary, research through the 1980s suggests this current view of the epidemiology of periodontal disease:

1. In cross-sectional surveys, only a small proportion of the adult population suffers from severe periodontitis, though moderate, site-specific periodontitis is common.
2. Gingivitis and periodontitis appear to have separate though not unrelated bacterial etiologies. Most gingivitis does not progress to periodontitis.
3. Although usually related to age in populations, periodontitis is not a natural consequence of aging.
4. Periodontitis is not the major cause of tooth loss in adults.

Nature of epidemiological data

In attempting to assess trends in periodontal diseases, we are still hampered by the necessity to compare modern data with PI data from a generation ago. The PI represented the current thinking of its time. The gingivitis-periodontitis continuum, as then perceived, was its philosophical underpinning, and all pockets of 3 mm. or more were considered pathological and given equal statistical weighting. (This approach was questioned by RAMFJORD as early as 1959).

The PI's use of group means is unsuitable for addressing research questions of susceptibility and host response. Uncertainties about the gingivitis-periodontitis relation raise validity questions; what can now be seen as the excessive weight given to gingivitis, even though RUSSELL (1956) considered the weighting "very little", could mask important differences between groups. Use of the PI without probing, as Russell recommended, might have led to underestimates in younger age-groups and overestimates in older groups. Perhaps the most significant long-term contribution of the PI was its ushering in the modern era of periodontal research; moving the field past the phase of observation and toward focussed research on natural history, etiology, and control.

There are still some public health applications where quick identification of problem groups is required. The ESI (Extent and Severity Index, CARLOS et al 1986), a half-mouth index based on probing measures, provides aggregated data for public health use. The CPITN (AINAMO et al 1982), also a partial recording index, was designed to quickly assess group treatment needs by scoring the worst conditions found. It is now routinely used by World Health Organization in planning dental services. Partial recording systems, which go back to RAMFJORD'S PDI (1959) have the advantage of being relatively quick, though they can underestimate the prevalence of serious disease (AINAMO and AINAMO 1985).

One goal of epidemiological research is to suggest etiological hypotheses, but such research in periodontal diseases has not gone much beyond the social and behavioral associations which were established a generation ago. Limitation of most field studies to cross-sectional designs has been one inhibiting factor. Most longitudinal studies are short-term clinical evaluations of therapies, necessarily restricted to diagnosed patients and therefore difficult to generalize from. Some have used designs which come close to the epidemiological case-control model (DZINK et al 1985), but use of active and inactive sites in the same periodontal patients seems to contravene the requirement for independent study and control groups. While clinical studies of patients are appropriate for comparison of treatment therapies and for testing agents for prevention and control, they are limited for testing etiological hypotheses because diseased people, by definition, cannot be grouped into those with and without disease, and those with and without exposure to the variable of interest. This is the essence of epidemiological study, without which some etiological questions just cannot be addressed.

Further research in periodontal epidemiology

Epidemiological studies need to be carried out on populations which include persons with and without disease. When the research questions are formulated, case-control studies can be a relatively quick first approach, in which persons with and without disease are contrasted for past exposure to hypothesized causes. "Exposure" could be defined as specific bacterial infection and host response factors.

On methodological issues, definition of what separates active from inactive disease might best be done through clinical research, but when this process is better understood it is likely that a "marker" for active disease could be developed for use in epidemiology. Ideally this would be a measure which does not require a high degree of training and expertise. With such a marker, prospective studies with general population groups would become far more practical, and basic questions such as types of bacterial infection, definition of different types of periodontitis, repair function in deep pockets, and the roles of plaque and calculus in etiology and progression, could be tested in field studies.

In terms of clinical measurements, assessment of four sites per tooth takes far too long for most field study purposes, an acceptable "sample" of sites is needed. There are controversies around all partial recording procedures, but it is hard to accept that appropriate specific sites could not be selected from current data. It would be even better if the difficulties associated with painstaking measurement in field studies were rendered moot by different approaches bases on new diagnostic technology. Measures such as DNA probes and immunofluorescent techniques, presuming that they can be adapted to field studies, would practically revolutionize epidemiological study in periodontal disease.

REFERENCES

AINAMO, J., BARMES, D., BEAGRIE, G., CUTRESS, T., and MARTIN, J. Development of the World Health Organization (WHO) Community Periodontal Index of Treatment Needs (CPITN). Int. Dent. J. 32: 281-291 (1982).

AINAMO, J., SARKKI, L., KUHALAMPI, M.L., PALOLAMPI, L., and PIIRTO, O. The frequency of periodontal extractions in Finland. Community Dent. Health 1: 165-172 (1984).

AINAMO, J., and AINAMO, A. Partial indices as indicators of the severity and prevalence of periodontal disease. Int. Dent. J. 35: 322-326 (1985).

BAELUM, V., FEJERSKOV, O., and KARRING, T. Oral hygiene, gingivitis, and periodontal breakdown in adult Tanzanians. J. Periodont. Res. 21: 221-232 (1986).

BAILIT, H.L., BRAUN, R., MARYNIUK, G.A., and CAMP, P. Is periodontal disease the primary cause of tooth extraction in adults? J. Am. Dent. Assoc. 114: 40-45 (1987).

BECK, J.D., LAINSON, P.A., FIELD, H.M., and HAWKINS, B.F. Risk factors for various levels of periodontal disease and treatment needs of Iowa. Community Dent. Oral Epidemiol. 12: 17-22 (1984).

BUCKLEY, L.A., and CROWLEY, M.J. A longitudinal study of untreated periodontal disease. J. Clin. Periodontol. 11: 523-530 (1984).

CAHEN, P.M., FRANK, R.M., and TURLOT, J.C. A survey of the reasons for dental extractions in France. J. Dent. Res. 64: 1087-1093 (1985).

CARLOS, J.P., WOLFE, M.D., and KINGMAN, A. The Extent and Severity Index: a simple method for use in epidemiologic studies of periodontal disease. J. Clin. Periodontol. 13: 500-505 (1986).

CHILTON, N.W. Some public health aspects of periodontal disease. Am. Dent. A. J. 40: 28-33 (1950).

CUTRESS, T.W., POWELL, R.N., and BALL, M.E. Differing profiles of periodontal disease in two similar South Pacific island populations. Community Dent. Oral Epidemiol. 10: 193-203 (1982).

DZINK, J.L., TANNER, A.C., HAFFAJEE, A.D., and SOCRANSKY, S.S. Gram negative species associated with active destructive periodontal lesions. J. Clin. Periodontol. 12: 648-659 (1985).

GREENWELL, H, and BISSADA, N.F. Variations in subgingival microflora from healthy and intervention sites using probing depth and bacteriologic identification criteria. J. Periodontol. 55: 391-397 (1984).

HALLING, A., and BJORN, A-L. Periodontal status in relation to age of dentate middle aged women. Swed. Dent. J. 10: 233-242 (1986).

HOOVER, J.N., and TYNAN, J.J. Periodontal status of a group of Canadian adults. J. Canad. Dent. Assoc. 52: 761-763 (1986).

HUGHES, J.T., ROZIER, R.G., and RAMSEY, D.L. Natural history of dental disease in North Carolina, 1976-77. (Durham, Carolina Academic Press, 1982).

HUGOSON, A., and JORDAN, T. Frequency distribution of individuals aged 20-70 years according to severity of periodontal disease. Community Dent. Oral Epidemiol. 10: 187-192 (1982).

ISMAIL, A.I., EKLUND, S.A., BURT, B.A., and CALDERONE, J.J. Prevalence of deep periodontal pockets in New Mexico adults age 27 to 74 years. J. Pub. Health Dent. 46: 199-206 (1986).

JAMISON, H.C. Prevalence and severity of periodontal disease in a sample of population. (Ann Arbor, University of Michigan dissertation, 1960).

KAY, E.J., BLINKHORN, A.S. The reasons underlying the extraction of teeth in Scotland. Brit. Dent. J. 160: 287-290 (1986).

LISTGARTEN, M.A, SCHIFTER, C.C., SULLIVAN, P., GEORGE, C., and ROSENBERG, E.S. Failure of microbial assay to reliably predict disease recurrence in a treated periodontitis population receiving regularly scheduled prophylaxes. J. Clin. Periodontol. 13: 768-773 (1986).

LÖE, H., THEILADE, E., and JENSEN, S.B. Experimental gingivitis in man. J. Periodont. 36: 177-187 (1965).

LÖE, H., ANERUD, A., BOYSEN, H., and SMITH, M. The natural history of periodontal disease in man; the rate of periodontal destruction before 40 years of age. J. Periodont. 49: 607-620 (1978).

LÖE, H., ANERUD, A., BOYSEN, H., and MORRISON, E. Natural history of periodontal disease in man. Rapid, moderate, and no loss of attachment in Sri Lankan laborers 14 to 46 years of age. J. Clin. Periodontol. 13: 431-440 (1986).

MILLER, A.J.,BRUNELLE, J.A., CARLOS, J.P.,BROWN, L.J., and LOE, H. Oral health of Unites States adults; the National Survey of Oral Health in U.S. employed adults and seniors:1985-1986. pp 3-11 (Washington, NIH Publ. No. 87-2868, 1987).

MOORE, W.E.C., HOLDEMAN, L.V., SMIBERT, R.M., GOOD, I.J., BURMEISTER, J.A., and RANNEY, R.R. Bacteriology of experimental gingivitis in young adult humans. Infect. Immun. 38: 651-667 (1982).

MOORE, W.E.C., HOLDEMAN, L.V., CATO, E.P., GOOD, I.J., SMITH E.P., RANNEY, R.R., and PALCANIS, K.G. Variation in periodontal floras. Infect. Immun. 46: 720-726 (1984).

NEWMAN, M.G. Current concepts of the pathogenesis of periodontal disease: microbiology emphasis. J. Periodontol. 56: 734-739 (1985).

PAGE, R.C. Current understanding of the aetiology and progression of periodontal disease. Int. Dent. J. 36: 153-161 (1986).

PILOT, T., and SCHAUB, R.M.H. Reappraisal of periodontal treatment needs. J. Dent. Res. 64: 260 (1985). Abstr No 770.

POWELL, R.N. The natural history of periodontal diseases. Ann. R. Austral. Coll. Dent. Surg. 8: 26-30 (1984).

RAMFJORD, S.P. Indices for prevalence and incidence of periodontal disease. J. Periodontol. 30: 51-59 (1959).

RUSSELL, A.L. A system of classification and scoring for prevalence surveys of periodontal disease. J. Dent. Res. 35: 350-359 (1956).

SELIKOWITZ, H-S., SHEIHAM, A., ALBERT, D., and WILLIAMS, G.M. Retrospective longitudinal study of the rate of alveolar bone loss in humans using bite-wing radiography. J. Clin. Periodontol. 8: 431-438 (1981).

SHEIHAM, A., SMALES, F.C., CUSHING, A.M., and COWELL, C.R. Changes in periodontal health in a cohort of British workers over a 14-year period. Brit. Dent. J. 160: 125-127 (1986).

SLOTS, J. The predominant cultivable microflora of advanced periodontitis. Scandinav. J. Dent. Res. 85: 114-121 (1977).

SLOTS, J. Bacterial specificity in adult periodontitis; a summary of recent work. J. Clin. Periodontol. 13: 912-917 (1986).

SOCRANSKY,S.S., HAFFAJEE, A.D., GOODSON, J.M., and LINDHE, J. New concepts of destructive periodontal disease. J. Clin. Periodontol. 11: 21-32 (1984).

WAERHAUG, J. Epidemiology of periodontal disease--review of literature; in: RAMFJORD, KERR, and ASH, eds, World workshop in periodontics; pp 181-211 (University of Michigan, Ann Arbor 1966).

WEINTRAUB, J.A., and BURT, B.A. Oral health status in the United States: tooth loss and edentulism. J. Dent. Educ. 49: 368-376 (1985).

Dr. B.A. Burt, School of Public Health, The University of Michigan, Ann Arbor, Michigan 48109-2029, USA

Periodontology Today. Int. Congr., Zürich 1988, pp. 77–85 (Karger, Basel 1988)

Can Treatment Needs be Defined on the Basis of Epidemiological Surveys?

Terence W. Cutress

Dental Research Unit, Medical Research Council, Wellington, New Zealand

Much confusion arises when clinicians, epidemiologists, investigators and planners meet in discussions. Definitions, motives and expectations tend to differ because the requirements and actions for guiding and implementing public health programmes call for 'convergent' thinking, whereas research and development is essentially a 'divergent' philosophy. The former concerns actions and behaviour related to "retaining the known, learning the predetermined and conserving what is", whereas the latter relates to, "revising the known, exploring the undetermined and constructing what might be"[11]. Planning and implementing health programmes require realistic, practical judgments based on empirical, objective and subjective experiences relevant to the times. Research, development, and field and clinical trials are inherently concerned with original ideas, hypotheses and conjecture.

Reasons for surveys of periodontal conditions are numerous. Surveys of treatment needs have pragmatic objectives. They estimate the magnitude of specific periodontal conditions in a population and relate them to appropriate categories of preventive and interceptive care. Assessment of treatment needs is hampered by recent advances in our understanding of the etiology, pathogenesis, and treatment of the diseases. The need to eliminate pockets or produce a plaque-free environment is doubted and the susceptibility of individuals to progressive disease is unpredictable. These and other imponderables confront the traditional approach to periodontal care[19].

It is well-established that gingivitis and periodontitis are common in most communities but these diseases do not inexorably lead to tooth loss. While, the significance of periodontal morbidity and its treatment are increasingly debated, there remains a responsibility at the public health level to evaluate the potential and real needs for care and act accordingly. Decisions cannot be held-over pending a maturing of recent concepts, opinions and research findings.

Defining Treatment Needs

The convergent approach of the epidemiologist and public health planner is to accept the clinical entities of gingivitis, periodontitis (with pocketing), calculus and microbial plaque as key elements in disease control and prevention. Because the potential for determining the rate of progression and disabling effects of periodontal diseases is unpredictable a blanket approach to prevention and control appears necessary. For surveys, predictions of 'at risk' potential or estimates of levels of disease activity are impractical and premature concepts[8]. A survey of treatment needs is essentially a population screening for prevalence and should not to be confused with predicting the 'at risk' potential of an individual[25].

Treatment Needs refer to the level of care considered appropriate for the control, reduction or cure of prevailing pathology. Categories of treatment needs are general rather than specific and are commonly identified at three levels[10,12,27]: (1) self-administered oral hygiene for minimising plaque formation at the gingival margin, (2) removal of plaque retentive factors (calculus, restoration defects), (3) complex periodontal care - which includes a wide range of procedures appropriate for managing deep periodontal pockets.

Requirements of treatment needs surveys proposed[23] several years ago remain relevant today, that is: the number of individuals needing treatment; type and extent of treatment; number of individuals needing preventive procedures; type and extent of preventive treatment; number and educational qualifications of personnel.

A screening survey is population, not individual, orientated. The distribution of the estimated treatment needs of a population sample will determine the magnitude and type of programmes required for the population. Each individual's assessed need locates him or her on a probable position on a scale of therapy but does not prescribe specific treatment.

The 1967 Workshop[17] on "Periodontal Needs" considered that data from general epidemiological surveys were not adequate for assessing treatment needs and that, anyhow, treatment procedures were empirical. An educated guess on the magnitude of (treatment) needs was believed to be impossible despite the abundance of data on the distribution and severity of the disease. Yet, reference was made to a report[13] on periodontal disease in the USA which found that about 1/3 of US adults were periodontally healthy; 1/3 had gingivitis only; 10% had early, 17% advanced, and 5% very advanced, disease. This appeared to be more than a guess on the needs of the population, particularly as the scope of the survey included data by age, socio-economic and other pertinent variables.

Present day aspirations are for realistic estimates of periodontal needs based on clinical conditions which pose a potential threat to lifelong retention of teeth. Such estimates should reveal the magnitude of needs and thereby provide a basis for sensible decision making.

Purpose of surveys of treatment needs

Surveys, by identifying the quantity of periodontal pathology and treatment needs in a population, provide the information necessary for determining the requirements for a population based approach to improving oral health. The reasons for promoting better periodontal health include, reducing the threat to tooth longevity, improved general oral health, personal esteem and social acceptability.

Objective assessment of treatment needs by surveys is essential for evaluating present and future requirements for preventive and curative programmes. Surveys provide guidance on effective deployment of resources such as manpower, offer a rational basis for setting of goals and provide the means to monitor changes in the prevalence of periodontal disease.

Surveys should be relevant to the prevention, reversal or containment of periodontal deterioration. Evaluation must identify the point prevalence of disease by individuals and teeth (or arch segments) for the respective periodontal criteria, should be age specific and recognise the influence of socio-economic and other pertinent factors on disease.

Clinical criteria

Although basic and clinical research into causes, progression and treatment of diseases have intensified, application of the new knowledge to survey methods appears impractical. Gingival inflammation, loss of periodontal attachment (with and without pocketing), and treatment to eliminate plaque and calculus remain the principal concerns for clinicians and epidemiologists alike. Causative factors directly or indirectly involve plaque and calculus without implicating them as diseases[15]. Use of tactile as well as visual observations is important to improve the objectivity of periodontal assessments. Expectations of more precise diagnosis by radiography, tooth mobility tests, microbial assay, exact measurement of pocket depths, gingival exudate composition, disease activity or disease progression rates are premature[8].

Preferred clinical criteria are those which discriminate between individuals with, no observed pathology, pathology limited to inflammatory conditions, pathological pocketing and calculus. These criteria remain the basis for diagnosis and treatment and will remain so until periodontal diseases are better defined clinically and diagnosis becomes more positive. Differentiating between 'marginal' and other forms of periodontitis appears impractical at the survey level despite its relevance to treatment need.

Indices suitable for identifying Treatment Needs

Any procedure which estimates, and discriminates between the prevalence of gingivitis, pocketing and plaque retentive factors has potential for assessing treatment needs. Classification of periodontal diseases was too general in most of the early studies. Lack of discrimination between gingivitis, early and advanced periodontitis, or number of teeth involved created a confused picture of disease distribution and severity, and hence needs. Because different levels of periodontal deterioration and disease severity require different treatment strategies, surveys which produced a single index figure have no value. When investigators reported their data in more detail a pattern of treatment needs emerged[4,6,13].

The value of a survey depends on the diagnostic criteria used, the epidemiological design, the data evaluation, and the relevance of the categories of need to the prevailing clinical conditions.

Indices which have been used for estimating treatment needs are the Periodontal Index (PI), Periodontal Status Index (PSI), Periodontal Treatment Needs System (PTNS) and Community Periodontal Index of Treatment Needs (CPITN). The most promising indices, the PTNS and CPITN, have features in common. However other indices have contributed towards the evolution of survey strategies which focus on treatment needs. For example, the PSI assessed plaque, calculus, intense gingivitis and advanced periodontal disease by segments, but used visual, non-tactile methodology. This may explain the differences in prevalence reported by several independent investigators (Table I).

Table I. Prevalence(%) of subjects and mean number of segments with gingivitis, periodontitis and calculus assessed by the Periodontal Status Index.

Age(years)	Gingivitis	Periodontitis	Calculus
	% (Mean)	% (Mean)	% (Mean)
Netherlands[21]			
15-24	62(1.9)	54(1.3)	79(3.2)
35-44	72(2.5)	67(2.1)	98(5.4)
>55	75(2.4)	81(2.8)	100(5.1)
New Zealand[4]			
15-19	48(1.3)	0(0)	50(0.6)
35-44	58(1.6)	5(0.1)	75(1.4)
55-64	65(1.8)	22(0.3)	80(1.4)
South Pacific[26]			
19	54(1.6)	1(0)	88(3.0)
35-44	81(3.6)	30(0.9)	88(4.7)
55-64	73(3.3)	34(1.1)	73(3.3)

Table II. Prevalence(%) of PI severity scores and mean PI scores of surveys in different geographic regions.

	Percentage of teeth scored:						Mean
	0	1	2	6	8	No. Subjects	PI Score
Pacific Region[7]							
6-44	59	29	7	5	0.6	428	0.8
	70	23	1	6	0.4	126	0.6
New Zealand[4]							
15-19	49	46	6	0	0	431	0.6
35-44	37	49	11	3	0.2	241	0.9
55-64	32	48	15	6	1	144	1.2
Africa[18]							
19-20	50	37	13	0	0	400	0.6
45-54	7	33	47	10	3	100	2.3
U.S.A.[13]							
18-24	33	58		10		945	0.5
35-44	27	47		26		1487	1.1

Periodontal Index

Use of mean PI scores to describe the relative periodontal status of populations found favour with many epidemiologists. However, single or mean scores are of no value in identifying treatment needs. Helpful statistics are those which provide information on the numbers of people and teeth with healthy periodontal conditions, those with gingivitis and those with periodontitis. Most reports on surveys using the PI do not provide this data. However, when prevalence rates by the separate clinical criteria are provided, the magnitude and type of population needs become apparent (Table II).

Prevalence data by numbers of individuals or teeth alone can produce a distorted pattern of needs. The 1976 and 1982 surveys (Table III) of the New Zealand population recorded prevalence of PI criteria by number of individuals (highest PI

Table III. Prevalence of PI severity scores for adults and teeth(shown in brackets) in New Zealand, 1976 and 1982[4,5].

	PI Score							
	0		1 or 2		6 or 8		Mean PI Score	
Age(years)	1976	1982	1976	1982	1976	1982	1976	1982
15-19	1	20	98	79	0.7	1	0.6	0.4
	(48)	(65)	(52)	(35)	(0)	(0.3)		
35-44	2	0	83	83	15	18	0.9	1.1
	(37)	(31)	(60)	(64)	(3)	(5)		

(No.of adults: 1976= 431,361; 1980= 267,263 for 15-19 and 35-44 year-olds respectively)

score) and teeth[4,5]. While the prevalence of subjects requiring care may be low the numbers of teeth involved may be high, or vice versa. (This set of data also show change over the six year period). Many other investigators, using the PI, have tempted our curiosity with their reports of mean PI values but limited our access to a 'Pandora's box' of potentially useful data on treatment needs. Other published PI data are more helpful on needs; e.g., the International Collaborative Study[1] reported several measures (PI) of periodontal health in ten populations.

Periodontal Treatment Needs System

Some of the earlier difficulties in conceptualizing treatment needs were overcome by rationalising levels of need in terms of the time required to provide the treatment[2,16]. The PTNS was a significant move away from the constraints of traditional academic epidemiology towards a pragmatic view of the relevance of periodontal morbidity and the need for, and feasibility of treatment programmes at the public health level.

Community Periodontal Index of Treatment Need

The CPITN has developed and promoted concepts similar to those of the PTNS. Numerous surveys have been reported which, by presenting uniform statistics on conditions and needs, have provided a substantial and relevant basis for appraising the epidemiological and public health significance of periodontal disease. Summaries of data are available in the literature[3,20]. Table IV shows typical CPITN profiles; extensive gingivitis at all ages, high prevalence of calculus, low to moderate prevalence of shallow pockets increasing with age, and a low to very low prevalence of deep pockets at all ages.

Two important findings have emerged from CPITN surveys: the relatively low prevalence of deep pocketing and the high prevalence of subgingival calculus in some populations. Both features are highly relevant to decisions taken at the community level, e.g.,it is obvious that massive deployment of resources to remove calculus are not feasible. If calculus control is an important factor then selfcare methods for prevention or removal become research priorities.

Table IV. Intercountry comparison of Community Periodontal Index of Treatment Needs data for 35-44 year olds.

	TNO %	TN1 %	TN2 % (Sext)	TN3 % (Sext)	No. Adults
Hong Kong[14]	1	99	99(1.2)	16(0.3)	668
New Zealand[5]	7	93	70(1.2)	8(0.2)	263
Queensland[22]	11	89	79(0.3)	4(0.1)	223
Sri Lanka[24]	5	93	92(4.2)	10(0.2)	1867
Philippines[9]	2	98	99(4.4)	1(.01)	640

% refers to subjects and ( ) to mean number of sextants.

Table V. Distribution of 46 surveys by their CPITN prevalence scores for 35-44 year olds.

Prevalence. Range, %	Highest CPITN Score 0	1	2	3	4
	No. Surveys				
0 - 10	40	40	2	3	24
11 - 20	5	4	3	4	15
21 - 30	0	1	6	10	2
31 - 40	1	1	13	14	3
41 - 100	0	0	22	15	2

Table VI. Distribution of 46 surveys by their mean CPITN sextant scores for 35-44 year olds.

No. Sextants. Range	Sextant CPITN score 0	1	2	3	4
	No. Surveys				
0 - 1	22	0	0	17	44
1.1 - 2	8	2	4	20	0
2.1 - 3	5	2	7	6	2
3.1 - 4	0	10	14	1	0
4.1 - 5	2	13	9	0	0
5.1 - 6	0	19	12	2	0

Tables V and VI have been calculated from a summary of 46 surveys[20]. They reveal a high prevalence (over 40%) of calculus (score 2) or shallow pockets(score 3) in 22 and 15 surveys respectively. Healthy(score 0) or gingivitis only (score 1) as highest score were uncommon, most surveys (40) reported a prevalence of 10% or less. Evaluation of the distribution of scores by sextants emphasised that deep pockets were associated usually with less than one sextant, whereas gingivitis and calculus exceeded three (often five and six sextants).

The partial mouth scoring (10 teeth)recommended for epidemiological surveys using the CPITN is a compromise which does not appear to significantly underestimate the prevalence of treatment needs, less so the distribution of individuals between categories of treatment needs.

Conclusions

Surveys of treatment needs are concerned with determining the distribution of periodontal conditions of a population for the purpose of implementing preventive and control measures. Within the limitations imposed by current clinical diagnostic procedures and treatment modalities, epidemiologists have developed screening procedures which provide estimates of the magnitude and severity of the periodontal treatment needs of population groups. Estimates of appropriate preventive and curative programmes and their feasibility in terms of costs and manpower requirements can be appraised.

It is recommended that estimates of treatment needs (by specified categories) obtained under epidemiological conditions be compared with clinical evaluations obtained using more detailed examination procedures.

References

1. ARNLJOT, H.J.; BARMES, D.E.; COHEN, L.K.; HUNTER, P.B.V. and SHIP, I.I.: Oral care systems. An international collaborative study. World Health Organization. (Quintessence Publishing Co. London 1985).
2. BELLINI, H.T. and GJERMO, P.: Application of the Periodontal Treatment Need System (PTNS) in a group of Norwegian industrial employees. Community Dent. Oral Epidemiol 1:22-29 (1973).
3. CUTRESS, T.W.: Periodontal health and periodontal disease in young people: global epidemiology. Int. dent. J. 36:146-151 (1986).
4. CUTRESS, T.W.; HUNTER, P.V.B. and HOSKINS, D.I.H.: Comparison of the Periodontal Index and the Community Periodontal Index of Treatment Needs (CPITN). Community Dent. Oral Epidemiol. 14:39-42 (1986).
5. CUTRESS, T.W.; HUNTER, P.V.B.; DAVIS, P.B.; BECK, D.J. and CROXSON, L.J.: Adult Oral Health and Attitudes to Dentistry in New Zealand 1976. (Wellington: Dental Research Unit, Medical Research Council of New Zealand 1979).
6. DAVIES, G.N.: Dental conditions among the Polynesians of Puka Puka. II. The prevalence of periodontal disease. J. dent. Res. 35:734-741 (1956).
7. DAVIES, G.N.; HOROWITZ, H.S. and WADA, W.:The assessment of periodontal disease for public health purposes. J. Periodontal Res. 9:62-70 (1974).
8. FINE, D.H. and MANDEL, I.D.: Indicators of periodontal disease activity: an evaluation. J. Clin. Periodontol. 13:533-546 (1986).
9. GARCIA, M.L. and CUTRESS, T.W.: A national survey of periodontal treatment needs of adults in the Philippines. Community Dent. Oral Epidemiol 14:313-316 (1986).
10. GJERMO, P.: Establishment of priorities in periodontal care; in SHANLEY, Efficacy of treatment procedures in periodontics; pp.317-324 (Quintessence Publishing Co., Inc. Chicago 1980).
11. GUILFORD, J.P.: The nature of human intelligence. (McGraw-Hill, New York 1967).
12. JOHANSEN, J.R., GJERMO, P. and BELLINI, H.T.: A system to classify the need for periodontal treatment. Acta Odontol.Scand. 31:297-305 (1973)

13. KELLY, J.E. and VAN KIRK, L.E.: Periodontal disease in adults. United States,1960-1962. National Center for Health Statistics. Series 11, No.12 (Washington: D.C., U.S. Department of Health, Education, and Welfare 1965).
14. LIND, O.P., EVANS, R.W., HOLMGREN, C.J., CORBET, E.F., LIM, L.P. and DAVIES, W.I.R.: Hong Kong Survey of Adult Oral Health 1984; (Department of Periodontology and Public Health, Faculty of Dentistry, University of Hong Kong 1986).
15. MANDEL, I.D. and GAFFAR, A.: Calculus revisited. A review. J. Clin. Periodontol. 13:249-257 (1986).
16. MARKKANEN, H.; RAJALA, M. and PAUNIO, K.:Periodontal treatment need of the Finnish population aged 30 years and over. Community Dent. Oral Epidemiol. 11:25-32 (1983).
17. O'LEARY, T.J.: Workshop Report "The Periodontal Needs of the United States Population". Am. Acad. Periodontol., (Chicago 1967).
18. OLSSON, B.: Periodontal disease and oral hygiene in Arussi province, Ethiopia. Community Dent. Oral Epidemiol. 6:139-145 (1978)
19. PILOT, T.: Analysis of the overall effectiveness of treatment of periodontal disease; in SHANLEY, Efficacy of treatment procedures in periodontics; pp.213-231 (Quintessence Publishing Co., Inc., Chicago 1980).
20. PILOT, T. and BARMES, D.E.:An update on periodontal conditions in adults, measured by CPITN. Int. Dent.J. 37:169-172 (1987).
21. PLASSCHAERT, A.J.M.; FOLMER, T.; VAN DEN HEUVEL, J.L.M.; JANSEN, J.; VAN OPIJNEN, L. and WOUTERS, S.L.J.: An epidemiological survey of periodontal disease in Dutch adults. Commmunity Dent. Oral Epidemiol. 6:65-70 (1978).
22. POWELL, R.N. and McENIERY, T.M.: Survey of Adult Dental Health 1984; (The Brisbane Statistical Division, University of Queensland, Australia 1985).
23. RAMFJORD, S.P.:Methodology for determining periodontal needs. J. Periodontol. 40:524-528 (1969).
24. SAPARAMADU, K.D.G.: National Oral Health Survey, Sri Lanka 1983-84; Ministry of Health; Dental Health Unit, Health Education Bureau, Colombo (1985).
25. SHEIHAM, A.: Screening for periodontal disease. J. Clin. Periodontol. 5:237-245 (1978)
26. SPEAKE, J.D. and MALAKI, T.: Oral health in Tuvalu. Community Dent.Oral Epidemiol. 10:173-177 (1982).
27. WHO: Epidemiology, etiology, and prevention of periodontal diseases; report of a WHO Scientific Group; Technical Report Series 621 (World Health Organization, Geneva 1978).

Dr. T.W. Cutress, Dental Research Unit, Medical Research Council, P.O. Box 27007, Wellington, New Zealand

Periodontology Today. Int. Congr., Zürich 1988, pp. 86–94 (Karger, Basel 1988)

Application of Statistical Modelling to Periodontal Diseases as Viewed by the Statistician

Jonathan Sterne

MRC Dental Research Unit, London, UK

1. Introduction

With the revolution in theories of the nature of periodontal diseases in recent years has come a revolution in the application of statistical methods to data from periodontal research (HAFFAJEE 1983a). The loss of periodontal attachment was seen as a slowly progressing, chronic, highly prevalent condition. The statistical models used attempted to associate mean disease levels in the mouth (the response variable) with mean levels of, for instance, plaque quantity or gingival inflammation (the explanatory variables). If, however, current views of these diseases are accepted then it is apparent that such statistical models are no longer appropriate. It is now believed that periodontal disease activity varies between disease sites in a mouth. Thus explanatory variables, which either may be measured at a site or may be subject characteristics, should be associated with the response variable at the individual site as well as the subject level, since differences may be obscured by simply comparing subject means. Periodontal diseases are no longer thought to progress at a slow, constant rate. Thus the response variable should be the measured loss of attachment, rather than the measured attachment level, since the latter reflects past disease history, rather than present disease activity. The aim of this paper is to describe currently available statistical techniques for the modelling of data from periodontal research, and to outline some possible pitfalls in the techniques currently being used.

A statistical model is a mathematical description of the relationship between the response and explanatory variables. It can generally be divided into a systematic part (for instance the relationship between the response and the nature of the micoflora at a site), and a random part, which is a probability model for that part of the variation not explained by the systematic part (for instance the distribution of the measurement error). All statistical tests depend on underlying models for the data, many of which make stringent assumptions which, if broken, render the test meaningless. In periodontal research the most obvious example is the incorrect assumption of independence between disease sites in the same subject.

In this paper I will show that it is possible both to formulate statistical models which describe data from periodontal research, and to estimate parameters from those models using computer software which is currently available.

2. The questions to be addressed

In order to discuss the application of statistical models to periodontal diseases it is necessary to be clear what questions the model is intended to answer. I shall attempt here to look at statistical models which can be used to associate the measured loss of attachment at a number of sites in a number of subjects with variables which are measured at the same sites or which are subject characteristics; either as predictors or markers of disease activity.

This approach does not prejudge the nature of the progression of periodontal diseases. If progression is slow and at a constant rate, then variables measured at baseline may correlate with the observed loss of attachment five years later. If an extreme version of the 'burst' theory is correct, then it may be necessary to measure explanatory variables on the same day as the disease episode in order to find those that may be associated with disease progression. The mathematical structure of the model in these two situations is the same.

I will not attempt here to assess the evidence that periodontal diseases progress in bursts of activity (SOCRANSKY 1982). If it is accepted that rates of disease progression may change (a far weaker and less controversial proposition) then it is apparent that the response variable must be the change in the attachment level at a site.

3. Measurement Error

The only way in which the loss of the connective tissue attachment to the tooth can currently be measured is by successive measurements made with a periodontal probe. The total attachment length is between 10mm and 15mm and, for most people in Western countries, this is not totally lost during an entire lifetime. Compared to this the magnitude of the measurement error, currently assumed have a standard deviation around 0.8mm for a single observation, is seen to be large in relation to the possible changes which may occur. Difficulty in accurately assessing the progression of periodontal diseases must be a major reason for the failure to identify aetiological agents.

It must be realised that the presence of measurement error cannot be removed by ingenious manipulation of the data. It is inevitable that the larger the error in measuring the response variable, the more difficult it is to detect an association with any explanatory variable.

Various approaches which attempt to allow firm conclusions to be drawn from periodontal disease data, despite the muddying effect of measurement error can be suggested. I attempt here to list some of the more obvious ones, and to point out possible pitfalls in current approaches.

3.1. Increasing the sample size

Any association, however small and whatever the measurement error, can be detected if the sample size is sufficiently great. The phrase "sample size" is ambiguous in periodontal terms. If there really were no subject effect, then to measure disease progression and corresponding explanatory variables at 100 sites in the same mouth would give the same size and power to statistical hypothesis tests as to measure one site in 100 subjects. The attractions in terms of cost of the former approach are obvious. If there is no variation whatsoever within a mouth other than measurement error, then measuring large numbers of different sites in the same mouth will yield no more information than making repeated observations at a single site. The problem in designing studies of periodontal disease is that the extent to which the disease is either host-based or site-based is unknown. Until more information is gained, the only safe course is to think of the sample size as the number of subjects in the study.

The number of subjects in studies of periodontal disease progression has been small compared with numbers participating in clinical trials. The small size of such studies, together with the large measurement error, may have meant that their power to detect associations has been insufficient.

3.2. Making repeated measurements

It is a basic arithmetical fact that if the standard deviation of a variable is σ, then the standard deviation of the mean of two independent such variables is $\sigma/\sqrt{2}$. Thus the simple recording of duplicate measurements of attachment levels at each examination will reduce the effect of measurement error by 30%. Repeat measurements are now routinely performed by many workers performing longitudinal studies (GOODSON 1986). The number of times which it is practically possible to repeat measurements is obviously limited by the danger of the periodontal probe causing trauma of the connective tissue, and of the examiner recalling the last measurement made at the site.

3.3. Improving measurement techniques

Various methods of reducing the error in measurement of attachment levels are under development, for instance by automatic detection of the cement-enamel junction (JEFFCOAT 1986). The substantial reducion of measurement error may well be the greatest possible contribution to the study of periodontal diseases.

3.4. Pitfalls in current approaches

3.4.1. The 'tolerance' method. This method (HAFFAJEE 1983a) for the detection of attachment loss divides sites into those where a large loss in attachment (usually 3mm or greater) was observed, and those where it was not. The aim of this procedure is to ensure that for most of those sites which are defined as diseased by this procedure, there is only a small probability that the observed change was due entirely to measurement error. It is recognised (HAFFAJEE 1983b, IMREY 1986) that such a procedure leads to high test specificity but low test sensitivity, but it is argued that this is reasonable because of the paramount need to detect periods of disease activity (SOCRANSKY 1987). It has also been argued (AEPPLI 1984) that a threshold value of 2mm rather than 3mm provides adequate specificity with much improved sensitivity.

It is important to recognise that the usefulness of this technique depends crucially on the unknown true distribution of periodontal disease progression. If the disease progresses uniformly, then disease sites and control sites will apparently be identified, when in reality differences are purely due to measurement error. If most sites do not experience any loss of attachment, but a few undergo disease activity, and wherever such disease activity occurs at least 3mm attachment is lost, then the tolerance method will distinguish between disease and other sites almost perfectly. The true distribution is unknown, and evidence for the truth of the latter scenario depends largely on techniques such as the tolerance method or the use of regression analysis which cannot, of their nature, distinguish between the latter extreme case and one where there is a range of true attachment losses at a larger number of sites (SOCRANSKY 1982, GOODSON 1982, MORRISON 1986).

3.4.2. Regression towards the mean. It has been pointed out (BLOMQVIST 1986) that because of measurement error there will be an inverse correlation between the measured attachment level at a site and subsequent change in attachment level. This can be illustrated as follows. Denote the true attachment level, the observed attachment level and the measurement error (which we suppose to have mean 0 and variance σ^2) at occasion i by a_i, y_i and e_i respectively. Thus $y_i = a_i + e_i$.

The change in observed attachment level on occasion 2 is given by $y_2 - y_1 = a_2 - a_1 + e_2 - e_1$. Thus the covariance of the initial attachment level with change in attachment level is given by $cov(y_1, y_1 - y_2) = cov(a_1 + e_1, a_2 - a_1 + e_2 - e_1) = cov(e_1, -e_1) = -\sigma^2$. Similarly the covariance between the observed change in attachment level on successive occasions is $cov(e_2 - e_1, e_3 - e_2) = cov(e_2, -e_2) = -\sigma^2$.

This means that the deeper the observed initial attachment level or the larger the observed initial loss of attachment, then the greater the likelihood that there is a subsequent observed increase in attachment level. The consequence is that deep sites will appear to get shallower, and, more seriously, if sites are selected for treatment on the basis of an observed loss of attachment, then they will appear to respond to treatment even if there is no treatment effect.

4. Currently available techniques for modelling periodontal disease data

It has repeatedly been emphasised by statisticians in recent years (IMREY 1986, OSBORNE 1987), that under no circumstances should significance tests be performed on data from many disease sites which has been grouped together without regard to a subject effect. This is because this practice makes the wholly unreasonable assumption that the progression of disease at a site is independent of that at any other site in the same mouth. Although this appears to have been accepted by biologists (SOCRANSKY 1986), their reluctance to accept it is perhaps illustrated by the recent appearance in the same issue of a periodontal journal of a paper in which significance tests were performed on data grouped over sites and subjects (MANDELL 1987), and a paper discussing the likely over-estimates of statistical significance produced by this practice (OSBORNE 1987). Statisticians have, however, been less readily able to explain satisfactory alternatives which allow explanatory variables measured at a site to be related to the response variable at that site in a satisfactory statistical model. This seems to have left the impression that there is a conflict between allowing for subject effects and allowing for site effects (SOCRANSKY 1987). This is not the case - we shall see that it is perfectly possible to perform statistical modelling which does both. I shall now discuss briefly some statistical techniques which can be applied to data from periodontal research.

4.1 Periodontal clinical trials

The aim of a periodontal clinical trial is to compare disease progression in subjects which undergo different treatments. The unit of observation is the disease site, so that the data consists of measurements of disease progression made at one or more sites in each subject. OSBORNE (1987) gives a simple method where the mean response for each subject, weighted by the number of observations for the subject, is used as the response to compare the treatments.

4.2 Variance components modelling

In many studies, the aim is to assess the effect of more than one explanatory variable; which may be measured at the site (eg collagen fragment levels) and/or subject (eg salivary IgA level). Statistical models which perform this task while allowing for non-independence of different sites in the same subject are now available. Variance Components, or Multilevel modelling (AITKEN and LONGFORD 1986, GOLDSTEIN 1986), was developed for the analysis of unbalanced data from educational surveys (pupil within class; class within school), and can equally be applied to data from periodontal research (disease site within subject; subject analysed on more than one occasion) (STERNE 1988) . This technique allows a response variable acting at the lowest level (i.e. site) to be related to explanatory variables acting at any level (site characteristics or subject characteristics measured on any occasion). Random subject effects are simultaneously estimated, thus avoiding the assumption of independence between sites in the same mouth. The FORTRAN code for 'VARCL', an interactive progamme which uses a fast scoring algorithm to calculate the maximum-likelihood estimates in variance components models, is commercially available either from the Centre for Applied Statistics, University of Lancaster, Cartmel College, Lancaster LA1 4YL, England; or from Dr. N. T. Longford, Educational Testing Service, Rosedale Road-22T, Princeton, New Jersey 08541, U.S.A.

4.3 An ad hoc method

It is relatively simple to perform a procedure that avoids the necessity for specialised software, but allows for variation in disease progression between subjects. A typical multiple regression model (which can be fitted by almost any statistical package, (for instance SPSS, SAS or MINITAB), with p explanatory variables, N subjects, and M_i sites measured in subject i can be written as:

$$y_{ij}=\sum_{k=1}^{p}\beta_k x_{ijk}+ e_{ij} \qquad (i=1,2,...,N;\ j=1,2,...,M_i)$$

where y_{ij}, x_{ijk} and e_{ij} are respectively the response at site j in subject i, the value of the kth explanatory variable at that site, and the error at that site; and $\{\beta_k\}$ (k=1,2,...,p) are the co-efficients of the explanatory variables (the larger the effect, the larger the co-efficient) and are estimated in fitting the model.

In order to allow for a subject effect, we now introduce N terms α_i (i=1,2,...,N) into the model, so that:

$$y_{ij}=\sum_{k=1}^{p}\beta_k x_{ijk}+ e_{ij} + \alpha_i$$

Again, this can easily be done by most statistical packages, and is equivalent to estimating the effect of N explanatory variables respectively equal to 1 at every site in subject i, 0 at every site in every other subject (i=1,...,N). In fitting the model we now estimate $\{\beta_k\}$ (k=1,2,...,p) and $\{\alpha_i\}$ (i=1,2,...,N).

We can interpret α_i as an estimate of the mean reponse for subject i, having allowed for the effect of the explanatory variables at each site. Thus the model above allows for differences in response between subjects. The estimates of the α's can then be related to subject level explanatory variables, such as the level of oral hygiene practised by the subject, or the subject's antibody response to a putative periodontal pathogen.

This method is equally applicable to Generalized Linear Modelling (for which the statistical package GLIM is designed), in which the response variable, rather than being normally distributed, may be, for example, binary (eg loss of attachment/no loss of attachment).

4.4. More than two measurements per site

In the above, I have been relating the change in attachment level, derived from successive measurements at a site, with explanatory variables measured once at the site or in the subject. In longitudinal studies we may have more than two successive measurements both of attachment levels and explanatory variables. Statistical models for such data must allow for correlation between the response on successive occasions.

Variance components models allow this to be done by adding a third level to the hierarchy. Thus at the top level is the subject, with explanatory variables such as gender, which do not change. At the second level is the subject data on a particular occasion, such as serum antibody levels to plaque bacteria, and at the third level the site data for that occasion, such as levels of a substance in gingival crevicular fluid.

As observed in section 3, there will be an inverse correlation between the loss of attachment on successive occasions, and between attachment level at examination i and the loss of attachment between examinations i and i+1. Thus any statistical model for longitudinal studies which has attachment loss as the response must allow for these random effects. Variance components modelling allows the specification of such random terms as explanatory variables.

5. Conclusions

The change in statistical methods used in periodontal research has arisen out of a valid desire to use methods appropriate to the nature of a disease process which varies in rate between different sites in the same mouth, and to associate disease progression at the site with explanatory variables measured at the same site. Unfortunately some of the methods adopted have not been statistically valid.

The chief disadvantage of the methods described in the previous section is their added complexity. Their generality means that many possible models could be chosen, so that care is needed in assessing their suitability both before and after data analysis. They ideally require both specialised software, and expert statistical advice in its use. Interpretation of the results of the fitting of these models is more difficult. However, such simple statements as "The levels of the organism Bacteroides intermedius were significantly elevated at sites showing subsequent loss of attachment" do have an equivalent, viz "The magnitude of the parameter β_5 relating the effect of Bacteroides intermedius to the response is significantly greater than zero".

However, the structure of data from periodontal research means that simple, easily interpreted procedures such as the t-test are either statistically invalid (if site data is pooled over subjects), or will lose information (if subject means are used). These general methods can be used on the unbalanced, hierarchical data sets which usually arise in periodontal research.

6. References

AEPPLI, D. M.; BOEN, J. R., and BANDT, C. L.: Measuring and Interpreting Increases in Probing Depth and Attachment Loss. J. Periodontol. 56: 262-264 (1984).

AITKEN, M., and LONGFORD N.: Statistical Modelling Issues in School Effectiveness Studies. J. R. Statist. Soc. A. 149: 1-43 (1986).

BLOMQVIST, N.: On the bias caused by regression towards the mean in studying the relation between change and initial value. J. Clin. Perio. 13: 34-37 (1986).

GOLDSTEIN, H. Multilevel mixed linear model analysis using iterative generalized least squares. Biometrika 73: 43-56 (1986).

GOODSON, J. M.; TANNER, A. C. R.; HAFFAJEE, A. D.; SORNBERGER, G. C., and SOCRANSKY, S. S.: Patterns of progression and regression of advanced destructive periodontal disease. J. Clin. Perio. 9: 472-481 (1982)

GOODSON, J. M.: Clinical measurements of periodontitis. J. Clin. Perio. 13: 446-455 (1986).

HAFFAJEE, A. D.; SOCRANSKY, S. S., and GOODSON, J.M.: Comparison of different data analyses for detecting changes in attachment level. J. Clin. Perio. 10: 298-310 (1983a).

HAFFAJEE, A. D., SOCRANSKY, S. S. and GOODSON, J. M.; Clinical parameters as predictors of destructive periodontal disease activity. J. Clin. Perio. 10: 257-265. (1983b).

IMREY, P. B.: Considerations in the statistical analysis of clinical trials in periodontitis. J. Clin. Perio. 13: 517-528 (1986).

JEFFCOAT, M. K.; JEFFCOAT, R. L.; JENS, S. C., and CAPTAIN, K.: A new periodontal probe with automated cemento-enamel-junction detection. J. Clin. Perio. 13: 276-280 (1986).

MANDELL, R. L.; EBERSOLE, J. L., and SOCRANSKY, S. S.: Clinical immunologic and microbiologic features of active disease sites in juvenile periodontitis. J. Clin. Perio. 14: 534-540 (1987).

MORRISON, E. C. and KOWALSKI, C. J.: Discussion: Clinical measurements of periodontitis. J. Clin. Perio. 13: 456-458 (1986).

OSBORNE, J.: The choice of computational unit in the statistical analysis of unbalance clinical trials. J. Clin. Perio. 14: 519-523 (1987)

SOCRANSKY, S. S.; HAFFAJEE, A. D.; GOODSON, J. M. and LINDHE, J.: New concepts of destructive periodontal disease. J. Clin. Perio. 11: 21-32 (1982).

SOCRANSKY, S. S.: General discussion: Considerations in the statistical analysis of clinical trials in periodontitis. J. Clin. Perio. 13: 530-531 (1986).

SOCRANSKY, S. S.; HAFFAJEE, A. D.; SMITH, G. L. F., and DZINK, J. L.: Difficulties encountered in the search for the etiologic agents of destuctive periodontal diseases. J. Clin. Perio. 14: 588-593 (1987).

STERNE, J. A. C.; JOHNSON, N. W.; WILTON, J. M. A.; JOYSTON-BECHAL, S., and SMALES, F. C.: Variance Components Analysis of Data from Periodontal Research. J. Perio. Res. (in press) (1988).

Address

Mr Jonathan Sterne, Medical Research Council Dental Research Unit, 32 Newark Street, London E1 2AA (UK).

Periodontology Today. Int. Congr., Zürich 1988, pp. 95–103 (Karger, Basel 1988)

Validity and Reliability of Clinical Measurements

Per Gjermo and Jostein Rise

Department of Periodontology and Institute of Community Dentistry, Dental Faculty, University of Oslo, Oslo

Introduction

In epidemiology the scores given to each person in a survey are not intended for making decisions on the individual level, but should as a sum reflect the disease status of the population. To this end a number of indicators have been suggested to reflect periodontal disease at various disease stages. Consequently, the degree to which these indicators really measure the disease (validity) and the degree to which we are able to record these indicators precisely (reliability) are of paramount importance when the results from epidemiologic and clinical studies are to be interpreted.

The present paper will initially address the definitions of validity and reliability and relate them to measurements of periodontal status and disease. Since several workshops have dealt with the problem of criterion validity (concurrent/ predictive) and how to improve reliability in terms of test-retest of the commonly used measurements of periodontal status (see for example CHILTON 1974, 1986), these aspects will not be discussed in detail. Our intention is to approach the problem of measuring the disease activity assuming this to be an unobservable process and emphasize the construction of valid and reliable indices for such purposes. Methods for assessing the reliability and validity of indicators and indices used will be suggested.

Definitions

The concepts of validity and reliability are usually defined separately, although they are not independent of each other.

Validity refers to the extent to which our measurements measure the characteristics we want to measure (or the marksman's ability to hit the bull's eye (figure 1 A)). For instance when we measure pocket depths we may wish to describe the damages caused by periodontal disease over time assuming that pocket depths reflect loss of attachment. On the other hand, if we measure the loss of attachment directly by measuring the distance from the cemento-enamel junction to the most coronal fibrous attachment the validity would be very high; the only problem being linked to the reliability of the measurements.

Reliability is an expression of 1) the stability which indicates the extent to which similar information is obtained with the methods employed for measurements of disease when the measurements are performed more than once; and 2) the equivalency which indicates the consistency between examiners and/or measurements performed at the same time. There are several sources for measurement errors:

1. For instance pocket depths may be measured with lack of constancy. This may be caused by a variety of conditions like variation in light source, variation in position of the examined person or examiner etc.

2. Lack of precision is another way of reducing the reliability of data. This will occur if variations in for example probing force result in different measurements of pocket depths in the same pocket. Variation in probing pocket depths due to use of instruments with for instance different thickness is called lack of congruency.

3. Variation in measurements may also be due to lack of objectivity by the examiner. The skill and experience differ between examiners and sometimes it may be difficult to assess whether or not bleeding occurs after probing or to assess "tendency" towards spontaneous bleeding. Moreover, in clinical trials or field experiments the examiner may be influenced by awareness of whether the examinee belongs to test or control group.

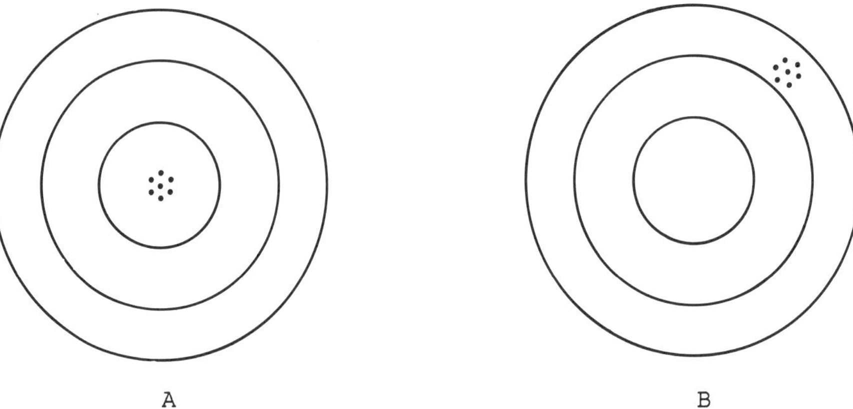

Fig. 1. A marksman's shots. A = High validity (and reliability). B = High reliability, but low validity.

The reliability of data in an investigation may thus be compared with a marksman's ability to hit at the same spot each time he fires, regardless of whether he hits the bull's eye or not (figure 1 B). However, there is a relationship between the two concepts, reliability and validity. In figure 2 this relationship is illustrated. The internal validity describes the validity of our operationalized variable as an expression of the characteristic we want to observe, the reliability describes the precision of our measurements and the external validity expresses the total validity of our data. This relationship may have different implications under different circumstances. For instance, if it is important to assess the exact disease status of a population in a cross-sectional survey or in a small scale intervention study high internal validity is a must (assuming that measurement errors (lack of precision) are random). In a longitudinal study where the objective is mainly to study changes in the condition, the reliability of the measurements may be more important for the external validity of the data.

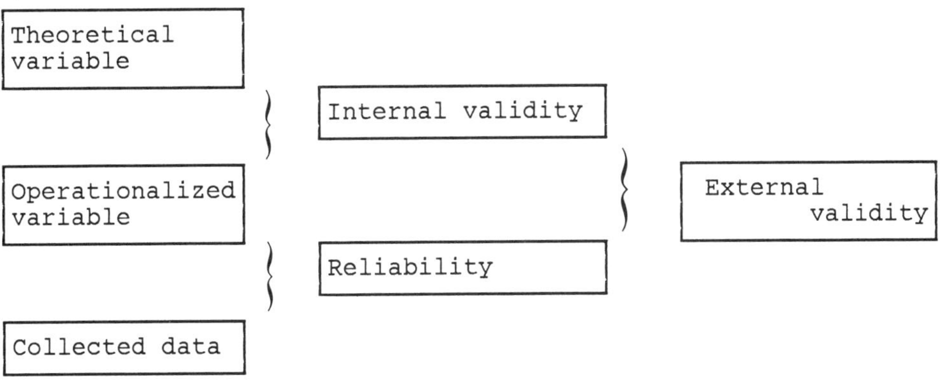

Fig. 2. The relationship between reliability and validity (after HELLEVIK 1980).

The validity and reliability of some periodontal disease measurements

Current methods of assessments of periodontal status have been developed when periodontitis was regarded as a slow and continuously progressing disease, starting with gingivitis which, in the course of time, would proceed to destructive periodontitis. Under such circumstances a fairly accurate picture of the status of the periodontal tissues would appear as a valid indicator of the activity of the disease. The challenge of periodontal clinical and epidemiologic research today is that the disease process itself with existing knowledge and accessible methods is non-observable (GOODSON 1986). According to the "random burst hypothesis" (SOCRANSKY, HAFFAJEE, GOODSON and LINDHE 1984) the periodontal status is a poor predictor of ongoing or future tissue destruction (predictive validity). The same seems to be the case for other traditionally used clinical predictors as degree of inflammation (bleeding), deep probeable pockets, suppuration and amount of supragingival plaque (BADERSTEN, NILVEUS and EGELBERG 1985, 1987, GOODSON 1986).

The internal validity (figure 2) of clinical assessments of diseases can easily be estimated if the phenomenon we want to describe can be observed directly. For instance the degree of inflammation, and the amount of accumulated loss of attachment can be assessed histologically (concurrent validity). However, when the phenomenon we want to measure is non-observable, as is periodontal disease activity (the process of tissue destruction) (GOODSON 1986), the validity can only be estimated by means of a theoretical model (MASTEKAASA 1987). This means that we will have to operationalize our unobservable variable by empirical indicators of the disease process. The validity of our data will then depend on to which extent our chosen indicator, or set of indicators if an index is used, reflects the unobservable phenomenon (disease activity) we want to obtain information about.

The validity of estimating cumulated effects of periodontal destruction by assessing the loss of attachment would from a clinical point of view seem satisfactory. Thus the external validity of the measurements would depend on the reliability of the measurements. However, the validity of measuring pocket depths for the same purpose has been questionned. Results from a recent study on the dental health of US adults indicated that retraction of the gingival margin may lead to underestimation of loss of attachment by measuring pocket depths (MILLER, BRUNELL, CARLOS, BROWN and LÖE 1987). However, such measurements may still be valuable for studying changes over time if high reliability of measures is obtained.

In their original study of clinical measurements of loss of attachment GLAVIND and LÖE (1967) reported high reproducibility after a period of intense calibration of the examiners. With their approach they used approximately 45 minutes per person to measure the loss of attachment, which is not acceptable in large scale studies. However, other investigators (HAFFAJEE, SOCRANSKY and GOODSON 1983) have used the same method in several longitudinal studies of periodontal disease. They found that differences between repeated measurements of loss of attachment were significant at the 1% level when the differences exceeded 2.46 mm, their measurement error taken into account.

Pocket depths are the basis for estimating the severity of periodontitis in currently used indices (RUSSEL 1956, AINAMO, BARMES, BEAGRIE, CUTRESS, MARTIN and SARDO-INFIRRI

1982). Both measurements of attachment loss and pocket depths require clinical procedures which may easily introduce measurement errors. Even if the periodontal probe is the same, the force used for probing, the direction of the probe and the condition of the tissue at the level of the fibrous attachment have been shown to be of importance (LISTGARTEN 1980, WATTS 1987) Therefore, standardized equipment and thourough training and calibration of examiners are very important when these methods are employed in order to obtain satisfactory reliability of the data.

Means and methods of improving validity and reliability of clinical measurements of periodontal disease

The validity of measurements depends on the strength of the association between the operationalized variable and the theoretical variable. Thus, the validity will usually be increased by using more than one indicator for assessment of the phenomenon, i.e. using an index. For large scale studies presence or absence decisions seem to be more reliable than do graded scales. Moreover, aggregating data (from surfaces to teeth or groups of teeth, or to subjects, and from subjects to groups of subjects) will increase reliability.

In the further discussion of validity and reliability we will use the functions of index construction as an organizing principle. Three purposes of indices can be identified in this context when separate scores for each indicator are added to arrive at one score for the individual (additive index):

1. Combining several individual variables into one index simplifies the data matrix and the subsequent empirical analysis without losing essential information at the aggregate levels in terms of averages or proportions.

2. The use of several variables combined to measure one phenomenon increases the possibility of capturing several aspects of the phenomenon under study and thus increase the validity.

3. By combining several measures into one, the error of each variable, provided it is random, will tend to cancel out in the total score and result in increased reliability.

Thus the use of well constructed indices will improve validity and reliability of the employed measurements.

Theoretical model for index construction

Assuming that periodontal disease is an unobservable phenomenon and therefore must be regarded as a theoretical concept which can be reflected (and presumably only approximated) by a number of empirical indicators, the construction of an index may be considered a mediating link between the theoretical and empirical levels. This relationship can be visualized in a measurement model (ZELLER & CARMINES 1985, MASTEKAASA 1987) (figure 3). The theoretical variable (w) which is denoted latent or unobserved is represented by several indicators (x_1 to x_t). The association between the theoretical variable and each empirical indicator is expressed by a coefficient of correlation (epistemic correlation; a_1 to a_t). If the variation in each variable is caused by variation in the theoretical variable (disease activity), there is also a positive correlation between the indicators, expressed in terms of internal consistency. This is the most common criterion to decide whether or not an indicator ought to be included in an index (NUNNALLY 1967). The stronger the association between the latent and the observed variables, the better the internal consistency, but the indicators will always be subject to some unreliability due to imperfect measuring. In figure 3 the expected correlation between x_1 and x_2 would be the product of $a_1 \times a_2$. It is assumed that the measurements of the indicators are subject to random error (u_1 to u_t).

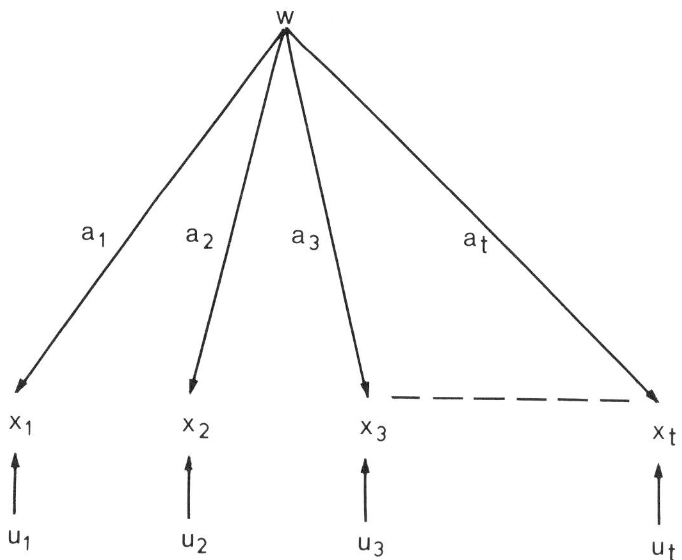

Fig. 3. A reflective model of index construction.

Models as described above are called reflective models and can be traced back to psychometric test-theory (see NUNNALLY 1967), using factor analysis for index construction (see KIM 1975). This method is able to detect those indicators which belong to the same dimension and thus can be used in an index by capturing the common factor of all indicators, and at the same time exclude what is unique to each of the variables. Thus both validity and reliability are enhanced. The factor loadings represent regression coefficients of factors to describe a given indicator and are similar to the epistemic correlations (KIM 1975). The factor loading may in this way be interpreted as one way of quantifying validity (GUILFORD and FRUCHTER 1973). The product of the factor loadings of 2 indicators provides an indication of the internal consistency of the model. However, the alpha coefficient (the mean of all possible split-half correlations) increases as the average correlations among the variables and the number of variables increase and is a better estimate of the internal consistency (CRONBACH 1951, McKENNEL 1977).The alpha coefficient also indicates how much of the observed variance is true variance and thus is an estimate of the reliability (GUILFORD and FRUCHTER 1973).

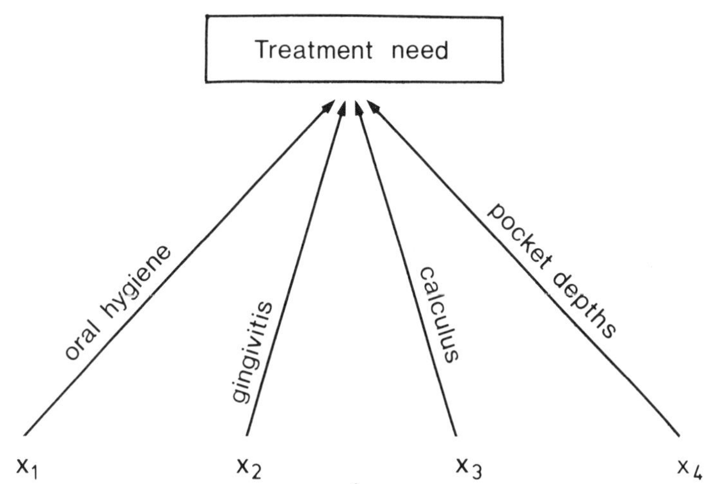

Fig. 4. A formative model for index construction.

There are other models for construction of indices than the reflective model. In the formative model (figure 4), where the variation in the phenomenon under study can be ascribed to variations in the indicators used, there is no need for internal consistency between the indicators. Formative models may be applied when the phenomenon we want to assess is observable, but at the same time is multifaceted. Treatment need may be regarded as such a multifaceted concept. For instance, gingivitis may call for another treatment approach than presence of calculus or pathologic pockets. If total treatment need can be expressed by a common unit of measurement (for example time requirements), different indicators of need for particular treatments may be combined in a formative index. Since no correlation among the indicators is required, internal consistency cannot be used as an estimate of reliability. In this case test-retest reliability appears to be the method of choice. Also, factor analysis cannot be used to estimate validity, but since the phenomenon (treatment need) in principle is observable, other and more direct methods are available.

Thus, the choice between a reflective and a formative model for constructing periodontal indices will depend on the phenomenon under study (observable versus non-observable) and the objective of the study.

References:

AINAMO, J., BARMES, D.E., BEAGRIE, G., CUTRESS, T., MARTIN, J. and SARDO-INFIRRI, J.: Development of the World Health Organization (WHO) Community Periodontal Index of Treatment Needs (CPITN). International dent. J. 32: 281-291 (1982).

BADERSTEN, A., NILVEUS, R. and EGELBERG, J.: Effect of non-surgical periodontal therapy. VII. Bleeding, suppuration and probing depth in sites with probing attachment loss. J. clin. Periodont. 12: 432-440 (1985).

BADERSTEN, A., NILVEUS, R. and EGELBERG, J.: Effect of non-surgical periodontal therapy. VIII. Probing attachment changes related to clinical characteristics. J. clin. Periodont. 14: 425-432 (1987).

CHILTON, N.W. (ed): Proceedings of the Conference on Clinical Trials of Agents used in the Prevention/Treatment of Periodontal Diseases. J. periodont. Res. 9: suppl. 14 (1974).

CHILTON, N.W. (ed): Conference on Clinical Trials in Periodontal Diseases. J. clin. Periodont. 13: (1986).

CRONBACH, I.J.: Coefficient alpha and the internal structure of tests. Psychometrica 16: 297-334 (1951).

GLAVIND, L. and LÖE, H.: Errors in the clinical assessment of destruction. J. periodont. Res. 2: 180-184 (1967).

GOODSON, J.M.: Clinical measurements of periodontitis. J. clin. Periodont. 13: 446-455 (1986).

GUILFORD, J.P. and FRUCHTER, B.: Fundamental statistics in psychology and education; pp. 407-434 (McGraw-Hill, New York 1973).

HAFFAJEE, A.D., SOCRANSKY, S.S. AND GOODSON, J.M.: Comparison of different data analyses for detecting changes in attachment level. J. clin. Periodont. 10: 298-310 (1983).

HELLEVIK, O. Forskningsmetode i sosiologi og statsvitenskap; 4th ed., p. 158 (Universitetsforlaget, Oslo 1980).

KIM, J.-O.: Factor analysis; in NIE, HULL, JENKINS, STEINBRENNER and BENT: SPSS statistical package for the social sciences; 2nd ed., pp. 468-514 (McGraw-Hill, New York 1975).

LISTGARTEN, M.: Periodontal probing. What does it mean? J. clin. Periodont. 7: 165-176 (1980).

MASTEKAASA, A.: Modellbruk, indekser og konsistenskriterier. Tidsskr. Samf.forskn. 28: 167-188 (1987).

McKENNEL, A.C.: Attitude scale construction; in O'MUIRCHEARTAIGH and PAYNE: The analysis of survey data; vol.1.: Exploring data structures; pp. 183-220 (John Wiley & Sons, Toronto 1977)

MILLER, A.J., BRUNELLE, J.A., CARLOS, J.P., BROWN, L.J. and LÖE, H.: Oral Health of United States Adults. (NIH Publication No. 87-2868, Bethesda 1987).

NUNNALLY, J.C.: Psychometric theory (McGraw-Hill, New York 1967).

RUSSEL, A.L.: A system of classification and scoring for prevalence surveys of periodontal disease. J. dent. Res. 35: 350-359 (1956).

SOCRANSKY, S.S., HAFFAJEE, A.D., GOODSON, J.M. and LINDHE, J.: New concepts of destructive periodontal disease. J. clin. Periodont. 11: 21-32 (1984).

WATTS, T.: Constant force probing with and without a stent in untreated periodontal disease: the clinical reproducibility problem and possible sources of error. J. clin. Periodont. 14: 407-411 (1987).

ZELLER, R.A. and CARMINES, E.G.: Measurement in the social sciences (Cambridge University Press, Cambridge 1980).

Per Gjermo, professor, dr. odont., Department of Periodontology, Dental Faculty, University of Oslo, P.O.B. 1109, Blindern, Oslo 3 (Norway)

Periodontology Today. Int. Congr., Zürich 1988, pp. 104–111 (Karger, Basel 1988)

What is a Periodontal Pathogen?

Jan Carlsson

Department of Oral Microbiology, University of Umeå, Umeå, Sweden

Pathogens and commensalism

The concept of a pathogen was introduced by Robert Koch more than 100 years ago when defining a bacterial species which causes a specific infectious disease. To apply this concept to periodontal diseases creates obvious problems. No bacterial species has so far been found to be able to colonize the periodontal pocket by itself and cause disease. The destruction of the periodontal tissues is always associated with complex bacterial communities in the periodontal pockets (SCHROEDER and ATTSTRÖM 1980, MOORE et al. 1985, SOCRANSKY et al. 1987). The organisms of these subgingival microbiotas are not only dependent on their host for their establishment, they also have to rely on each other for such important ecological determinants as adherence and supply of nutrients (GIBBONS and VAN HOUTE 1975).

Many sites of the human body are colonized by bacterial communities. In most sites there is a commensal relationship. The bacteria derive benefits from the human body, but they do not inflict the body any harm (ALEXANDER 1971). This commensalism is possible thanks to various defense systems, which prevent the bacteria from invading the tissue of their host. One very important part of this defense is the epithelial lining of the human body and the continuous shedding of the superficial epithelial cells (GIBBONS and VAN HOUTE 1975). In the dentogingival area, however, the epithelial lining and the shedding of the epithelial cells do not work as an efficient defense, because the tissue is in close contact with bacteria firmly anchored to the solid tooth surface. The body, therefore, has to rely on some other defense strategy to prevent a bacterial invasion. That defense - the inflammation - is put into action as soon as bacteria accumulate on the teeth (LÖE et al. 1965).

Inflammation - tissue destruction and repair

Inflammation is characterized by recruitment of phagocytes, lymphocytes and plasma proteins into an irritated extravascular site. When bacteria are involved, inflammation may lead to inducement of specific immune responses, to complement-mediated bacteriolysis, and to phagocytosis and killing of the bacteria. The inflammation is mediated by substances formed in many independent systems. Some of these systems and their interactions are illustrated in figure 1.

Bacteria initiate inflammation in various ways. Bacterial products are chemotactic for neutrophils, activate the plasma proteinase cascade systems, trigger mast cells to release biogenic amines, and stimulate inflammatory cells and resident tissue cells to form cytokines, platelet activating factor (PAF) and prostanoids (FEARON 1981, BACH 1982, SUNDSMO and FAIR 1983, MARCEAU et al. 1983, DAYER and DEMCZUK 1984, HANAHAN 1986, NEEDLEMAN et al. 1986, WILKINSON 1987, PROCTOR 1987, SAMUELSSON et al. 1987). Cytokines of special interest in host defense are interleukin 1 (IL-1) and tumor necrosis factor (TNF) (DINARELLO 1986, BEUTLER and CERAMI 1986, OLD 1987).

The defense mobilized by the inflammation is primarily aimed at preventing a bacterial invasion. Some effectors of this defense may, however, also damage the host (figure 2). Oxygen products from inflammatory cells injure tissue cells (FANTONE and WARD 1982), and proteases from both inflammatory cells and resident tissue cells degrade components of the extracellular tissue matrix (TAICHMAN et al. 1966, TAICHMAN et al. 1984, SAKSELA 1985, MEIKLE et al. 1986). In the periodontal tissues it is of special interest that mediators of inflammation such as prostanoids, cytokines, bradykinin and thrombin directly or indirectly activate osteoclasts and initiate bone resorption (CENTRELLA and CANALIS 1986, DINARELLO 1986, LERNER et al. 1987).

With tissue injury follows repair and remodelling of the tissue (figure 2). At an inflamed site this repair is orchestrated by cytokines like IL-1 and TNF, and growth factors such as platelet-derived growth factor (PDGF), and transforming growth factors, alpha (TGF-α) and beta (TGF-β) (DINARELLO 1986, BEUTLER and CERAMI, 1986, SPORN and ROBERTS 1986, SPORN et al. 1986, TERRANOWA and WIKESJÖ 1987).

The defense systems mobilized by inflammation are usually efficient against bacteria which accidentally penetrate the epithelial lining of our body. The defense appears to be less suited for its purpose when used against a microbiota more or less permanently established in the host such as the microbiota of the periodontal pocket.

"A periodontal pathogen" - a misconception

It is important to realize that inflammation is not a unique defense system against a few types of specific bac-

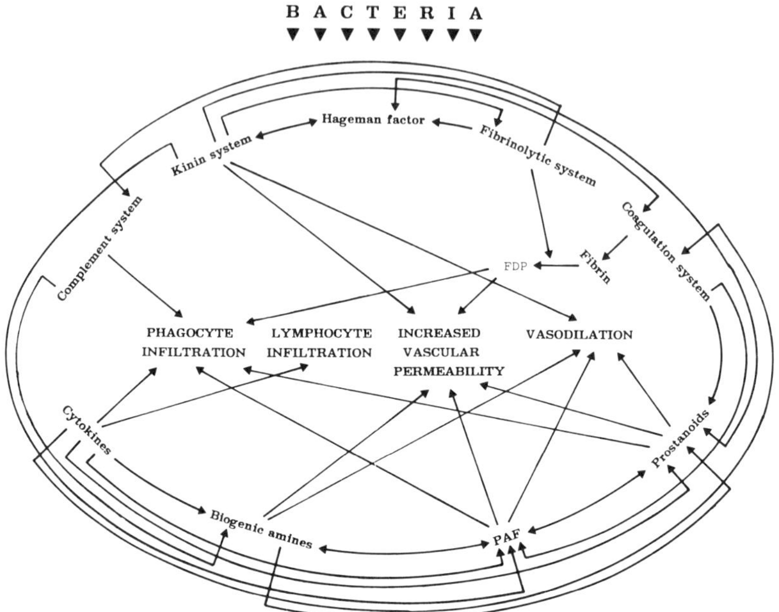

Figure 1. Schematic illustration of how bacteria may initiate an inflammation, which is characterized by vasodilation, increased vascular permeability, and accumulation of phagocytes and lymphocytes. There are both plasma- and cell-derived mediators of inflammation. The plasma-derived mediators are formed in the complement, kinin, fibrinolytic and coagulation systems (the plasma proteinase cascade systems). Fibrin degradation products (FDP) may also work as inflammatory mediators. Cell-derived mediators are cytokines (e.g. IL-1 and TNF), biogenic amines (e.g. histamine), platelet activation factor (PAF) and prostanoids (e.g. prostaglandins, prostacyclins, leukotriens and lipoxins). The cell-derived mediators are formed by inflammatory cells such as platelets, neutrophils, basophils, macrophages and lymphocytes and by resident tissue cells like epithelial cells, mast cells, fibroblasts and osteoblasts. The formation of the inflammatory mediators is sometimes initiated by an activation of the Hageman factor (WIGGINS and COCHRAN 1979, KAMATA et al. 1985), but bacterial products may trigger the formation of the inflammatory mediators on all levels of the various mediator systems. Arrows in the figure show the extensive interactions among the various mediator systems.

teria. The defense is engaged as soon as any bacterium or its products come in contact with the subepithelial tissues. It is likely that most members of the subgingival microbiota have the capacity to initiate inflammation and in that way contribute to the periodontal tissue injury. From this follows that

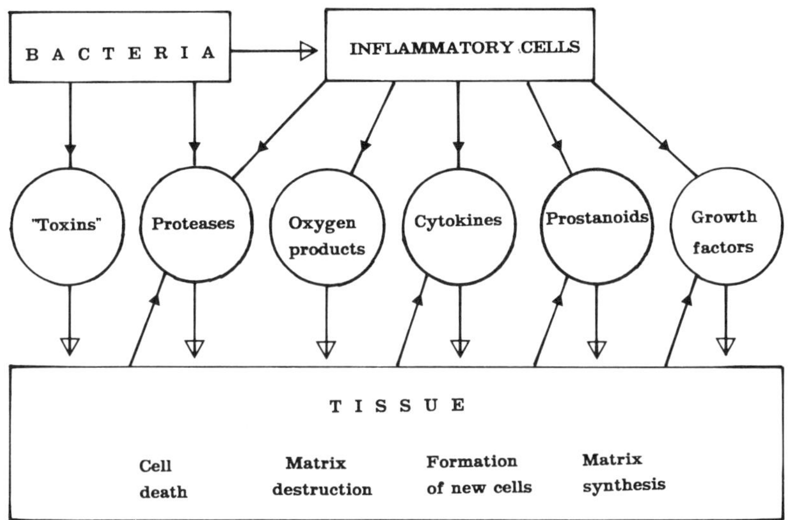

Figure 2. Schematic illustration of the interaction among bacteria, inflammatory cells and tissue in periodontal disease. In the inflamed tissue there is not only an injury of cells and destruction of extracellular tissue matrix, but also formation of new cells and synthesis of new tissue matrix. The damage and the repair of the tissue are initiated by bacteria, inflammatory cells and resident tissue cells. It should be noted that the proteases, cytokines, prostanoids and growth factors are derived both from inflammatory cells and resident tissue cells.

all bacteria of the subgingival microbiota could be considered "pathogens".

The defense against the subgingival microbiota is often achieved with a minimum of tissue loss. There may, however, be situations where this will not be the case. The commensal organisms of the microbiota may reach such high numbers that the defense systems of the host will not be able to cope with them. The microbiota may also harbor organisms which specifically perturbe the defense strategies of the host (figure 3).

One may choose to restrict the designation "periodontal pathogens" to those bacteria which have specific mechanisms to perturbe the host defense and in that way cause an accelerated destruction of periodontal tissues. It should be remembered, however, that such a "pathogen" will never work in isolation. It is always a member of a complex bacterial community, and it will not fulfill the criteria of Koch's postulates. To call such a member of a complex microbiota a "pathogen" creates obvious conceptual difficulties, not only from a scientific point of view but also when applied to the treatment of periodontal diseases.

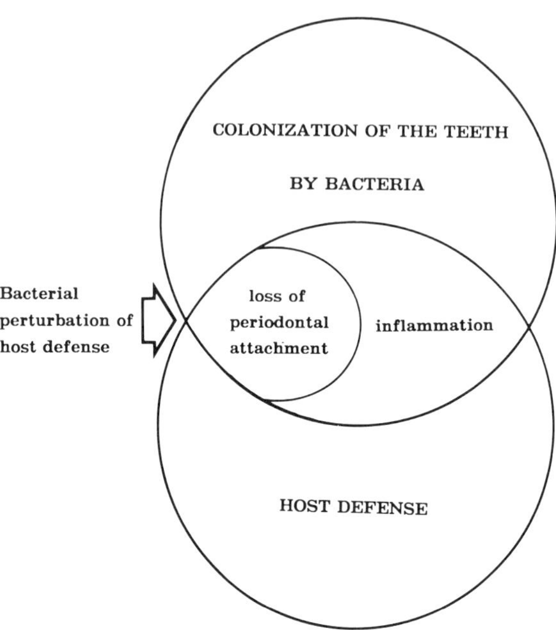

Figure 3. Host-parasite interaction in periodontal disease. Bacteria colonizing the teeth cause inflammation in the periodontal tissues. The inflammatory reaction is a defense against the microbiota colonizing the periodontal pocket. The host defense may be perturbed when the commensal subgingival microbiota becomes so large that the host defense cannot cope with it. Some bacteria of this subgingival microbiota may also have specific virulence factors which perturbe the host defense. This results in loss of periodontal attachment.

An important breakthrough in the area of periodontal microbiology was the finding that a single member of a subgingival microbiota could have a specific virulence factor. Actinobacillus actinomycetemcomitans produces a toxin which kills the most important cell of the host defense, the neutrophil (BAEHNI et al. 1979, VAN DYKE et al. 1985). This has been an impetus to a search for other virulence factors among the members of the subgingival microbiota (see reviews by SLOTS and GENCO 1984, CARLSSON et al. 1986, THEILADE 1986, BROOK 1987 and LISTGARTEN 1987). By necessity, the virulence factors, the organisms of the complex microbiotas, and the tissue reactions related to periodontal diseases have to be studied in isolated systems. Each system gives its own "keyhole" perspective on the disease. "Keyholes" next door may give different views. In recent years there has been a tendency for each enthusiastic research worker to guide the clinicians from his own "keyhole". The concept of a "periodontal pathogen" has encouraged this type of guidance. The clinicians may lose confidence in the research endeavors, if that will go on.

We should realize that the concept of "pathogen" was originally deviced for specific microorganisms which caused specific diseases. This does not seem to apply to periodontal diseases. It may therefore be advisable to abandon the concept of "periodontal pathogen" for these diseases. "Pathogenic microbiota" should be preferred. With the concept of a "pathogenic microbiota" we acknowledge the fact that periodontal diseases have a polymicrobial etiology, and that a multitude of defense systems have to be mobilized by the host against these infections. This may not mean any major change in the direction of our present research efforts, but it asks for a more careful and humble acknowledging of the multifactoral etiology of the periodontal diseases, when the research results are presented, and when these results are put into practice in the treatment of periodontal diseases.

References

ALEXANDER, M.: Microbial ecology; pp. 207-388 (John Wiley & Sons, Inc., New York 1971).

BACH, M.K.: Mediators of anaphylaxis and inflammation. Annu. Rev. Microbiol. 36: 371-413 (1982).

BAEHNI, P., TSAI, C-C., McARTHUR, W.P., HAMMOND, B.J., AND TAICHMAN, N.S.: Interaction of inflammatory cells and oral microorganisms. VIII. Detection of leukotoxic activity of a plaque-derived gram-negative microorganism. Infect. Immun. 24: 233-243 (1979).

BEUTLER, B., and CERAMI, A.: Cachectin and tumour necrosis factor as two sides of the same biological coin. Nature 320: 584-588 (1986).

BROOK, I.: Role of encapsulated anaerobic bacteria in synergistic infections. Crit. Rev. Microbiol. 14: 171-193 (1987).

CARLSSON, J., NILSSON, T., and SUNDQVIST, G.: Effect of proteinases from black-pigmented Bacteroides on human plasma proteins; in LEHNER, T. and CIMASONI, G., The borderland between caries and periodontal disease III; pp.99-123 (Editions Médecine et Hygiène, Genève 1986).

CENTRELLA, M., and CANALIS, E.: Local relulators of skeletal growth: A perspective. Endocr. Rev. 6: 544-551 (1986).

DINARELLO, C.A.: Multiple biological properies of recombinant human interleukin 1 (beta). Immunobiology 172: 301-315 (1986).

DAYER, J-M., and DEMCZUK, S.: Cytokines and other mediators in rheumatoid arthritis. Springer Semin. Immunopathology 7: 387-413 (1984).

FANTONE, J.C., and WARD, P.A.: Role of oxygen-derived free radicals and metabolites in leukocyte-dependent inflammatory reactions. Am. J. Pathol. 107: 397-418 (1982).

FEARON, D.T.: Complement as a mediator of inflammation. Clin. Immunol. Allergy 1: 225-242 (1981).

GIBBONS, R.J., and van HOUTE, J.: Bacterial adherence in oral microbial ecology. Annu. Rev. Microbiol. 29: 19-44 (1975).
HANAHAN, D.J.: Platelet activating factor: A biologically active phosphoglyceride. Annu. Rev. Biochem. 55: 483-509 (1986).
KAMATA, R., YAMAMOTO, T., MATSUMOTO, K., and MAEDA, H.: A serratial protease causes vascular permeability reaction by activation of the Hageman factor-dependent pathway in guinea pigs. Infect. Immun. 48: 747-753 (1985).
LERNER, U.H., JONES, I.L., and GUSTAFSON, G.T.: Bradykinin: A new potential mediator of inflammation-induced bone resorption. Studies of the effects on mouse calvarial bone and articular cartilage in vivo. Arthritis Rheum. 30: 530-540 (1987).
LISTGARTEN, M.A.: Nature of periodontal diseases: Pathogenic mechanisms. J. Periodontal Res. 22: 172-178 (1987).
LÖE, H., THEILADE, E., and BÖRGLUM JENSEN, B.: Experimental gingivitis in man. J. Periodontol. 36: 177-187 (1965)
MARCEAU, F., LUSSIER, A., REGOLI, D., and GIROUD, J.P.: Pharmacology of kinins: Their relevance to tissue injury and inflammation. Gen. Pharmac. 14: 209-229 (1983).
MEIKLE, M.C., HEATH, J.K., REYNOLDS, J.J.: Advances in understanding cell interactions in tissue resorption. Relevance to the pathogenesis of periodontal diseases and a new hypothesis. J. Oral Pathol. 15: 239-250 (1985).
MOORE, W.E.C., HOLDEMAN, L.V., CATO, E.P., SMIBERT, R.M., BURMEISTER, J.A., PALCANIS, K.G., and RANNEY R.R.: Comparative bacteriology of juvenile periodontitis. Infect. Immun. 48: 507-517 (1985).
NEEDLEMAN, P., TURK, J., JAKSCHIK, B.A., MORRISON, A.R., AND LEFKOWITH, J.B.: Arachidonic acid metabolism. Annu. Rev. Biochem. 55: 69-102 (1986).
OLD, L.J.: Tumour necrosis factor. Polypetide mediator network. Nature 326: 330-331 (1987).
PROCTOR, R.A.: Fibronectin: An enhancer of phagocyte function. Rev. Infect. dis. 9: 412-419 (1987).
SAKSELA, O.: Plasminogen activation and regulation of pericellular proteolysis. Biochim. Biophys. Acta 823: 35-65 (1985).
SAMUELSSON, B., DAHLÉN, S-E., LINDGREN, J.Å., ROUZER, C.A., and SERHAN, C.N.: Leukotrienes and lipoxins: Structures, biosynthesis, and biological effects. Science 237: 1171-1176 (1987).
SCHROEDER, H.E., and ATTSTRÖM, R.: Pocket formation; An hypothesis; in LEHNER, T. and CIMASONI, G., The borderland between caries and periodontal disease II; pp. 99-123 (Academic Press, London 1980).
SLOTS, J., AND GENCO R.J.: Microbial pathogenicity. Black-pigmented *Bacteroides* species, *Capnocytophaga* species, and *Actinobacillus actinomycetemcomitans* in human periodontal disease: Virulence factors in colonization, survi-

val, and tissue destruction. J. Dent. Res. 63: 412-421 (1984).
SOCRANSKY, S.S., HAFFAJEE, A.D., SMITH, G.L.F., and DZINK, J.L.: Difficulties encountered in the search for the etiologic agents of destructive periodontal diseases. J. Clin. Periodontol. 14: 588-593 (1987).
SPORN, M.B., and ROBERTS, A.B.: Peptide growth factors and inflammation, tissue repair, and cancer. J. Clin. Invest. 78: 329-332 (1986).
SPORN, M.B., ROBERTS, A.B., WAKEFIELD, L.M., ASSOIAN, R.K.: Transforming growth factor-β: Biological function and chemical structure. Science 233: 532-534 (1986).
SUNDSMO, J.S., FAIR, D.S.: Relationships among the complement, kinin, coagulation, and fibrinolytic systems. Springer Semin. Immunopathol. 6: 231-258 (1983).
TAICHMAN, N.S., FREEDMAN, H.L., and URIUHARA, T.: Inflammation and tissue injury - I. The response to intradermal injections of human dentogingival plaque in normal and leukopenic rabbits. Arch. Oral Biol. 11: 1385-1392 (1966).
TAICHMAN, N.S., TSAI, C-C., SCHENKER, B.J., and BOEHRINGER, H.: Neutrophil interactions with oral bacteria as a pathogenic mechanism in periodontal diseases. Adv. Inflam. Res. 8: 113-142 (1984).
TERRANOVA, V.P., and WIKESJÖ, U.M.E.: Extracellular matrices and polypeptide growth factors as mediators of functions of cells of the periodontium. J. Periodontol. 58: 371-380 (1987).
THEILADE, E.: The non-specific theory in microbial etiology of inflammatory periodontal diseases. J. Clin. Periodontol. 13: 905-911 (1986).
VAN DYKE, T.E., LEVINE, M.J., and GENCO, R.J.: Neutrophil function and oral disease. J. Oral Pathol. 14: 95-120 (1985).
WIGGINS, R.C., and COCHRANE, C.G.: Hageman factor and the contact activation system; in HOUCK, J.C., Chemical messengers of the inflammatory process; pp. 179-196 (Elsevier/North-Holland Biomedical Press, Amsterdam 1979).
WILKINSON, P.C.: Leukocyte locomotion and accumulation: The contributions of cell polarity and cell growth; in MOVAT, H.Z., Leukocyte emigration and its sequelae; pp. 1-13 (Karger, Basel 1987).

Jan Carlsson, Department of Oral Microbiology, University of Umeå, S-901 87 Umeå, Sweden.

Periodontology Today. Int. Congr., Zürich 1988, pp. 112–122 (Karger, Basel 1988)

Are there Convincing Animal Models for Periodontal Diseases?

Roy C. Page

Departments of Periodontitis, School of Dentistry, and Pathology, School of Medicine, and the Research Center in Oral Biology, University of Washington, Seattle, Washington, USA

Introduction

The nature of human periodontal disease has been investigated intensively for more than two decades. Since the early 1970s, in vitro studies using modern concepts and techniques of cellular and molecular biology have been performed. Progress has been made in identifying and characterizing bacteria that cause human periodontitis, and numerous hypothetical pathways and mechanisms through which bacteria, by provoking a particular host response, can potentially induce destruction of host tissues have been proposed. Knowledge has now developed to the point that well-characterized animal models of human periodontitis are required to demonstrate that mechanisms worked out in vitro are in fact operative in vivo, and to further elucidate normal structure and function.

For almost a hundred years, clinicians and investigators have observed and studied spontaneously occurring and induced periodontal diseases in animals in an effort to better understand these diseases in humans. The first report appears to have been that of TALBOT (1899), who described periodontitis in mongrel dogs. Since that time, periodontal diseases have been studied in many species including mice, rats, hamsters, mink, dogs, sheep, and several nonhuman primate species. A wealth of dependable data about periodontitis in species other than man now exists. The purpose of the present paper is to consider whether there exist convincing animal models of the periodontal diseases as they are currently understood to occur in humans. Because of space limitations, only rodents, dogs, and nonhuman primates are considered.

Data on animal models published prior to 1982 have been summarized and reviewed previously, and readers are referred to that publication for more details and references (PAGE AND SCHROEDER 1982). Only more recent key references are provided here.

Criteria for Assessment of Animal Models

The most convincing animal model would be one in which all aspects of the disease are analogous to periodontitis in man. The data make abundantly clear, however, that while many of the manifestations of periodontal diseases in humans are observed to some degree in other species, no analog of human diseases exists, nor is it likely that one will ever be found. A reasonable approach to determining whether convincing models exist, therefore, would be to compare periodontal diseases in various animal species to the disease as it is observed in humans, and to thereby illuminate features and aspects held commonly and those that differ. It must be noted at the outset that whether a given model is convincing is, in the final analysis, dependent upon the question or questions for which answers are being sought.

Determinants of Patterns of Disease

A great deal of progress has been made recently in our understanding of inflammatory diseases in general, and several basic principles have been elucidated. These principles are important in understanding the relationships between periodontitis in humans and in other mammalian species. First, terrestrial mammals have only a finite number of systems with which to fend off microbial challenge and to respond to injury. In general, the same systems exist in all, and when considered individually they operate in a rather consistent, predictable manner in all species. There are differences, but they are relatively minor. Second, the systems which provide protection to fend off infection are the same systems that participate in tissue destruction. It is clear that activation of any host defense system, be it the immune response, acute inflammation, the complement cascade, the phagocytic leukocytes, or various combinations of these, creates the potential for a great deal of tissue damage as well as for potentially lifesaving protection. In most cases the damage created can readily be repaired, and the price paid in terms of tissue damage is small relative to the protection provided. Third, factors determining whether or not tissue damage will occur, and if so how much, and the duration of the destructive process, are only poorly understood. It is clear, however, that the nature of the driving force is important. All chronic inflammatory diseases continue so long as the driving force remains present, and all tend to resolve when the driving force (in the case of periodontitis, bacteria) is inactivated or removed. In addition to the nature of the driving force, the systems which are called into play, the exact manner in which they are activated, and the magnitude of their participation, determines the type and extent of tissue damage. This can vary greatly from one species to another, from one disease to another, and from one stage of a given disease to another. Consequently, one might expect many features of periodontal disease to be held commonly among species, while important differences would also be expected to exist. This conclusion is consistent with observations.

With some exceptions the essential features of periodontitis are held in common by all mammalian species. Periodontitis is, without exception, a destructive disease characterized by growth and apical extension of bacteria between the periodontal tissues and the tooth surface with the formation of gingival and periodontal pockets, changes in junctional and associated epithelia, inflammation, destruction of periodontal attachment, degradation of alveolar bone.

In spite of the features held in common among species, periodontal disease in each manifests unique features. Uniqueness can be expected because mammals differ in size, lifespan, diet, habits, rates of growth, and to a lesser extent structure of the teeth and their surrounding tissues. Animal size is extremely important. Microbial plaque has a finite radius of effectiveness. When plaque extends to within 0.5 mm of the bone surface, osteoclastic resorption occurs and will continue until the bone surface is 1.5 to 2.5 mm removed (see PAGE and SCHROEDER, 1982). At sites in humans and other large animals where the alveolar housing is very thin, extension of microbial plaque apically causes destruction of the entire thickness of the alveolar process; angular craters form in bone in the interdental and interradicular regions thicker than 2.5 mm. In small animals, the teeth, alveolar housing, and soft tissues are really of minute dimensions, i.e., the distance from one root surface to that of the neighboring tooth, although containing the same structural elements organized in a manner similar to humans, is but a fraction of a millimeter. The interdental space and col region or even a small gingival pocket of an animal such as a mouse can accommodate very small amounts of plaque before a state of microbial overgrowth is reached. The range of effectiveness of bacteria under these conditions relative to the available tissue volume will be enormous relative to that occurring in larger animals and man. One really cannot expect the formation of periodontal pockets as typically seen in humans to be the same in small species such as rodents, nor in very large animals such as in cattle and horses.

Size considerations, although important, are overshadowed in some species such as rodents where the lifespan is short. The teeth and indeed the whole jaws undergo somewhat drastic physiological changes throughout the life of the animal.

Structural details of tissues surrounding the teeth are surprisingly consistent among species, especially in light of extreme size differences; minor differences exist, and can be major determinants of lesion morphology and location.

Features of Models

Rodents

Periodontal disease occurs in rodents and it has been studied in considerable detail in mice, rats, and hamsters (see PAGE and SCHROEDER, 1982). Pathologic features include alterations in epithelia, destruction of connective tissue of the gingiva and periodontal ligament, and resorption of alveolar bone and in some cases tooth roots. Although these features are very similar to pathologic alterations in humans and other mammals, mechanisms underlying them differ greatly from those operative in humans. The disease can be induced by monoinfection or by diets that greatly enhance overgrowth of components of the flora. Any of a very large number of microbial species, many not related etiologically to periodontitis in humans, can induce periodontal destruction in rodents as monoinfectants. The disease presents clinically and histologically as a highly acute inflammatory lesion with vasculitis and very large numbers of transmigrating neutrophilic granulocytes. Tissue destruction can progress to the point of tooth exfoliation in the absence of an infiltrate of macrophages, lymphocytes, and plasma cells. In these regards, the disease differs completely from that observed in dogs, sheep, nonhuman primates, and humans. Because of the minute thickness of the alveolar bone and the radius of effectiveness of plaque, the entire alveolar process and sometimes the roots of the teeth are destroyed.

The nature and course of periodontal destruction in rodents are influenced by the unique construction of the periodontal tissues. The keratinizing sulcal epithelium extends apically lateral to the junctional epithelium and produces a stratum granulosum joined to the junctional epithelium. As microbial overgrowth occurs, this structural arrangement permits the gingiva to be displaced laterally, resulting in the formation of large, bulbous gingival pockets filled with rapidly proliferating bacteria, hair, and debris. A pocket epithelium as seen in other species does not form.

A second important determinant is the highly interrelated changes resulting from a short lifespan, a single dentition, rapid growth of the jaws, occlusal wear, and continuous eruption of molar teeth. These result in shifting of the molars in vertical and horizontal planes, and thus in continuous change in tooth position relative to the alveolar process and the entire jaw throughout the life of the animal. As a consequence, there is an increasing distance from the cementoenamel junction to the alveolar bone margin on the palatal and lingual aspects of the molars. The pathologic changes of periodontal disease are superimposed on these dynamic, rapidly changing tissue relationships. Therefore, observed alterations result not only from active destruction of tissue, but also from direct inhibiting effects on tissue growth and apposition.

Dogs

Spontaneously occurring and induced periodontal destruction have been studied in more detail in dogs, especially in Beagles, than in any other nonhuman species, and the dog is currently the most widely used experimental animal (see PAGE and SCHROEDER, 1982). Many features of spontaneous lesions in dogs closely resemble human periodontitis, although there are important differences. Dogs used in periodontal research are relatively large in size, have a lifespan counted in years rather than months, and have a primary and a permanent dentition. Consequently, rapid jaw growth and shifting of the teeth as occurs in rodents are not significant factors in dogs, and morphology of the bone lesions can be very similar to those seen in humans.

Two anatomic details are of importance. Dogs whose teeth have not been subjected to routine toothbrushing for plaque control frequently do not have a gingival sulcus, and the earliest pathologic alteration occurs in the most coronal portion of the connective tissue of the marginal gingiva rather than lateral and apical to the bottom of the gingival sulcus, as occurs in humans. Secondly, the furca of multi-rooted teeth may not be completely covered by bone, and in contrast to humans, bone destruction usually is seen first and most severely in furca regions rather than in interproximal areas.

The infectious nature of gingivitis and periodontitis in dogs is firmly established, and the overall process of pocket formation and tissue alteration is very similar to that observed in humans. Microbial plaque forms on the surfaces of the crowns of the teeth, then extends apically along the root surface. A gingival pocket forms with a pocket epithelium, and the infiltrate is predominated by plasma cells, lymphocytes, and neutrophilic granulocytes. The connective tissue of the gingiva and periodontal ligament are destroyed, and the alveolar bone undergoes osteoclastic resorption. Mechanisms of tissue destruction in dogs are probably similar to those occurring in humans.

Spontaneously occurring periodontitis is seen with a high prevalence in domestic dogs, higher in some species such as poodles than in others, and with a much lower, albeit highly variable, prevalence in dogs residing in colonies. In domestic dogs, destructive lesions may be seen randomly on any of the teeth, and pockets and craters may be narrow, deep, and tortuous as are the pockets occurring frequently in humans. In marked contrast, in colony dogs periodontal destruction is seen mostly around premolars, and to a lesser extent first molars, with incisors, canines, and second molars usually remaining unaffected. As inflammation worsens, tissues of the marginal gingiva begin to proliferate and to convert to a form of highly inflamed granulation tissue that gradually extends apically and replaces the attached gingiva. Deep pockets may form, or alternatively the gingival tissue and alveolar bone may retreat apically as the disease worsens, such that teeth near exfoliation may manifest little or no probing depth. Large accumulations of hair near the gingival margin are usually associated with advancing destruction in colony animals.

Otherwise normal dogs fed a soft diet without any means of plaque control develop gingivitis within a few weeks, and may manifest attachment loss after months or years. It is of considerable interest that even though all of the animals have plaque and calculus and gingivitis, and they are partially inbred, commonly housed, and fed the same diet, approximately 20% do not develop periodontitis. In animals that do develop disease, the pattern is irregular, bone loss is of the horizontal type without formation of bone craters or angular defects, and the rate of periodontal tissue breakdown varies considerably from one dog to another, and from one experimental time to another.

Generally speaking, microbial species considered to be pathogenic for humans are also associated with periodontal destruction in dogs. With worsening of gingival inflammation, the predominant cultivable bacteria in the supragingival deposits are _Actinomyces_, especially _A. viscosus_ and other anaerobic rods. In subgingival deposits _Bacteroides gingivalis_, _Fusobacterium nucleatum_, assorted coccobacilli, and _Capnocytophaga_ are found. _B. fragilis_ and _F. nucleatum_ appear to be significantly and positively correlated with frequency of ulcerations in pocket epithelium and with the size of inflammatory lesions.

Nonhuman Primates

Gingivitis and periodontitis have been studied to a very limited extent in a variety of nonhuman primates. Spontaneously occurring gingivitis is present in virtually all animals, but the prevalence of periodontitis is very low. Clinical and histopathologic features of gingivitis in wild and colony-maintained monkeys, as well as features associated with eating soft diets without toothbrushing, have been studied in _Macaca speciosa_, _M. mulatta_, and _M. fascicularis_. Clinical manifestations are the same as in humans. Some investigators describe an inflammatory cell infiltrate predominated by macrophages, while others observed a predominance of lymphocytes and plasma cells as is seen in humans (BRECX et al., 1985; NALBANDIAN et al., 1985). Studies have been performed both on wild-caught and colony-maintained marmosets (Saguinus oedipus and Callithrix jacchus). Clinically the disease is a highly acute inflammation. Microscopically, the inflammatory infiltrate contains large numbers of neutrophilic granulocytes and numerous round cells presumed to be macrophages but in marked contrast to humans, plasma cells and lymphocytes are not found. In spite of the unusual nature of the inflammatory infiltrate, periodontal destruction progresses to very advanced stages. Clinical and histopathologic features of gingivitis and periodontitis in baboons (Popio anubis and Theropithecus gelada) closely resemble those seen in human disease.

Of all the species studied so far, spontaneously occurring gingivitis and periodontitis in the chimpanzee (Pan troglodytes) most closely resemble these diseases in humans; however, prevalence is low, the degree of attachment loss, even in very old animals with massive amounts of coronal and root calculus and plaque, is not severe, and the gingival tissue manifests a great deal more thickening, scarring, and fibrosis than is seen in humans or other species. Histologic and ultrastructural features of the lesions are identical to those seen in humans, including an inflammatory infiltrate containing large numbers of transmigrating neutrophilic granulocytes, but predominated by lymphocytes and plasma cells. A disease identical to localized juvenile periodontitis as seen in humans has been reported in one animal (see PAGE and SCHROEDER, 1982).

Ligature-Induced Periodontitis

Periodontal destruction can be induced in a fairly controlled manner by placement of silk or cotton ligatures around the necks of the teeth in the gingival sulcus. Such ligatures serve to cause ulceration of the sulcal wall and to trap and enhance growth of microbial plaque. Severe acute inflammation develops, and periodontal destruction manifested as loss of periodontal attachment and resorption of alveolar bone ensues. The ligature-induced lesion, first described in rats, has been studied in dogs and in nonhuman primates (see PAGE and SCHROEDER, 1982; HOLT et al., 1987; OFFENBACHER et al., 1988). The pathologic alterations resemble closely, but are not identical to, those observed in spontaneously occurring lesions in the same species with regard to composition of the inflammatory infiltrate and destruction of the connective tissue and bone. Further, the bacterial species strongly linked to human periodontitis are associated with the ligature-induced lesions in dogs and nonhuman primates.

In dogs, immediately following subgingival ligature placement, ulceration of the junctional epithelium occurs, the flora becomes predominantly gram-negative and anaerobic with high proportions of Bacteroides species, and microbial plaque extends subgingivally. Within 4 to 7 days, the tissues become swamped with neutrophilic granulocytes and connective tissue destruction occurs; within 2 to 3 weeks, osteoclast-mediated alveolar bone resorption is observed. Subsequently, the lesions begin to subside unless the ligature is moved apically. Extracts of gingival tissue harvested during the period of acute inflammation induce bone resorption _in vitro_, and administration of anti-inflammatory drugs such as indomethacin, suppresses and delays the acute inflammation and blocks bone resorption, indicating a role for agents such as prostaglandins.

In the squirrel monkey (_Saimiri sciureus_), the junctional epithelium becomes ulcerated and bacteria accumulate and extend between the ulcerated surface and the ligature within the first 3 days. Within 1 to 2 weeks, the flora consists almost exclusively of filaments and rods with many spirochetes. The numbers of leukocytes in the gingival tissue increase dramatically, with neutrophilic granulocytes accounting for about 76% and macrophages for 34% of the total. Proportions of lymphocytes and plasma cells remain exceedingly small. By 10 weeks, the population of neutrophilic granulocytes decreases and relative proportions of round cells, presumably macrophages, increase. Bone resorption and apical migration of the junctional epithelium are seen for the first 2 weeks, and continue from week 2 to week 10 but at a greatly reduced rate. No further progression occurs from week 26 to week 52.

Ligature-induced lesions have been created in _Macaca fascicularis_ at sites already manifesting chronic gingivitis but without pocket formation or bone loss. Prior to placement of ligatures, the sites were populated with _B. intermedius_, _B. gingivalis_, and _Camphylobacter sputorum_. Within 1 to 3 weeks following ligation, gram-negative rods increase. Active loss of periodontal attachment and bone destruction occur at weeks 4 to 7, during which 77% of the flora is made up of gram-negative rods with _B. gingivalis_ accounting for about 34% of the total, and the tissues are infiltrated by neutrophilic granulocytes, lymphocytes, and plasma cells (BRECX et al., 1985; NALBANDIAN et al., 1985). By 8 to 17 weeks, signs of acute inflammation decrease, manifestations of periodontal destruction cease, and the flora tends to shift back toward baseline values. In _M. mulatta_ mean attachment loss observed 3 months after placement of ligatures was 0.92 mm, and at 6 months 1.06 mm. These values were significantly reduced by administration of a nonsteroidal anti-inflammatory drug (OFFENBACHER et al., 1988).

Are There Convincing Models of Human Periodontal Diseases?

Yes, there are convincing models, but there exists no analog of human periodontal diseases. Whether a given model is convincing is dependent upon its specific characteristics and the requirements of the model needed for solution of the problem under consideration. A rather large variety of models, characterized to varying degrees of completeness, is available to us. Because pathways of host defense and tissue destruction are, by and large, shared by terrestrial mammals, all hold in common the essential features of periodontitis. These are extension of microbial plaque apically between the tooth and periodontal tissues with initiation and perpetuation of destructive inflammation, formation of gingival and periodontal pockets, and destruction of gingival tissue, periodontal attachment, and alveolar bone. Furthermore, in all species, periodontitis is an infectious process, and in some species, especially in dogs and nonhuman primates, the species of bacteria involved appear to be the same as in human disease. On the other hand, forms of periodontitis are, in one or more respects, unique from one species to another and from these diseases in humans. The disease in chimpanzees comes closest to being analogous to human periodontitis, but even in these animals, progression seems exceedingly slow relative to the disease in man, even in the presence of massive amounts of microbial deposits, and the degree of gingival fibrosis is much greater than in humans.

The existence in various animals of forms of periodontitis manifesting a rather large variety of characteristics and features is a benefit, not a handicap, for investigators using animal models. Comparisons among species have yielded new insights into the nature of human periodontitis. For example, the fact that a form of periodontitis with all the essential pathologic tissue alterations occurs in rodents and progresses to tooth exfoliation in the absence of a local infiltrate of lymphocytes, macrophages, and plasma cells is extremely informative with regard to the nature of mechanisms responsible for tissue destruction and bone resorption. Existence of several models with differing characteristics permits investigators to choose the one model most appropriate for the problem under consideration. Our real problem is not variety, but rather the lack of a sufficient degree of characterization in any species, even in dogs, to ensure correct use as a model.

Mice, rats, and hamsters have been and continue to be widely used in periodontal research for a variety of purposes such as assessment of the pathogenicity of various species of bacteria, elucidation of details of tissue alterations such as bone resorption, and determination of the role of humoral and cell-mediated immunity in the course of periodontitis.

In light of the multiplicity of microbial species that can induce periodontal destruction in these animals, complexity of the pathogenic mechanisms resulting from superimposition of pathologic alteration on rapidly changing tissues, and lack of an immunopathologic infiltrate at the site of the lesion, interpretation of results of such experiments becomes exceedingly complicated. On the other hand, rodents present an excellent opportunity for investigation of normal tissue structure and function, production and turnover of connective matrix components, and elucidation of the role of components of acute inflammation, such as neutrophilic granulocytes, in tissue destruction.

A considerable amount of useful information has been obtained from dogs in which periodontal destruction has been induced by feeding a soft diet. However, the development of a progressive and destructive periodontal disease by this means is not entirely predictable; the rate of breakdown varies considerably from one dog to another and from one experimental period to another, and plaque-induced gingivitis does not always progress to destructive periodontitis. Further, months to years are required to induce disease. Use of dogs with spontaneously occurring periodontitis is made difficult by the extreme variation from one strain to another and among animals of the same strain, and the long period of time required for the disease to appear.

The high degree of similarity between the teeth and periodontal structures of human and nonhuman primates, and similarity of the oral flora and host-parasitic interactions, makes primates ideal for many types of investigation. The great variation in size presents numerous advantages. For example, some primates such as the marmoset are no larger than a mature rat and can be used for studies requiring labeling with radioactive compounds, while other species such as the chimpanzee are of sufficient size that periodontal surgery and other therapeutic manipulations can be performed. The oral flora of nonhuman primates has not been thoroughly studied but the limited information available indicates that types of bacteria associated with healthy periodontal tissues, and those associated with gingivitis and periodontitis, are very similar to species found in humans. Prevalence of spontaneously occurring periodontitis in nonhuman primates seems, however, to be very low.

Ligature-induced periodontal destruction in dogs and nonhuman primates may provide the best models currently available for a large variety of studies, especially those relating to microbial etiology, mechanisms of tissue destruction, assessment of the roles of various cells comprising the inflammatory infiltrate, the role of humoral and cell-mediated immune responses, and testing efficacy of chemotherapeutic agents. The procedure causes microbial colonization of the subgingival area and induces severe inflammation, attachment loss, and alveolar bone resorption. The technique employed is simple, but standardization is difficult. Ligatures can be positioned initially and secured, but soft tissue may shift over time relative to the ligature because of gingival swelling or recession, and the ligatures may be lost. Unless ligatures are moved apically over time, only a single episode of destructive activity is seen.

Features of ligature-induced lesions differ in significant ways from spontaneously occurring periodontitis in humans. For example, in dogs, extensive connective tissue and bone destruction can occur without formation of a periodontal pocket or detachment of the supracrestal collagen fibers from the root surface. Once the ligatures are removed, lesions tend not to progress but rather to heal (JANSEN et al., 1982). Although bone destruction and periodontal attachment loss appear to occur rather rapidly in dogs and in squirrel monkeys, weeks and months seem to be required in some other primates, such as Macaca. In spite of these shortcomings, ligature models are now coming into wide use.

References

BRECX, M.C.; NALBANDIAN, J.; OOYA, K.; KORNMAN, K.S., and ROBERTSON, P.B.: Morphological studies on periodontal disease in the cynomolgus monkey. II. Light microscopic observations on ligature-induced periodontitis. J. Periodont. Res. 20:165 175 (1985).

HOLT, S.; FELTON, J.; BRUNSVOLD, M.; EBERSOLE, J., and KORNMAN, L.: Implantation of B. gingivalis initiates periodontitis in monkeys. J. Dent. Res., Spec.Issue (Abs. 1873) 66:341 (1987).

JANSEN, J., von DISK, J.; and PILOT, T.: Artificial periodontal defects around incisor teeth of beagle dogs. A clinical and histometrical analysis. J. Periodont. Res. 17:210-218 (1982).

NALBANDIAN, J.; BRECX, M.C.; OOYA, K.; KORNMAN, K.S., and ROBERTSON, P.B.: Morphological studies on periodontal disease in the cynomolgus monkey. I. Light microscopic observations on gingivitis. J. Periodont. Res. 20:154 164 (1985).

OFFENBACHER, S.; BRASWELL, L.D.; LOOS, A.S.; JOHNSON, H.G.; HALL, C.M.; McCLURE, H.; ORKIN, J.L.; STROBERT, E.A.; GREEN, M.D., and ODLE, B.M.: Effects of flurbiprofen on progression of periodontitis in Macaca mulatta. J. Periodont. Res., in press (1988).

PAGE, R.C., and SCHROEDER, H.E.: Periodontitis in man and other animals. A comparative review; 330 pp. (S. Karger, Basel, 1982).

TALBOT, E.S.: Interstitial gingivitis or so-called pyorrhea alveolaris; Chapter I, pp. 1-19 (S.S. White Dental Mfg. Corp., Philadelphia, 1899).

Dr. R.C. Page, Center for Research in Oral Biology, SM-42, University of Washington, Seattle, Washington 98195, USA

Periodontology Today. Int. Congr., Zürich 1988, pp. 123–131 (Karger, Basel 1988)

Is the Specific Plaque Hypothesis still Tenable?

Anne Tanner

Department of Microbiology, Forsyth Dental Center, Boston, Mass. USA

The specific plaque hypothesis suggests that periodontal infections resemble other infections in that specific species cause different periodontal or gingival diseases. If the validity of this hypothesis is questioned, then the alternative hypothesis requires examination.

Non-Specific Plaque Hypothesis

The non-specific plaque hypothesis suggested that periodontal diseases resulted from overgrowth of plaque microorganisms, with any species having the possibility of causing destructive disease. This hypothesis explained previous clinical experiences when investigators linked the universal presence of gingival inflammation and periodontal pocket formation with the apparently ubiquitous presence of abundant dental plaque.

Epidemiological and microbiological data appeared to give scientific credence to a non-specific plaque hypothesis. Subjects with abundant plaque demonstrated increased amounts of alveolar bone loss compared to subjects with less dental plaque (good tooth brushers) (28). Darkfield microscopy revealed no differences in bacterial morphotypes from six different gingival or periodontal states (26). Little difference was detected in groups of gram positive and negative rods and cocci in pooled plaque samples cultured from subjects showing little or advanced alveolar bone loss (5). Animal models were not available that would support oral implantation of human periodontal isolates (25).

It seems possible that the non-specific plaque hypothesis may have dominated as a result of clinical observations. Treatment regimens (toothbrushing by the patient; scaling, curettage, and different forms of periodontal surgery by the dental practitioner) were directed towards a non-specific reduction in plaque amount. These procedures would have at least a temporary effect on gingival inflammation. If these were the only treatments available, and plaque reduction with resolution of gingivitis the only result, one could imagine how tempting it was to suggest, "non-specific plaque reduction resulted in successful periodontal therapy, hence, periodontal disease is a non-specific infection!" The non-specific plaque hypothesis was re-evaluated and rejected by many investigators in the 1970's and 1980's.

Specific Plaque Hypothesis

Data that supported a specific plaque hypothesis included additional epidemiological surveys, use of animal models that supported specific oral infections, and most importantly, the clear differences in the microorganisms associated with health and periodontal diseases.

Epidemiological data indicated that populations in Norway (28) and Sri Lanka (18) had much plaque and alveolar bone loss, whereas, other populations in Sri Lanka (18), South Africa (24), Tanzania (1), and Kenya (2) had abundant plaque and calculus, but little or no periodontal attachment loss. Thus, bacterial masses on teeth did not inevitably result in loss of periodontal attachment. Epidemiologic studies indicated that only certain individuals or sites exhibited destructive periodontal disease, a fact which would be explained by differences in infection.

Transmission of dental diseases in animal models, especially rodents, conclusively demonstrated the bacterial etiology of periodontal infections. Early evidence of bacterial specificity in periodontal infections was demonstrated by induction of disease only by certain species of either animal or human origin, and not by other species. This was done by super-infecting individual species into the oral cavities of conventional (11), or gnotobiotic animals (11, 33; tables I and II).

Certain animal models of periodontal disease have alveolar bone loss and subgingival species which appear similar to those seen in the human oral cavity. Furthermore, as has been observed in human periodontal infections, only a finite number of species appear associated with periodontal infections. Suspected periodontal pathogens in beagle dogs and two species of monkeys have included black-pigmented *Bacteroides*, and *Capnocytophaga* species (14, 15).

The demonstration of different microbiotas in periodontal health and disease in humans depended upon the recognition that periodontal disease is a site localized disease, and that diseased sites may not be continuously progressing, but demonstrated periods of activity and quiescence. Differentiation of health and disease related microbiotas has also required use of improved microbiological methods to culture and identify the species isolated (32).

For a valid non-specific plaque hypothesis, one would expect random association of species with destructive disease. Each species found in health (or possibly gingivitis) would be equally distributed among disease sites. When single site samples, instead of samples pooled from several (or all) teeth, were analyzed the data indicated that different species were not randomly associated with disease, but that distinct subsets of species were related to health and different diseases (11).

The microbiota of healthy (supragingival) sites consisted mainly of gram positive species, including facultative streptococci and actinomyces, *S. epidermidis* and *Rothia dentocariosa.* The major difference between healthy sites and diseased sites was the introduction, and increasing dominance, of gram negative and anaerobic species.

The microbiota of experimental gingivitis (19) was associated with an increase in microorganisms, and sequential colonization of fusiforms, motile species and spirochetes. Culturally species associated with experimental gingivitis included *A. viscosus, A. naeslundii, F. nucleatum, V. parvula,* and *Treponema* species (22). Species cultured from long standing, chronic gingivitis have included *Campylobacter* species, *F. nucleatum, Veillonella,* and *B. intermedius.*

Evidence indicates that two periodontal (or gingival) diseases, acute necrotizing ulcerative gingivitis (ANUG) and juvenile periodontitis, represent clearly distinct clinical entities, with individual specific etiological gram negative species. ANUG lesions were associated with tissue invasive medium sized spirochetes (17). Many cases of juvenile periodontitis seemed to result from an *Actinobacillus actinomycetemcomitans* infection (3, 15, 21, 30, 36) with a high probability of tissue invasion of this species in destructive phases of the infection (3, 6, 21, 27).

Table I. Isolates from humans that which induced alveolar bone loss in mono-infected gnotobiotic rats

Species	Dental Source
Actinomyces naeslundii & viscosus	Gingivitis
Bacillus cereus	Gingivitis
Streptococcus sanguis	Gingivitis
Streptococcus mutans	Dental Caries
Streptococcus salivarius	Tongue
A. actinomycetemcomitans	Juvenile Periodontitis
Capno. gingivalis & ochracea	Juvenile Periodontitis
Eikenella corrodens	Juvenile & Adult Periodontitis
Selenomonas flueggeii	Papillon Lefevre
Bacteroides gingivalis & forsythus	Adult Periodontitis
Fusobacterium nucleatum	Adult Periodontitis
Capnocytophaga sputigena	Adult Periodontitis

Table II. Isolates from humans that implanted but **failed** to induce alveolar bone loss in mono-infected gnotobiotic rats

Species	Dental Source
Staphylococcus epidermidis	Health
Streptococcus mitis & milleri	Health
Streptococcus sanguis	Health
Actinomyces israelii & odontolyticus	Gingivitis
Arachnia propionica	Gingivitis
Bacteroinema matruchotii	Gingivitis
Propionebacterium acnes	Gingivitis
Rothia dentocariosa	Gingivitis
anaerobic *Streptococcus*	Gingivitis
Bacteroides oralis	Gingivitis
Campylobacter sputorum	Gingivitis
Leptotrichia buccalis	Gingivitis
Fusobacterium nucleatum	Gingivitis & Periodontitis

Of equal importance to site specificity for adult periodontitis was the demonstration and measurement of progressive or "active" phases of periodontal attachment loss (10), and that phases of "activity" appear to be relatively rare events (31). Thus, in those subjects with progressive "active" disease, instead of all sites having a similar disease experience, there may be truly healthy sites, gingivitis sites in the presence or absence of alveolar bone loss, in addition to those sites showing "active" periodontal attachment loss.

Furthermore, "adult periodontitis" appears to include several different diseases associated with different (etiological) species (34). While the separation of disease types and assignment of specific pathogens has yet to be accomplished, in a recently completed study of 33 subjects (4), *W. recta, B. intermedius, F. nucleatum, B. gingivalis,* and *B. forsythus* were elevated more often in active sites, whereas, *S. mitis, C. ochracea, S. sanguis II, V. parvula* and an unnamed *Actinomyces* species were elevated in inactive sites. It was determined in the same study that a site was more likely to be active if *B. forsythus, B. gingivalis, P. micros, A. actinomycetemcomitans, W. recta,* or *B. intermedius* was detected in that site, and less likely to be active if certain gram positive species were detected.

The microbiology data of the last 10 years conclusively demonstrated that periodontal attachment loss was not related to species associated with healthy sites. The ability to distinguish species related to active and inactive lesions indicated that not all species found in subgingival sites were equally likely to be related to attachment loss. These data indicated that only a specific plaque hypothesis was tenable.

Contrary to a previous suggestion that periodontal treatment was always successful, subjects were found with "intractable" disease, (continued periodontal attachment loss) despite repeated debridement, including surgical procedures (13, 29). Thus, non-specific plaque reduction failed to arrest periodontal destruction and could no longer justify a non-specific plaque hypothesis.

When periodontal diseases were recognized as specific infections, treatment regimens were designed to eliminate specific species. Specific diagnosis of juvenile periodontitis included clinical characterization of the disease, with detection of *A. actinomycetemcomitans* in diseased sites (15, 21, 30, 36). Treatment frequently consisted of surgical debridement (or curettage) with adjunctive systemic tetracycline (15, 21, 30, 36) . Treatment was considered sufficient only with clinical resolution of lesions and failure to detect *A. actinomycetemcomitans* (15, 21, 36).

Why Might The Specific Plaque Hypothesis Be Questioned?

Perhaps the most difficult microbiota to define and understand, especially considering specificity and non-specificity, is that of gingivitis. With better descriptors of healthy, experimental gingivitis, and active periodontal lesions, "gingivitis" appears to have become the "wastebasket" state for all sites that do not fit any of the above categories. Thus, "gingivitis" sites include inflamed inactive sites from subjects that may never have experienced periodontal destruction, as well as sites from subjects who have had, or are currently undergoing periodontal attachment loss.

Every species that has been isolated in health, experimental gingivitis or destructive periodontal diseases has at one time or another been isolated from "inactive, gingivitis" sites. It seems likely that the lack of clear distinction between active and inactive sites could lead to questioning of a specific plaque hypothesis.

Two areas that might suggest re-assessment, in 1988, of a specific plaque hypothesis because of overlap of species in active and inactive sites are:

1) The presence of suspected periodontal pathogens in inactive sites.
2) The absence of suspected pathogens in active sites.

"Specific" treatment regimens similar to those devised for juvenile periodontitis have been applied to "adult" periodontitis. Success has been mixed. Some cases did indeed show resolution of progressive disease (8, 12, 29). Clinical data here could justify a specific plaque hypothesis. Other diseased sites did not respond to therapy (12, 29) and were either unchanged or demonstrated accelerated alveolar bone loss. It seems possible that this failure of a "specific" therapy could prompt a revival of a non-specific plaque hypothesis to disease: "if a specific treatment did not work, maybe it was a non-specific infection".

Thus, a third reason to suspect a specific plaque hypothesis is:

3) The failure of "specific" antibiotic treatment to stop progression of disease.

1) Presence Of Suspected Periodontal Pathogens In Inactive Sites

The "carrier state" is an expected outcome if disease progresses with periods of exacerbation and remission. After an acute episode of destruction, it seems unlikely that the pathogen will "spontaneously" disappear from the periodontal pocket. In addition, inaccurate clinical measurements may misdiagnose active lesions. Some subjects harbor suspected periodontal pathogens in multiple sites (table III).

The ubiquitous presence of *B. forsythus, W. recta* and *F. nucleatum* suggests that these species may actually "spill over" from active sites rather than existing in a carrier state. It may thus be necessary to reconsider "gingivitis" sites, depending on the disease activity state of the subject. In subjects with active disease, there may be pathogens in undiseased sites as species are transmitted within an oral cavity and thus reflect the disease state of the subject. However, it seems possible that in subjects who have never experienced periodontal loss, and appear stable, the "gingivitis" sites may more closely resemble those of experimental gingivitis which does not usually (if ever) progress to attachment loss. This latter microbiota might be a realistic goal of successful periodontal treatment. Comparison of these "gingivitides" has yet to be done.

Table III. Microbiota of subject with multiple active sites at two time periods (% of isolates)

	Inactive Sites			Active Sites					
Species	ra	rb	rc	rd	re	rf	rg	rh	ri
F. nucleatum	40	4	0	18	2	0	6	6	2
B. forsythus	12	16	48	4	14	36	42	4	o
W. recta	8	6	6	16	10	20	24	6	3

2) Absence Of Suspected Pathogens In Active Sites.

Table IV. Species isolated from subjects with "active" disease (15 sites, 13 active)

	# Sites Isolated	# Isolates	Mean %
Fusobacterium nucleatum	12	33	4.4
Wolinella recta	8	13	1.7
Eikenella corrodens	8	10	1.3
Bacteroides oris	**7**	**14**	**1.9**
Bacteroides forsythus	6	25	3.3
Selenomonas noxia	**6**	**25**	**3.3**
Fusobacterium periodonticum	**6**	**18**	**2.4**
Bacteroides gracilis	6	14	1.9
Bacterides buccae	**6**	**7**	**0.9**
Capnocytophaga ochracea	5	8	1.1
Bacteroides gingivalis	4	40	5.3
Capnocytophaga gingivalis	4	10	1.3
Bacteroides intermedius	4	9	1.2
Bacteroides capillosus	**4**	**7**	**0.9**
Bacteroides oralis	**4**	**4**	**0.5**
Campylobacter concisus	3	4	0.5
Selenomonas sputigena	3	4	0.5
Selenomonas flueggeii	**2**	**3**	**0.4**
Selenomonas artemidis	**2**	**3**	**0.4**

In a recent series of subjects examined with active lesions (table IV), many sites did not harbor gram negative species previously associated with recent attachment loss (4, 11, 29, 34). Were these sites then representative of a non-specific infection?

Periodontal attachment loss just before sampling ranged from 0 mm (2 sites) to over 6 mm. Correlation coefficients were determined seeking species that might relate to amount of attachment loss (table V).

Table V. Correlation coefficients of gram negative species with amount of attachment loss (15 sites)

Species	R	# sites	# strains
Selenomonas noxia	0.72	6	25
Selenomonas flueggeii	0.56	2	3
Bacteroides capillosus	0.42	4	7
Bacteroides buccae	0.36	6	7
Fusobacterium periodonticum	0.27	6	18

In this set of subjects neither black-pigmented *Bacteroides* species isolated was associated with attachment loss.

The minimal number of species that together would best account for increased attachment loss was then sought.

Attachment loss = 1.95 + (0.37) *Selenomonas noxia* + (1.2) *Selenomonas flueggeii*

$R^2 = 0.62$

As *S. noxia* was detected in only 6 of 13 active sites, this species was not associated with, or could account for, all the attachment loss. However, the association of *S. noxia* with the more aggressively destructive sites (sites with more mm of recent attachment loss), suggests that this species may be a periodontal pathogen.

These data (and communications from frustrated clinicians using diagnostic services in the US that report "no pathogens detected" from aggressively progressive disease sites) indicate that not all pathogens have been recognized, and sites with "no recognizable pathogens" may harbor unrecognized pathogens, including uncultivated or new species. Thus, with revised taxonomies of subgingival species, one can seek new species before resorting to calling sites with few previously recognized pathogens, non-specific infections.

3)The Failure Of "Specific" Antibiotic Treatment (Tetracycline) To Stop Progression Of Disease.

Table VI. Microbiota of sites before and 6 months after local delivery of tetracycline (% of Isolates)

Patient K	Site 124		Site 323
Species	Before	After Treatment	(Before, Untreated)
Selenomonas noxia	22	0	2
Bacteroides forsythus	0	24	12
Bacteroides intermedius	0	24	4
Fusobacterium nucleatum	4	14	2

Specific intensive local antibiotic treatment to individual sites (9), can, in the short term, dramatically suppress the microbiota in that site (8), with subsequent periodontal attachment gain. Localized suppression of species however, does not guarantee that sites cannot become re-infected from other sites in the same oral cavity (table VI).

In site 124, local tetracycline therapy (9), achieved long term suppression of *S. noxia.* However, three suspected periodontal pathogens increased in proportions after therapy. *F. nucleatum* was detected in the site before therapy and may never have been eliminated. However, two species, *B. forsythus* and *B. intermedius* were undetected in the treated site before therapy. As these species were isolated from untreated site 323 before therapy, the data suggests that *B. forsythus* and *B. intermedius* may have originated from another site. Transmission of species after treatment has been suggested in humans (21, 30) and in monkeys from diseased (ligated) to previously healthy (non-ligated) sites (14).

Thus, it seems possible that treatment of specific infections may require treatment to the whole mouth, to prevent transmission of pathogenic species harbored in untreated sites to treated sites. This generalized therapy to eradicate pathogens however, should not be confused with non-specific types of treatment (20).

Furthermore, it is possible that the clinical effects seen *in vivo* following tetracycline therapy may be non-specifically mediated. Non-bacterial activity of tetracycline has been demonstrated to include inhibiting collagenase (7), anti-inflammatory activity (23), and as a root conditioning agent (35).

Thus, it seems possible that a specific antibacterial agent may fail because its activity may not be effective against the pathogen causing the disease, or, it may just appear to fail if post-treatment sites become reinfected from other oral sites. These observations however should not detract from the specificity of periodontal infections, but rather suggest that improved treatment regimens need to be devised.

Conclusion

The reasons that dental infections might be considered to be non-specific infections, were elegantly summarized by Loesche (20).

1) The lack of bacterial invasion of the tissues;
2) their apparent non-specific nature;
3) their chronicity, which prevented the documentation of the natural history of the infection(s) and,
4) their universality, as all people have such an infection at some time in their life.

Bacterial invasion has been demonstrated in periodontal infections, they do not appear to be non-specific, acute phases of disease progression have been demonstrated and periodontal disease has not been found to be a universal experience. This manuscript proposes that these findings, with the proposed solutions to possible reservations, demonstrate that a specific plaque hypothesis is still tenable.

Key questions to be asked at the conference

Why do certain researchers and clinicians prefer a non-specific (rather than a more normal specific) plaque hypothesis for periodontal infections?

How would the believers in non-specific infections propose to test this entirely unique hypothesis?

What is considered to be the most effective form of therapy: local treatment, generalized treatment or a combination of both?

References

1. BAELUM, V.: Pattern of periodontal breakdown in adult Tanzanians. Scand. J. Dent. Res. 95: 221-228 (1987).
2. BAELUM, V.; FEJERSKOV, O., and MANJI, F.: Periodontal diseases in adult Kenyans. J. Clin. Periodontol. (1988) in press.
3. CHRISTERSSON, L.A.; ALBINI, B.; ZAMBON, J.J.; WIKESJO, U.M., and GENCO, R.J.: Tissue localization of *Actinobacillus actinomycetemcomitans* in human periodontitis. I. Light, immunofluoresence and electron microscopic studies. J. Periodontol. 58: 529-539 (1987).
4. DZINK, J. L.; HAFFAJEE, A.D., and SOCRANSKY, S.S.: The predominant cultivable microbiota of active and inactive periodontal lesions. J. Clin. Periodontol. (1988) in press.
5. GIBBONS, R.J.; SOCRANSKY, S.S.; SAWYER, S.; KAPSIMALIS, B., and MACDONALD, J. B.: The microbiota of the gingival crevice area of man. II. The predominant cultivable organisms. Arch. Oral. Biol. 8: 281-289 (1963).
6. GILLETT, R. and JOHNSON, N. W.; Bacterial invasion of the periodontium in a case of juvenile periodontitis. J. Clin. Periodontol. 9: 93-100 (1982).
7. GOLOB, L.M.; GOODSON, J.M.; LEE, H.M.; VIDAL, A.M.; MCNAMARA,T.F., and TAMAMURTHY, A.M.: Tetracyclines inhibit tissue collagenases. Effects of ingested low-dose and local delivery systems. J. Periodontol. 56: (11 suppl) 93-97 (1985).
8. GOODSON, J.M.; HOGAN, P.E., and DUNHAM, S.L.: Clinical responses following periodontal disease treatment by local drug delivery. J. Periodontol. 56: 81-87 (1985).
9. GOODSON, J.M.; OFFENBACHER, S.; FARR, D.H., and HOGAN, P.E.: Periodontal treatment by local drug delivery. J. Periodontol. 56: 265-272 (1985).
10. GOODSON, J.M.; TANNER, A.C.R.; HAFFAJEE, A.D.; SORNBERGER, G.C., and SOCRANSKY, S.S.: Patterns of progression and regression of advanced destructive periodontal diseases. J. Clin. Periodontol. 9:472-481 (1982).
11. GRANT, D.A.; STERN, I.B., and LISTGARTEN, M.A.: Periodontics in the traditions of Gottleib and Orban. 6th ed., pp.165-197 (C.V. Mosby, St. Louis 1988).
12. HAFFAJEE, A.D.; SOCRANSKY, S.S.: DZINK, J.L.; TAUBMAN, M.A., and EBERSOLE, J.L.: Clinical, microbiological and immunological features of subjects with refractory periodontal diseases. J. Clin. Periodontol. (1988) in press.
13. HIRSCHFELD, L. and WASSERMAN, B.: A long-term survey of tooth loss in 600 treated periodontal patients. J. Periodontol. 49: 225-237 (1978)
14. KEIL, R.A.; KORNMAN, K.S., and ROBERTSON, P.B.: Clinical and microbiological effects of localized ligature-induced periodontitis on non-ligated sites in the cynomolgus monkey. J. Periodont. Res. 18: 200-211 (1983).
15. KORNMAN, K.S. and ROBERTSON, P.B.: Clinical and microbiological evaluation of therapy for juvenile periodontitis. J. Periodontol. 56: 443-446 (1985).
16. KORNMAN, K.S.; SEIGRIST, B.; SOSKOLNE, W.A., and NUKI, K.: The predominant cultivable subgingival flora of beagle dogs following ligature placement and metronidazole therapy. J. Periodont. Res. 16: 251-258 (1981).
17. LISTGARTEN, M.A.: Electron microscopic observation of the bacterial flora of acute necrotizing ulcerative gingivitis. J. Periodontol. 36: 328-339 (1965).
18. LOE, H.; ANERUD, A.; BOYSEN, H., and MORRISON, E.: Natural history of periodontal disease in man. Rapid, Moderate and no loss of attachment in Sri Lankan laborers 14 to 46 years of age. J. Clin. Periodontol. 13: 431-445 (1986).

19. LOE, H.; THEILADE, E., and JENSEN, S.B.: Experimental gingivitis in man. J. Periodontol. 36: 177-187 (1965).
20. LOESCHE, W.J.: Chemotherapy of dental plaque infections. Oral Sci. Rev. 9: 65-107 (1976).
21. MANDELL, R.L.; TRIPODI, L.S.; SAVITT, E.; GOODSON, J.M., and SOCRANSKY, S.S.: The effect of treatment on *Actinobacillus actinomycetemcomitans* in localized juvenile periodontitis. J. Periodontol. 57: 94-99 (1986)
22. MOORE, W.E.C.; HOLDEMAN, L.V.; SMIBERT, R.M.; GOOD, I.J.; BURMEISTER, J.A.; PALCANIS, K.G., and RANNEY, R.R.: Bacteriology of experimental gingivitis in young adult humans. Infect. Immunol. 38: 651-667 (1982).
23. PLEWIG, G. and SCHOPF, E.: Anti-inflammatory effects of antimicrobial agents: an in vivo study. J. Invest. Dermatol. 65: 532-536 (1975).
24. REDDY, J.; AFRICA, C.W., and PARKER, J.R.: Darkfield microscopy of sub-gingival plaque of an urban black population with poor oral hygiene. J. Clin. Periodontol. 13: 578-582 (1986).
25. ROSEBURY, T.: Recent developments in fusospirochetal and related infections. J. Periodontol. 17: 121-125 (1946).
26. ROSEBURY, T.; MACDONALD, J.B., and CLARKE, A.R.: A bacteriologic survey of gingival scrapings from periodontal infections by direct examination, guinea pig inoculation, and anaerobic cultivation. J. Dent. Res. 29: 718-731 (1950).
27. SAGLIE, F.R.; CARRANZA, F.A., and NEWMAN, M.G.: The presence of bacteria within the oral epithelium in periodontal disease. 1. Scanning and transmission electron microscopic study. J. Periodontol. 56: 618-624 (1985).
28. SCHEI, O.; WAERHAUG, J.; LOVDAHL, A., and ARNO, A.: Alveolar bone loss as related to oral hygiene and age. J. Periodontol. 30: 7-16 (1959).
29. SLOTS, J.; BRAGD, L.; WIKSTRÖM, M,, and DAHLÉN, G.: The occurrence of *Actinobacillus actinomycetemcomitans*, *Bacteroides gingivalis* and *Bacteroides intermedius* in destructive periodontal disease in adults. J. Clin. Periodontol. 13: 570-577 (1986).
30. SLOTS, J. and ROSLING, B.G.: Suppression of the periodontopathic microflora in localized juvenile periodontitis by systemic tetracycline. J. Clin. Periodontol. 10:465-486 (1983).
31. SOCRANSKY, S.S.; HAFFAJEE, A.D.; GOODSON, J.M.,and LINDHE, J.: New concepts of destructive periodontal disease. J. Clin. Periodontol. 11: 21-32 (1984).
32. SOCRANSKY, S.S.; HAFFAJEE, A.D.; SMITH, G.L.F., and DZINK, J.L.: Difficulties encountered in the search for the etiologic agents of destructive periodontal diseases. J. Clin. Periodontol. 14: 588-593 (1987).
33. TANNER, A.C.R.: A study of the bacteria associated with advanced periodontal disease in man. Ph. D. Thesis, University of London. (1981).
34. TANNER, A.C.R.; HAFFER, C.; BRATTHALL, G.T.; VISCONTI, R.A., and SOCRANSKY, S.S.: A study of the bacteria associated with advancing periodontal disease in man. J. Clin. Periodontol. 6: 278-307 (1979).
35. TERRANOVA, V.P.; FRANZETTI, L.C.; HIC, S.; DIFLORIO, R.M.; LYALL, R.M.; WIKESJO, U.M.; BAKER, P.J.; CHRISTERSSON, L.A., and GENCO, J.J.: A biochemical approach to periodontal regeneration: tetracycline treatment of dentin promotes fibroblast adhesion and growth. J. Periodont. Res. 21: 330-337 (1986).
36. ZAMBON, J.J.; CHRISTERSSON, L.A., and GENCO,R.J.: Diagnosis and treatment of localized juvenile periodontitis. J. Am. Dent. Assoc. 113:195-199 (1986).

Dr. A. Tanner, Forsyth Dental Center, 140 Fenway, Boston, MA 02115, USA

Periodontology Today. Int. Congr., Zürich 1988, pp. 132–140 (Karger, Basel 1988)

Does the Analysis of the Subgingival Flora Have Value in Predicting Periodontal Breakdown?

J. Slots, N.S. Taichman, J. Oler and M.A. Listgarten

School of Dental Medicine, University of Pennsylvania, Philadelphia, PA, USA

Introduction

The development of appropriate tests for predicting destructive periodontal disease is a major challenge for current periodontal research. Such measurements may be based on clinical, microbiological, immunological and gingival crevice fluid determinations. This paper will discuss some fundamental statistical issues in diagnostic testing (3) and will provide initial data on the capability of *Actinobacillus actinomycetemcomitans* to predict localized juvenile periodontitis and progressive adult periodontitis.

Statistics

The *Bayesian decision theory* (4) represents a valuable means of revising probabilities of events ("prior probabilities") based on additional information ("empirical evidence"). Table I illustrates this statistical approach for evaluating the efficacy of a test for progressive periodontitis. This theory can be applied to periodontal disease by utilizing the data published by Listgarten et al. (9). These investigators studied 92 adults for recurring periodontitis and found that only 1% of the teeth demonstrated an increase in pocket depth over a period of 11 months (prior probability column; Table I). One would anticipate even lower disease activity in individuals with a history of little or no periodontal disease.

We then contemplate that a test can be developed to predict active periodontitis with a nosologic sensitivity of 96% (the probability of a positive test result, given that the patient or the tooth will get the disease) and a nosologic specificity of 95% (the probability of a negative test result, given that no disease will develop; 1 - nosologic

Table I. Bayes' theorem calculation for test of periodontal disease activity[a)]

Events A_i	Prior probabilities (given) $P(A_i)$	Likelihoods (empirical evidence) $P(B/A_i)$	Joint probabilities $P(A_i)\ P(B/A_i)$	Posterior probabilities $P(A_i/B)$
A_1: Has active disease	0.01	0.96	0.0096	$\frac{0.0096}{0.0591} = 0.16$
A_2: Does not have active disease	0.99	0.05	0.0495	$\frac{0.0495}{0.0591} = 0.84$
	1.00		$P(B) = 0.0591$	1.00

a) Bayes' theorem formula for two basic events, A_1 and A_2:

$$P(A_1/B) = \frac{P(A_1)\ P(B/A_1)}{P(A_1)\ P(B/A_1) + P(A_2)\ P(B/A_2)}$$

B denotes the event "test indicates active disease"

specificity = 0.05). The nosologic indexes are presented in the empirical evidence column in Table I. This certainly is not a poor diagnostic performance compared to available tests. However, the indexes which are most informative to the clinician pertain to the predictive accuracy of a positive test result ("diagnostic sensitivity", i.e., the probability of getting the disease, given a positive outcome in the diagnostic test) and a negative test result ("diagnostic specificity", i.e., the probability of not getting the disease, given a negative outcome in the diagnostic test). The diagnostic efficacy indexes in our example are given in the posterior probability column in Table I. The probability is 16% that a tooth will experience progressive periodontitis given that the test indicates active disease. Although the posterior probability is 16 times higher than the prior probability, 16% is still a low probability of correctly predicting progressive periodontitis. This disappointing result stems from the fact that a relatively large number of teeth are being encountered which will not experience breakdown but for which the test has indicated (falsely) the likelihood of further destruction. Stated another way, the diagnostic difficulty arises because progressing periodontitis occurs at a low frequency in the general population and because a nosologic specificity of 95% is not sufficiently high for diseases of low incidence. Since we face a trade-off between nosologic specificity and sensitivity, the sensitivity of a given test may be seriously compromised by pushing the specificity value close to 100%. Thus, the prospect is not promising for developing a reasonably accurate test for screening of active periodontitis in the general population.

Algebraically, we can improve the efficacy of a diagnostic test by increasing the disease incidence. Clinically, this can be done by testing high-risk individuals. Assuming that a disease has a frequency of 50% in a selected group of individuals, the test described in Table I will give rise to respectable posterior probabilities of 0.950 (diagnostic sensitivity) and 0.050 (diagnostic specificity = 0.950). The discussion which follows will demonstrate how this approach can be applied to three groups of periodontal patients.

Localized juvenile periodontitis

Children who have parents or older siblings with localized juvenile periodontitis have about a 50% risk of developing the disease (5). Since *A. actinomycetemcomitans* is the major putative bacterium in localized juvenile periodontitis (11), we have initiated a study to determine whether this or other organisms are predictors of the disease. Presently, 32 unaffected children (6-13 years of age) from 20 families with localized juvenile periodontitis are enrolled in the study. Subgingival bacterial samples are obtained every 3 months from the mesial surfaces of first permanent molars (target sites where the disease is most likely to develop) and from the first maxillary premolars (control sites). Table II summarizes the microbiological findings in a 12 year old girl who "converted" from health to disease at 3 molar target sites.

Table II. Maximum percent of organisms during conversion from periodontal health to localized juvenile periodontitis

Organisms	Sites[a)]					
	Control 1-4	Target 1-6	Control 2-4	Target 2-6	Target 3-6	Target 4-6
A. actinomycetem-comitans	1.9	6.9	0.2	15.4	92.5	77.1
B. gingivalis	0	0	0	0	0	0
B. intermedius	<0.1	7.8	0	4.5	0.2	8.7
E. corrodens	2.3	<0.1	0.2	0.8	<0.1	0.2
Capnocytophaga	0	<0.1	0.3	1.5	0.5	<0.1
Fusobacterium	<0.1	<0.1	0	0.1	<0.1	0.1
Wolinella	0	0	0	0	<0.1	0
Spirochetes[b)]	1.0	16.0	0	2.0	0	0
Motile rods[b)]	4.0	31.0	7.0	10.0	54.0	54.0

a) Sites 1-6, 3-6 and 4-6 converted from periodontal health to periodontitis.

b) Determined by phase-contrast microscopy

At 3-6 months prior to clinically detectable breakdown, sites 1-6, 3-6 and 4-6 yielded A. actinomycetemcomitans in proportions of 6.9%, 69.5% and 49.7%, respectively. At time of "initial" clinical breakdown, the organism constituted 4.4%, 92.5% and 77.1% of total isolates. During this observation period, A. actinomycetemcomitans did not exceed 2% of the cultivable microflora in any of the control sites. Bacteroides intermedius was the only other species which appeared to be associated with the periodontal destruction but it was recovered in markedly lower proportions when compared to A. actinomycetemcomitans (Table II).

In contrast to the above risk group, testing for A. actinomycetemcomitans in the general population offers little in predicting localized juvenile periodontitis. A. actinomycetemcomitans may occur in the oral cavity of about 25% of young Americans (13) and localized juvenile periodontitis affects less than 1% of the population (8). Accordingly, only 4% of young children colonized by A. actinomycetemcomitans may develop the disease. If other bacteria also can cause localized juvenile periodontitis, bacterial testing is even less efficacious.

Adult periodontitis

Subjects with "refractory" periodontitis constitute another high-risk patient group. We are presently conducting a longitudinal study to determine the capacity of subgingival A. actinomycetemcomitans, Bacteroides gingivalis and B. intermedius to predict periodontal breakdown in refractory adult periodontitis. The investigation is designed as a two-group repeated measures study with both within-subject (internal) and independent (external) controls. At baseline, 86 adult periodontitis patients were grouped as 62 target patients (revealed at least 1 of the 3 test bacteria above threshold proportions in at least 3 periodontal sites) and 24 control patients (revealed no test organism above threshold proportions in any of 12 periodontal sites examined). Three target and 3 control sites were followed in each target patient and 6 sites were followed in each control patient. The thresholds used were 0.01% for A. actinomycetemcomitans, 0.1% for B. gingivalis and 2.5% for B. intermedius (1). The patients were placed on maintenance care and examined clinically and microbiologically every 3 months. Further periodontal breakdown was defined as an increase of 2 mm or more in probing pocket depth or probing attachment level. The microbiological examination routinely included the 3 test bacteria and a number of other potential periodontal pathogens.

The explanatory capability of baseline microbiological measures on changes in probing pocket depth was examined using a multiple regression stepwise selection procedure to determine the best predictors from (1) the proportions of the studied bacteria and (2) the number of teeth positive for these organisms. Both sets of potential regressors were examined to determine normalizing, variance stabilizing transformations. The bacterial proportions were rightly skewed. Natural logarithm, square root and negative reciprocal transformations down the ladder of powers (Tukey) improved fit to model assumptions. The number of positive teeth were only selectively skewed, with suitable transformations made when indicated.

At 6 months, 21 target and 12 control patients showed from 1 to 6 teeth (target, control and other teeth) with ongoing periodontal destruction. The best explanatory bacterium was A. actinomycetemcomitans, showing two-tailed P-values from 0.04 to 0.08 in the various analyses performed. The diagnostic contribution of B. gingivalis could not be established because it occurred in only 9 patients. B. intermedius did not explain changes in clinical measurements. Other bacteria which were positively associated with periodontal breakdown included Bacteroides forsythus (7) and Eikenella corrodens. Capnocytophaga species tended to be negatively correlated with destructive periodontitis.

Periodontal treatment

Microbiological diagnosis may be very valuable in evaluating the prognosis after treatment of progressive periodontitis. The microbiological test is here used together with a clinical diagnosis ("active periodontitis", determined, for example, by longitudinal clinical measurements). The individual diagnostic procedures then become contributory. Microbiological diagnosis before and after treatment provides information about the pathogen(s) which have to be eradicated and about the effectiveness of treatment. The clinical diagnosis establishes that the individual is indeed susceptible to disease and not merely a "carrier" of the organism(s).

However, only a few studies have been carried out to determine the efficacy of diagnostic microbiology in periodontal treatment. Slots and Rosling (12) treated 20 localized juvenile periodontitis lesions in 6 patients. Before treatment, all lesions yielded A. actinomycetemcomitans. Tetracycline therapy resulted in the elimination of the organism from 12 lesions and was accompanied by gains of probing attachment from 0 to 4.5 mm. Two sites continued to harbor very small amounts of the organism and also gained 1-2 mm in attachment level. Another 2 sites demonstrated relatively high numbers of A. actinomycetemcomitans and a stable attachment level. Four sites with high posttreatment counts of A. actinomycetemcomitans were the only sites which continued to lose attachment after therapy. This investigation and other studies by Christersson et al. (2) and Kornman and Robertson (6) suggested that monitoring subgingival A. actinomycetemcomitans may be useful in determining treatment effectiveness and prognosis of localized juvenile periodontitis.

Slots (10) described 10 adult patients who demonstrated ongoing loss of periodontal attachment despite comprehensive surgical therapy and professional tooth cleaning every 3 months. Nine deep periodontal pockets in 4 patients revealed

A. actinomycetemcomitans. After systemic tetracycline therapy, these lesions became free of detectable A. actinomycetemcomitans. The removal of the pathogenic microflora paralleled a decrease in probing pocket depth of 2 mm or more and a radiographically detectable gain of crestal alveolar bone.

Summary and concluding remarks

A single and accurate test to demonstrate etiologic agents and predict outcome disease in the general population may not be developed in periodontics. Difficulties arise because of a low incidence of active periodontitis and a requirement for a test with high nosologic specificity. The latter may be unattainable because of the multimicrobial etiology of periodontitis and the high proportion of individuals carrying periodontal pathogens without experiencing disease.

However, microbiological diagnosis may be very helpful in predicting destructive periodontal disease in high-risk patients. These may include young children in families with localized juvenile periodontitis, adults with refractory periodontitis, AIDS patients, individuals with neutrophilic defects, etc.. A. actinomycetemcomitans seems to be a good predictor organism for certain types of periodontitis. With increased knowledge about periodontal pathogens, other organisms will likely be useful prognosticators. Moreover, diagnostic efficacy may be improved by combining a number of diagnostic tests including, for example, clinical and immunologic measurements.

In addition to the problems with low disease incidence, a diagnostic test should be evaluated for technical difficulty of performance. The test should also be subjected to a "cost-benefit" analysis in order to determine the balance between the test's financial cost, its clinical discomfort, and its clinical benefits. These and other issues need to be addressed in diagnostic periodontics.

References

1. BRAGD, L.; DAHLEN, G.; WIKSTROM, M., and SLOTS, J.: The capability of Actinobacillus actinomycetemcomitans, Bacteroides gingivalis and Bacteroides intermedius to indicate progressive periodontitis; a retrospective study. J. Clin. Periodontol. 14: 95-99 (1987).

2. CHRISTERSSON, L.A.; SLOTS, J.; ROSLING, B.G., and GENCO, R.J.: Microbiological and clinical effects of surgical treatment of localized juvenile periodontitis. J. Clin. Periodontol. 12: 465-476 (1985).

3. FEINSTEIN, A.R.: Clinical epidemiology: The architecture of clinical research; (W.B Saunders Company, Philadelphia 1985).

4. FLEISS, J.L.: Statistical methods for rates and proportions; 2nd ed., pp. 1-18 (John Wiley & Sons, New York 1981).

5. GENCO, R.J.; VAN DYKE, T.E.; LEVINE, M.J.; NELSON, R.D., and WILSON, M.E.: Molecular factors influencing neutrophil defects in periodontal disease. J. Dent. Res. 65: 1379-1391 (1986).

6. KORNMAN, K.S. and ROBERTSON, P.B.: Clinical and microbiological evaluation of therapy for juvenile periodontitis. J. Periodontol. 56: 443-446 (1985).

7. LAI, C.-H.; LISTGARTEN, M.A.; SHIRAKAWA, M., and SLOTS, J.: Bacteroides forsythus in adult gingivitis and periodontitis. Oral Microbiol. Immunol. 2: 152-157 (1987).

8. LINDHE, J. and SLOTS, J.: Periodontal disease in children and young adults; in LINDHE, Textbook of clinical periodontology; 2nd ed. (Munksgaard, Copenhagen 1988) (in press).

9. LISTGARTEN, M.A.; LEVIN, S.; SCHIFTER, C.C.; SULLIVAN, P. EVIAN, C.I., and ROSENBERG, E.S.: Comparative differential dark-field microscopy of subgingival bacteria from tooth surfaces with recent evidence of recurring periodontitis and from nonaffected surfaces. J. Periodontol. 55: 398-401 (1984).

10. SLOTS, J.: Microbiology in periodontics. Tandlaegebladet 90: 794-798 (1986).

11. SLOTS, J. and LISTGARTEN, M.A.: Bacteroides gingivalis, Bacteroides intermedius and Actinobacillus actinomycetemcomitans in human periodontal diseases. J. Clin. Periodontol. 15: (1988) (in press).

12. SLOTS, J. and ROSLING, B.G.: Suppression of the periodontopathic microflora in localized juvenile periodontitis by systemic tetracycline. J. Clin. Periodontol. 10: 465-486 (1983).

13. SWEENEY, E.A.; ALCOFORADO, G.A.P.; NYMAN, S., and SLOTS, J.: Prevalence and microbiology of localized prepubertal periodontitis. Oral Microbiol. Immunol. 2: 65-70 (1987).

Acknowledgments

These studies were supported by grants from the National Institutes of Health (DE 06085, DE 07118, RR 00040 and RR 01224).

Author's address

JORGEN SLOTS, D.M.D., Ph.D., M.A., M.S. Department of Periodontics and Periodontal Diseases Research Center, School of Dental Medicine, University of Pennsylvania, 4001 Spruce Street, Philadelphia, PA 19104 (USA).

Periodontology Today. Int. Congr., Zürich 1988, pp. 141–149 (Karger, Basel 1988)

Sources of Variations in the Evaluation of the Subgingival Microbiota

Gunnar Dahlèn and Maude Wikström

Department of Oral Microbiology, University of Göteborg, Göteborg, Sweden

The subgingival microbiota is composed of 250-300 different bacterial species (MOORE et al, 1982) present in various numbers and proportions in different sites of different individuals from different parts of the world. Our knowledge of the subgingival microbial composition is based on single samples, hopefully representing the existing microbiota, evaluated with different methods. A proper comparison of studies carried out in different laboratories is very difficult to make, due to our limited information of the importance of different sources of variation. In an attempt to illustrate the magnitude of different sources of variation this presentation consider the presence of three bacterial species; Actinobacillus actinomycetemcomitans, Bacteroides gingivalis, and Bacteroides intermedius in subgingival samples from individuals with different health and periodontal status analyzed with the same technique. The sources of variations have been divided into measurement errors and biological variations (COLTON, 1974).

1. Measurement errors

   Measurement errors refers to all those sources of variation caused by the sampling and the sampling method and the microbial cultivation and identification techniques.

2. Biological variations

   a. Temporal variations are ment the variations caused by interactions between bacteria and between bacteria and the host resulting in a continous reorganisation of the subgingival microbiota.

b. Intra-individual variations include the microbial variations between sites in the same individual due to the location of the site in the jaw, anatomic factors, dental restorations, pocket depth and periodontal status.

c. Inter-individual variations refer to the microbial variations due to common health status, age, sex, genetical factors, geographic domicile, habits, diet, etc.

Material and Methods

In the studies referred to, all samples were taken with paper point technique and analysed at the same conditions. After careful supragingival cleaning with sterile scaler and cotton pellets, three stiff points were inserted to the bottom of the pocket for 10 secs. The points were transferred to the laboratory in a vial containing 3 ml transport medium VMGA III (MÖLLER, 1966), prepared and stored under oxygenfree gas, and 15 glass beads 3 mm in diameter. The sample reached the laboratory within 1-24 hrs. It was dispersed on a Vortex mixer at maximal setting for 10 secs and diluted to 10^{-2} and 10^{-4} in VMG I (MÖLLER, 1966). A volume of 0.1 ml transport medium and dilutions were uniformly spread on Brucella blood agar plates (BBL, Microbiological Systems, Cockeysville, MD) enriched with 0.5% hemolyzed horse blood and $5 \cdot 10^{-5}$% menadione and on TSBV-agar plates (SLOTS, 1982). The Brucella blood agar plates were incubated in jars with 95% H_2 and 5% CO_2, using the hydrogen combustion method, at $37^{\circ}C$ for 7 days and the TSBV-agar plates in jars with 10% CO_2 and 90% air at $37^{\circ}C$ for 5 days.

Total viable count was calculated from the Brucella blood agar plates and expressed as the number of colony forming units (CFU) per ml transport medium.

B. gingivalis was identified on the Brucella blood agar plates as green-black pigmented colonies not giving fluorescence under long-wave UV light (SLOTS and REYNOLDS, 1982).

B. intermedius was identified on the Brucella blood agar plates as black-pigmented colonies giving red fluorescence under long-wave UV light and ability to produce indol and ferment sugars.

A. actinomycetemcomitans was identified on the TSBV-agar plates as small, star-shaped, adherent and catalase positive colonies.

Measurement errors

Measurement errors could be divided into those giving false positive and those giving false negative results. The risk to obtain false positive results with the used method is neglectable. At a more extended characterization of 62 strains of B. gingivalis, 51 strains of B. intermedius and 50 strains of A. actinomycetemcomitans, isolated from subgingival samples and preliminary classified according to the criteria given above (WIKSTRÖM and DAHLEN; unpublished, DAHLEN et al. I; unpublished) only one strain, a strain classified as B. intermedius, was found to belong to the B. melaninogenicus group.

The sensitivity of the method has been calculated from duplicate samples, taken one week apart, of 106 untreated sites of 16 subjects (DAHLEN et al. II; unpublished) and was found to be 0.84 for B. gingivalis, 0.88 for B. intermedius and 0.83 for A. actinomycetemcomitans. The reproducibility was evaluated by means of kappa statistics (HUNT, 1986) on results obtained from duplicate samples from the untreated as well as from hygienist treated sites. This showed good or excellent agreement both for total CFU numbers and the proportions of A. actinomycetemcomitans and B. gingivalis, while the values obtained for B. intermedius showed less agreement. The B.intermedius results could be explained by the lower proportions of this species in the subgingival microbiota compared to that of B. gingivalis, and by the use of unselective medium for cultivation of B. intermedius when compared to the results obtained for A. actinomycetemcomitans. The same trend was obtained in samples from pockets $\geq$9 mm and $\leq$6 mm and in samples with a total viable count $\geq 200 \cdot 10^5$ and $\leq 5 \cdot 10^4$ and in samples obtained from treated sites. A comparison between the variance due to laboratory processing and that due to sampling showed that almost all variance was due to the sampling procedure (WIKSTRÖM et al. unpublished). Laboratory processing contributed to 6% of the total variance obtained for A. actinomycetemcomitans, 11% for B. gingivalis and 2% for B. intermedius. The variance of the sampling procedure using the paper point technique is suggested to contain unrelevant bacteria from the upper portion of the pocket which increases the dilution factor and by that risk of false negative results. Furthermore it is not known to what extent this technique really gets access to the discrete zones. Most investigators agree, however that sampling the loosely adherent plaque with paper points gives a high recovery of black-pigmented *Bacteroides* (MOORE et al. 1982, TANNER and GOODSON, 1987).

Temporal variations

In an analysis of variance of short time variation (repeated sampling 15 min apart) compared to longtime (5 repeated samplings during 5 weeks) it was found that 77% of the total variation for *B. gingivalis*, 100% *B. intermedius*, and 86% *A. actinomycetemcomitans* variation was dependent on the short time variation, i.e. the sampling procedure *per se* WIKSTRÖM et al. unpublished).

In a study by WENNSTRÖM et al. (1987) 46 periodontal diseased sites with bleeding on probing of 30 patients were left without any form of treatment during 12 months. In 12 *A. actinomycetemcomitans* positive sites the bacteria were recovered in 9 one year later. Furthermore 5 sites were positive for *B. gingivalis* and 17 sites for *B. intermedius* at baseline.of these, 3 and 12, respectively were still positive after 12 months and 4 new sites for both *Bacteroides* species were positive. All 16 sites that were negative for all of the three species at baseline were also negative one year later. It was suggested that most of the variations obtained were due to methodological errors, even if some could be explained by a temporal variations.

Intra-individual variations

Since many microorganisms have very strict requirements for colonization and growth, the pocket depth and the presence of inflammation exudate probably are the most important factors for the pocket milieu and thereby determining the composition of the subgingival flora (SLOTS, 1979). It would therefore be possible to recover similar bacteria from sites with similar pocket depth and inflammation, provided that the pockets are continously exposed to the bacteria.

Table 1. Intraindividual variations in three different types of studies. Presence of A. actinomycetemcomitans, B. gingivalis and B. intermedius in periodontal sites.

Study	Total no of patients	Periodontal condition	Site selection	Bacteria	No of patients with indicated bacteria – percent of sites ≤ 25	> 25 - 50	> 50 - 75	>75 - 100
1[a)]	22	gingivitis	16, 24 31, 45	A. actinomycetemcomitans	2	1	0	0
				B. gingivalis	0	0	0	0
				B. intermedius	6	7	3	3
2[b)]	63	periodontitis	deepest pocket in each quadrant ≥ 4 mm	A. actinomycetemcomitans	4	1	3	7
				B. gingivalis	6	7	7	8
				B. intermedius	8	14	13	12
3[c)]	22	periodontitis	all pockets with 6 mm or more pocket depth 4 - 9 pockets	A. actinomycetemcomitans	1	2	0	7
				B. gingivalis	1	0	2	9
				B. intermedius	1	4	3	14

a) WIKSTRÖM (unpublished)

b) combined data from ROSLING and DAHLÉN (unpublished) and THORSTENSSON et al. (I) (unpublished)

c) combined data from DAHLÉN et al. (unpublished) and WIKSTRÖM et al. (unpublished)

Table 1 shows the baseline recovery of A. actinomycetemcomitans, B. gingivalis and B. intermedius in 5 different ongoing studies in which samples have been taken from 4 or more sites in each patient. There was throughout a higher probability to find the three bacterial species in the majority of the sites with deep pockets than in just one or two. This tendency was not found in the gingivitis group. There is also a clinical experience of having typical B. gingivalis or A. actinomycetemcomitans patients. However, systematic studies on the inter-individual distribution of these bacteria in relation to site characteristics are lacking.

Inter-individual variations

There are som evidences of a various prevalence of microorganisms due to inter-individual factors. Higher prevalence of A. actinomycetemcomitans has been reported from Panama (EISENMAN et al. 1983) compared to North America (ZAMBON et al. 1983) and Scandinavia (AISKAINEN et al. 1986). A higher prevalence seems also be present for both A. actinomycetemcomitans and B. gingivalis in nonperiodontitis adults in Kenya compared to a similar group in Sweden (Table 2). Since systematic epidemiological studies are few, it can not fully be ruled out whether there are certain racial differences or if the differences obtained reflect socio-economic or geographical distributed subpopulations.

The colonization of black-pigmented Bacteroides are stimulated by hormones in the gingival crevice (SLOTS and GENCO, 1984) suggesting the puberty as critical for the change in prevalence of B. gingivalis and B. intermedius in children compared to adults. The prevalence of A. actinomycetemcomitans, B. gingivalis and B. intermedius has been investigated in adults with different medical background compared to healthy individuals with different periodontal conditions (Table 2). No obvious differences could be seen between these groups, except that adult diabetic patients have a higher frequency of B. gingivalis compared to age and sex matched controls. No B. gingivalis was detected in the juvenile diabetic individuals.

Conclusions

Using the same methodology in a number of studies it has been

Table 2. Interindividual variation. Frequency of A. actinomycetemcomitans, B. gingivalis and B. intermedius (% of individuals) in different groups of individuals (at least two sites sampled).

Group of individuals	No of individuals	Periodontal condition	A. actino-mycetem-comitans	B. gingivalis	B. intermedius	Study
Healthy Swedish adults	22	gingivitis	14	0	86	a
Healthy Kenyan adults	20	gingivitis	40*	70**	100	b
Healthy Swedish adults	63	periodontitis $\geq$ 4 mm pockets	24	44	75	c, d
Healthy Swedish adults	22	periodontitis $\geq$ 6 mm pockets	45	54	100	e, f
Reumatoid arthritis adults	11	gingivitis periodontitis	45	36	100	g
Hypogammaglobulinaemia or IgG subclass deficiency (adults)	11	gingivitis	18	0	36*	h
Diabetes (adults)	31	gingivitis periodontitis	26	55***	77	i
Age and sex matched controls	34	gingivitis periodontitis	18	24	68	i
Diabetes (juvenile)	10	healthy gingiva, gingivitis	30	0	60	j

* $p < 0.05$ compared to healthy Swedish adults
** $p < 0.001$ compared to healthy Swedish adults
*** $p < 0.001$ compared to age and sex matched controls

a) WIKSTRÖM (unpublished)
b) DAHLEN et al. (1988)
c) ROSLING and DAHLEN (unpublished)
d) THORSTENSSON et al. (I) (unpublished)
e) DAHLEN et al. (unpublished)
f) WIKSTRÖM et al. (unpublished)
g) LAURELL and DAHLEN (unpublished)
h) GAHNBERG et al. (1988)
i) THORSTENSSON et al. (II) (unpublished)
j) RYLANDER and DAHLEN (unpublished)

possible to evaluate the most important factor that might influence on the recovery of A. actinomycetemcomitans, B. gingivalis and B. intermedius. In adults it seems that the pocket depth and degree of inflammation together with the sampling procedure are responsible for the major variation. It might be argued that the high reproducibility in our studies is a result of insensitive techniques and limited to only a few bacterial species. On the other hand the high recovery rate of these bacteria, which is similar or even higher than that obtained in other studies, tells for a high reliability of the methods.

References

ASIKAINEN, S.; JOUSIMES-SOMES, H.; KANERVO, A., and SUMMANEN, P.: Certain bacterial species and morphotypes in localized juvenile periodontitis and in matched controls. J. Periodont. 58: 224-230 (1987).

COLTON, T.: Statistics in medicine. Little, Brown and Company, Boston, Mass, (1974).

DAHLEN, G.; MANJI, F.; BAELUM, V., and FEJERSKOV, O.: Presence of Actinobacillus actinomycetemcomitans, Bacteroides gingivalis and Bacteroides intermedius in Kenyan adult population. Submitted to J. Clin Periodontol. (1988).

EISENMANN, A.C.; EISENMANN, R.; SOUSA, O., and SLOTS, J.: Microbiological study of localized juvenile periodontitis in Panama. J. Periodont. 54: 712-713 (1983).

GAHNBERG, L.; DAHLEN, G.; BJÖRKANDER, J.; SLOTS, J., and HANSSON, L-Å.: Periodontal disease and dental caries in relation to primary hypogammaglobulinaemia and IgG subclass deficiencies. Submitted to Infect. Immun. (1988).

HUNT, R.J.: Percent agreement Pearson's correlation, and kappa as measures of inter-examiner reliability. J. Dent. Res. 65: 128-130 (1986).

MOORE, W.E.C.; RANNEY, R.R., and HOLDEMAN, L.V.: Subgingival microflora in periodontal disease: cultural studies: in GENCO and MERGENHAGEN, Host-parasite interactions in periodontal diseases; pp 13-26 (American Society for Microbiology, Washington D.C. 1982).

MÖLLER, Å.J.R.: Microbiological examination of root canals and periapical tissues of human teeth. Thesis. Odontol. Tidskr. 74: 1-380 (1966).

SLOTS, J.: Selective medium for isolation of Actinobacillus actinomycetemcomitans. J. Clin. Microbiol. 15: 606-607 (1982).

SLOTS, J.: Subgingival microflora and periodontal disease. J. Clin. Periodontol. 6: 351-382 (1979).

SLOTS, J., and GENCO, B.: Black-pigmented Bacteroides species, Capnocytophaga species, and Actinobacillus actinomycetemcomitans in human periodontal disease: Virulence factors in colonization, survival and tissue destruction. J. Dent. Res. 63: 412-421 (1984).

SLOTS, J., and REYNOLDS, H.S.: Longwave UV-light fluorescence for identification of black-pigmented Bacteroides spp. J. Clin. Microbiol. 16: 1148-1151 (1982).

TANNER, A.C.R., and GOODSON, J.M.: Sampling of microorganisms associated with periodotal disease. Oral. Microbiol. Immunol. 1: 15-20 (1986).

WENNSTRÖM, J.L.; DAHLEN, G.; SVENSSON, J., and NYMAN, S.: Actinobacillus actinomycetemcomitans, Bacteroides gingivalis and Bacteroides intermedius, predictors of attachment loss? Oral Microbiol. Immunol. 2: 00-00 (1987). In press.

ZAMBON, J.J.; CHRISTERSSON, L.A., and SLOTS, J.: Actinobacillus actinomycetemcomitans in human periodontal disease: prevalence in patient groups and distribution of biotypes and serotypes within families. J. Periodont. 54: 707-711 (1983).

Dr. G. Dahlèn, Department of Oral Microbiology, University of Göteborg, Guldhedsgatan 10, 413 46 Göteborg, Sweden

Periodontology Today. Int. Congr., Zürich 1988, pp. 150–159 (Karger, Basel 1988)

Is Microbial Tissue Invasion a Reality during Periodontal Breakdown?

Robert M. Frank

Centre de Recherches. Unité INSERM U 157. Faculté de Chirgurie Dentaire, Université Louis Pasteur, Strasbourg, France

1. Introduction :

The microbial flora associated with the development of periodontal diseases is highly complex. According to a review by MOORE (27) 325 distinct bacterial species have been found in the human gingival crevice and our knowledge is far from complete since many bacterial species have never been formally described or have even been ignored. Although it is generally recognized that bacteria of the subgingival plaque are the etiologic agents of periodontodal diseases (21,29,30,40), it was widely accepted that the microorganisms confined to the periodontal pocket did not invade the surrounding soft tissues and that the periodontal breakdown was mainly induced by diffusion of bacterial products (enzymes, toxins, antigens and/or mitogens) into the surrounding epithelial and connective tissue environment. Only one exception was recognized to this general concept. This was the invasion of spirochetes in cases of acute necrotizing ulcerative gingivitis (ANUG) (23).

The ultrastructural studies of TAKARADA et al (41), FRANK (14), ALLENSPACH-PETRZILKA and GUGGENHEIM (2,3), GILLETT and JOHNSON (6), SAGLIE et al. (33,35), CARRANZA et al (7) and MANOR et al. (26), established the possibility of bacterial tissue invasion in periodontal diseases, despite the fact that LIAKONI et al. (22) in a transmission electron microscopic study of human adult and juvenile periodontitis and ERICSSON et al. (13) in experimental periodontitis induced in the beagle dog, failed to find bacteria in the pocket epithelium and gingival connective tissue.

It is intended in the present paper to review the concept of bacterial invasion in various human periodontal diseases and in animal models and to analyze the results obtained with culture techniques, in light, transmission and scanning electron microscopy and immunofluorescence and immunocytochemical electron microscopy. In addition original results will be presented.

2. Bacterial Invasion In Acute Necrotizing Ulcerative Gingivitis (ANUG) :

Penetration of spirochetes into the periodontal tissues in cases of ANUG have been reported since the beginning of the century (6,12,39). By transmission electron microscopy (TEM), LISTGARTEN and SOCRANSKY (24), LISTGARTEN (23), HEYLINGS (20) and COURTOIS et al. (11) confirmed in ulcerated areas of ANUG the presence of spirochetes, easily recognizable by their typical axial filaments and their undulating shape, in the intercellular spaces of the epithelium and in the underlying connective tissue. Other types of bacteria were also noted (11,20).

Using an animal model, MALTHA et al. (25) were able to reproduce ANUG in beagle dogs and observed in light microscopy the invasion of the sulcular epithelium by spirochetes thus playing a role in the creation of a portal of entry into gingival tissue for other bacteria and bacterial products.

3. Bacterial Invasion In Cases Of Juvenile Periodontitis :

Various microorganisms and especially *Haemophilus actinomycetemcomitans* (*Actinobacillus actinomycetemcomitans* = Aa), classically associated with juvenile periodontitis (27,45) have been localized by different convergent techniques within the soft periodontal tissues. The invading bacteria penetrated in the periodontal connective tissue through the pocket epithelium (7,16,34,35) (site 1 figure 1). However SAGLIE et al. (36) showed the presence of Gram-positive and Gram-negative bacteria in the intercellular spaces of the outer gingival epithelium (site 2 figure 1).

Using light, scanning and transmission electron microscopy Gram-negative fusiform, coccobacilli and spirochetes as well as some mycoplasma (28) were found in the invaded tissues (7,35).

The intratissular presence of Aa was further confirmed by use of specific antibaterial sera with fluorescent light microscopy (8,9,36) completed by TEM studies and cultures on selective medium of minced, surface-disinfected sections of gingival biopsies (8,9).

4. Bacterial Invasion In Chronic Periodontitis :

In chronic periodontitis the presence of bacteria in gingival tissues was first postulated by GOADBY (17) and described in light microscopy by TURNER and DREW (43), BECKWITH et al. (15) and HABERMAN (19). However the penetration of microorganisms into the tissues was only seriously considered after the ultrastructural studies of TAKARADA et al. (41), FRANK and VOEGEL (15), FRANK (14), ALLENSPACH-PETRZILKA and GUGGENHEIM (2,3), SAGLIE et al. (33,35), CARRANZA et al. (17) and MANOR et al. (26).

Fig. 1 : Bacterial penetration in the lamina propria either through the pocket epithelium (site 1) or through the gingival epithelium (site 2). En = enamel. De = dentine. Ce = cementum.

Fig. 2 : Presence of numerous microorganisms and spirochetes in the enlarged intercellular spaces of the pocket epithelium in a case of human chronic periodontitis . X 9000.

Fig. 3 : Microorganisms in a cell of the pocket epithelium. Chronic human periodontitis with root exposure. X 10000

Fig. 4 : Filamentous microorganisms in an epithelial cell belonging to the pocket wall. X 38000.

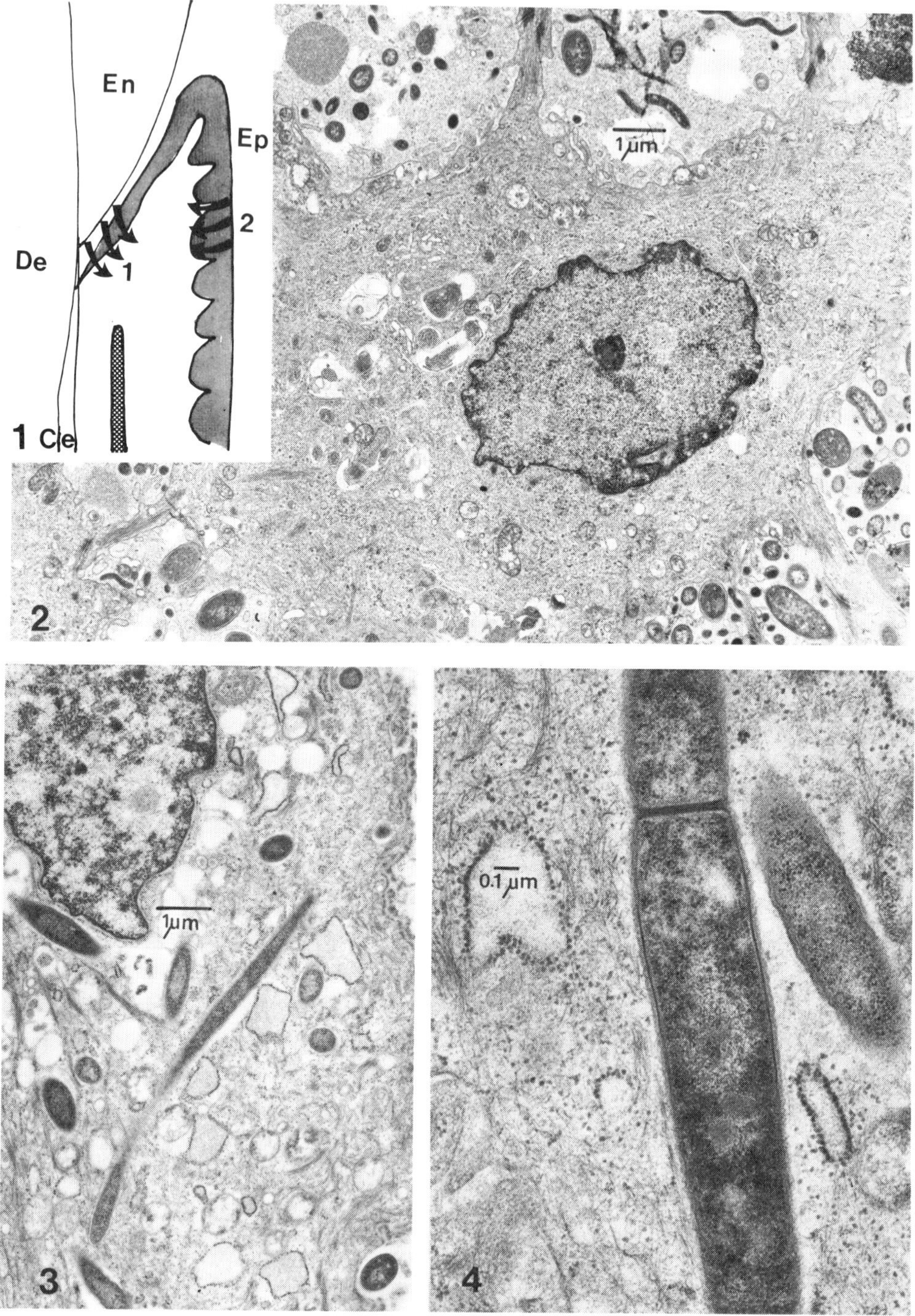
En
Ep
De
Ce
1
2
1
1 µm
2
1µm
3
0.1 µm
4

Gram-negative and Gram-positive coccoid, rod-shaped and filamentous bacteria as well as typical spirochetes were seen penetrating the connective tissue of the lamina propria through the pocket epithelium (Figure 1, site 1). The bacteria were further observed in contact with and within the alveolar bone (15) or invading the radicular dentine and pulp of periodontally diseased caries free human teeth (1).

Bacterial penetration through the outer gingival epithelium (figure 1, site 2) in the case of chronic periodontitis initially described in light microscopy by PEKOVIC and FILLERY (31), was confirmed by SAGLIE et al. (35,36) and PERTUISET et al. (32). With an immunoperoxidase technique, SAGLIE et al. (37) found in this location a higher numbers of Langerhans cells associated with epithelial bacterial invasion.

Bacterial identification was also assessed by Gram staining in light microscopy (31) and fluorescence microscopy. The intragingival presence of Bacteroides melaninogenicus and its products was demonstrated by immunofluorescence (10,42). The gingival penetration of Actinomyces viscosus, A.naeslundii, B.gingivalis and to a lesser extent B. ss. intermedius was confirmed by a double staining immunofluorescence technique (31). The penetrating bacteria were always associated with antibodies and frequently also with complement. With the peroxidase immunocytochemical technique, SAGLIE et al. (37) localized in the gingival B.gingivalis and to a lesser extent Capnocytophaga gingivalis.

Finally bacterial penetration into soft periodontal tissues has been demonstrated in two different animal models. In gnotobiotic rats, ALLENSPACH-PETRZILKA and GUGGENHEIM (2) found an intragingival invasion of B.melaninogenicus ss intermedius after oral inoculation, whereas SALLAY et al. (38), in ligature induced periodontitis and immunosuppressed rats (after treatment with cyclophosphamide) observed bacterial invasion of the gingiva. No bacterial penetration was observed in the control rats with experimental periodontitis which were not immuno-suppressed.

5. Original Observations In Transmission Electron Microscopy :

In this study, buccal gingival biopsies in 5 cases of advanced human chronic periodontitis (patients aged 46 to 60 years) with pocket depths between 6 to 10mm, were prepared and observed in a Jeol 100B TEM as previously described (14). In addition, buccal gingival areas adherent to 5 extracted human teeth of 3 patients aged 51 to 58 years were studied

Fig. 5 : Bacterial penetration in a superficial cell (Ec) of the pocket epithelium connected to an amorphous organic pellicle (Pe) by numerous hemi-desmosomes (arrows). Ce = cementum surface. Po = pocket space. X 11000.

Fig. 6 : Presence of Gram-negative bacteria in an inner pocket epithelial cell connected to the cementum (Ce) by hemi-desmosomes (arrows) and an extracellular space (i). X 35000.

Fig. 7 : Presence of a layer of polymorphonuclear neutrophils between the pocket epithelium and the subgingival plaque (Pl). X 11000.

Fig. 8 : Inner part of the layer of PMNs adjacent to epithelial cells of the pocket epithelium (Ep). H = red cell. X 5000.

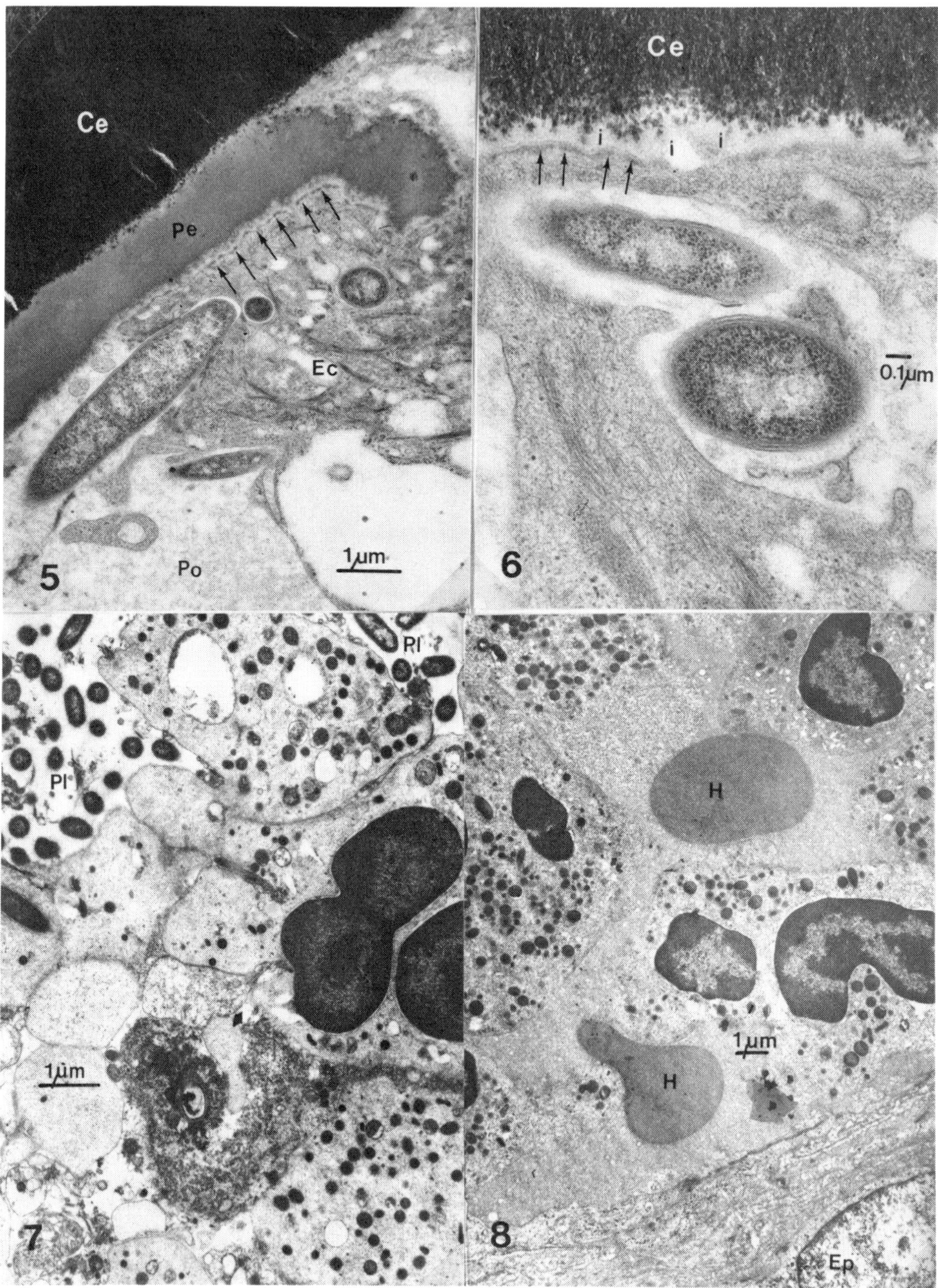
Ce
Pe
Ec
Po
1µm
5
Ce
i
i
i
0.1µm
6
Pl
Pl
1µm
7
H
H
1µm
8
Ep

with TEM on non-decalcified sections made with a diamond knife. The roots of these 5 teeth with chronic periodontitis were exposed for at least 2mm in an apical direction measured from the enamel-cementum junction to the outer gingival level. The root surface exposed to the oral cavity presented superficial cemental caries.

Bacterial invasion of the pocket epithelium and the underlying connective tissue was observed in 3 out of the 5 advanced cases of chronic periodontitis. The same proportion was noted in the teeth with retracted periodontal tissues and cemental caries. The previous observations made by FRANK (14) were largely confirmed. Bacterial invasion of the pocket epithelium occurred either through the enlarged intercellular spaces (figure 2) or through intracellular penetration of the microorganisms (figures 3, 4, 5, 6). Various types of coccoid, filamentous and rod-shaped predominantly Gram-negative bacteria were found in the cytoplasm of the non-keratinized epithelial cells, where they seemed to be well-tolerated judging from the unaltered aspect of cytoplasmic organelles and matrix. The epithelial penetration of filamentous bacteria seemed to occur through a progressive invagination of the microorganism in the cell (figure 5). This intracellular bacterial penetration can even reach the deep parts of the junctional epithelium adjacent to the cementum surface (figure 6).

A very important feature was the presence of a multilayered zone of polymorphonuclear neutrophilic leukocytes (PMNs) located between the subgingival plaque occupying the pocket and the surface of the pocket epithelium (figures 7, 8, 9, 10). Some PMNs were intact with numerous intracellular granules (figure 8). Superficial PMNs in contact to the subgingival plaque were sometimes degranulated (figure 7, to the left) or presented phagocytosed bacteria (figure 9). Severely altered and degranulated superficial PMNs surrounded by numerous microorganisms were also seen (figure 10). When present, important alterations of the PMNs layer with numerous engulfed bacteria were noted in those cases where bacterial invasion occurred through the pocket epithelium.

6. Discussion and Conclusion :

From all the evidences available, it appears that microbial tissue invasion during periodontal breakdown in cases of ANUG, juvenile and chronic periodontitis has now been established. Since bacterial invasion is generally observed in advanced cases, it is probably not a prerequisite for the development of periodontal disease, but constitutes certainly an important part of the pathological processes. It is also apparent that the types of invading bacteria can be different for each periodontal disease and further investigations are necessary for precise identification of the intratissular bacterial associations involved.

The microorganisms can invade the soft periodontal tissues through the pocket epithelium or the outer gingival epithelium. The epithelial invasion can occur through enlarged intercellular spaces or by cell penetration. These invading bacteria contribute to the destruction of the epithelial and connective tissues and even of the crestal alveolar bone (15).

Local host defense mechanisms are essential for the development of bacterial tissue invasion which occurs only when these mechanisms are compromised. An experimental demonstration has been presented by SALLAY et al. (38). Using ligature induced periodontal lesions in normal and immunosuppressed rats after cyclophosphamide injections, bacterial invasion of the soft periodontal tissues was observed only in the latter group. It is likely that the reduction in PMNs and mononuclear cells resulted in increased susceptibility to bacterial invasion.

From our electron microscopic investigations, we are convinced that bacterial penetration is strongly dependent on the behaviour of the superficial layer of PMNs located between the subgingival plaque and the pocket epithelium (figures 7,8,9,10). Bacterial invasion seemed to occur when the microorganisms were able to cross the PMNs layer.

These superficial PMNs are able to release lysozomal enzymes (4) to phagocytose and destroy intracellularly as well as extracellularly the plaque bacteria. But the invading microorganisms are also able to kill the PMNs (figure 10) and in such conditions the barriers of PMNs is insufficient to prevent bacterial invasion. The precise conditions of bacterial invasion have to be further investigated, but it is now well-known that these bacteria are able to produce collagenase as well as trypsin-like proteases (18,44). Finally it must be mentioned that bacterial penetration in junctional epithelium is however possible in absence of PMNs (figure 5).

Fig. 9 : The superficial PMNs adjacent to the subgingival plaque located in the periodontal pocket present numerous phagocytosed bacteria. X 11000.

Fig. 10 : Severely altered and degranulated superficial PMN surrounded by numerous microorganisms within the apical part of the periodontal pocket. X 8000.

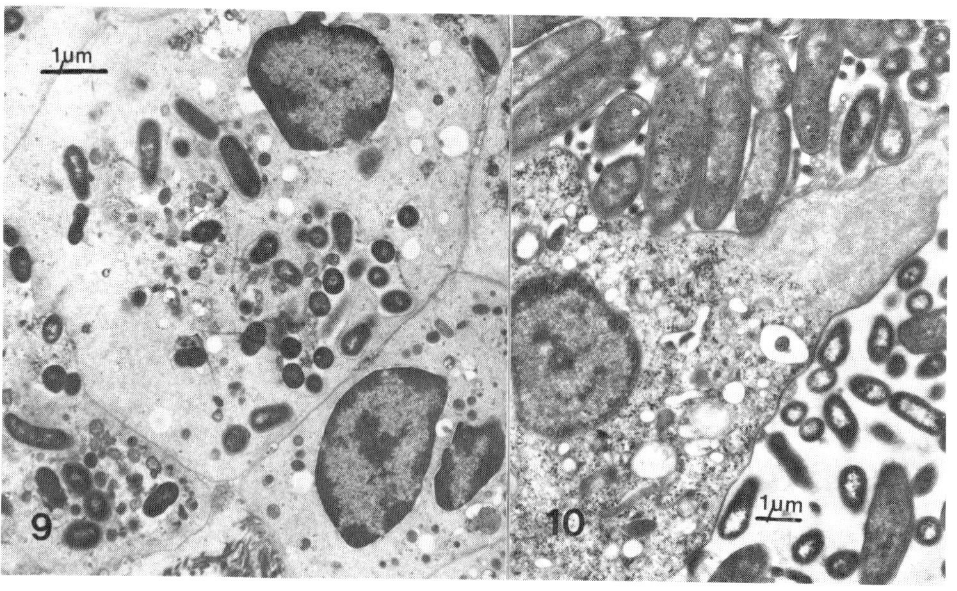

7. References :

1. ADRIAENS, P.A. ; LOESCHE, W.J. and BOEVER, J.A. de : Bacteriological study of the microbial flora invading the radicular dentine of periodontally diseases caries-free human teeth ; in LEHNER and CIMASONI, The borderland between caries and periodontal disease III ; pp.383-390 (Med. Hyg., Genève 1986).
2. ALLENSPACH-PETRZILKA, G.E. and GUGGENHEIM, B. : Bacteroides melaninogenicus ss intermedius invasion of rat gingival tissue. J. Periodont. Res. 17 : 456-459. (1982).
3. ALLENSPACH-PETRZILKA, G.E. and GUGGENHEIM, B. : Bacterial invasion of the periodontium : an important factor in the pathogenesis of periodontitis. J. Clin. Periodont. 10 : 609-617. (1983).
4. BAEHNI, P. ; TSAI, C.C. ; TAICHMAN, N.S. and McARTHUR, W. : Interaction of inflammatory cells and oral microorganisms. J.Periodont. Res. 13 : 333-348 (1978).
5. BECKWITH, T. ; SIMONTON, F.V. and WILLIAMS, A. : A histologic study of the gum in pyorrhea. J. Am. Dent. Ass. 12 : 129-153 (1925).
6. CAHN, L.R. : The penetration of the tissue by Vincent's organisms. A report of a case. J. Dent. Res. 9 : 695-698 (1929).
7. CARRANZA, F.A.,jr ; SAGLIE, R. ; NEWMAN, M.G. and VALENTIN, P.L. : Scanning and transmission electron microscopic study of tissue invading microorganisms in localized juvenile periodontitis. J. Periodont. Res. 54 : 598-617 (1983).
8. CHRISTERSSON, L.A. ; ALBINI, B. ; ZAMBON, J.J., WIKESJO, U.M.E. and GENCO,R.J.Tissue localization of Actinobacillus actinomycetemcomitans in human periodontitis. I. Light, immunofluorescence and electron microscopic studies. J. Periodont. 58 : 529-539 (1987a).
9. CHRISTERSSON, L.A. ; WIKERJO, U.M.E. ; ALBINI, B. ; ZAMBON, J.J. and GENCO,R.J.Tissue localization of Actinobacillus actinomycetemcomitans II. Correlation between immunofluorescence and culture techniques. J. Periodont. 58 : 540-545 (1987b).
10. COURANT, P. and BADER, H. : Bacteroides melaninogenicus and its products in the gingiva of man J. Periodontics. 4 : 131-136 (1966).
11. COURTOIS, G.J. ; COBB, C.M. and KILLOY, W.J. Acute necrotizing ulcerative gingivitis.A transmission electron microscope study. J.Periodont 54 671-679 (1983).
12. ELLERMAN, V. Zur Kenntniss der Spindelbazillen. Ztschrft. Hyg. und Infektionkrankh. 56 : 452-461 (1907).
13. ERICSSON, I. ; LINDHE, J. ; LILJENBERG, B. and PERSSON, A.L. Lack of bacterial invasion in experimental periodontitis. J.Clin. Periodont. 14 : 478-485 (1987).
14. FRANK, R.M. : Bacterial penetration in the apical pocket wall of advanced human periodontitis. J. Periodont. Res. 15 : 563-573 (1980).
15. FRANK, R.M. and VOEGEL, J.C. Bacterial bone resorption in advanced cases of human periodontitis. J. Periodont. Res. 13 : 251-261 (1978).
16. GILLETT, R. and JOHNSON, N.W. : Bacterial invasion of the periodontium in a case of juvenile periodontitis. J. Clin. Periodont. 9 : 93-100 (1982).

17. GOADBY, K.W. : Erasmus Wilson's lecture on pyorrhea alveolaris.Lancet. 1 : 633-638 (1907).
18. GRENIER, D. and MAYRAND, D. : Functional characterization of extracellular vesicles produced by Bacteroides gingivalis. Infect.Immunity 55 : 111-117 (1987).
19. HABERMAN S. : Inflammatory and non-inflammatory responses to gingival invasion by microorganisms. J. Periodont. 30 : 190-195 (1959).
20. HEYLINGS, R.T. : Electron microscopy of acute ulcerative gingivitis (Vincent's type). Brit. Dent. J. 122 : 51-56 (1967).
21. JORDAN, H.V. and KEYES, P.H. : Periodontal lesions in the syrian hamster. II. Findings related to an infections and transmissible component. Archs oral Biol. 9 : 372-400 (1964).
22. LIAKONI, H. ; BARBER, P. and NEWMAN, H.N. : Bacterial penetration of pocket soft tissues in chronic adult and juvenile perodontitis cases. An ultrastructural study. J. Clin. Periodont. 14 : 22-28 (1987).
23. LISTGARTEN, M.A. : Electron microscopic observations of the bacterial flora of acute necrotizing ulcerative gingivitis. J. Periodont. 36 : 328-339 (1965).
24. LISTGARTEN, M.A. and SOCRANSKY, S.S. : Ultrastructural characteristics of a spirochete in the lesion of acute necrotizing ulcerative gingivostomatitis (Vincent's infection).Archs oral Biol. 9 : 95-96 (1984).
25. MALTHA, J.C., MIKX, F.H.M. and KUIJPERS, F.J. : Necrotizing ulcerative gingivitis in beagle dogs. III. Distribution of spirochetes in interdental gingival tissue. J. Periodont. Res. 20 : 522-531 (1985).
26. MANOR, A. ; LEBENDIGER, M. ; SHIFFER, A. and TOVEL, H. : Bacterial invasion of periodontal tissues in advanced periodontitis in humans. J. Periodont. 55 : 567-573 (1984).
27. MOORE, W.E.C. : Microbiology of periodontal disease. J. Periodont.Res. 22 : 335-341 (1987).
28. NEWMAN, M. ; SAGLIE, R. ; CARRANZA, F.A.jr. and KAUFMAN, K. Mycoplasma in periodontal disease. Isolation in juvenile periodontitis. J. Periodont. 55 : 574-580 (1984).
29. PAGE, R.C. and SCHROEDER, H.E. : Periodontitis in man and other animals. A comparative review ; pp. 17-21 (Karger, Basel, 1982).
30. PALENSTEIN HELDERMAN, W.H. van : Microbial etiology of periodontal disease. J. Clin. Periodont. 8 : 261-280 (1981).
31. PEKOVIC, D.D. and FILLERY, E.D.: Identification of bacteria in immunopathological mechanisms of human periodontal diseases. J. Periodont. Res. 19 : 329-351 (1984).
32. PERTUISET, J.H., SAGLIE, R. ; LOFTHUS, J. ; REZENDE, M. and SANZ, M. : Recurrent periodontal disease and bacterial presence in gingiva. J. Periodont. 58 : 553-558 (1987).
33. SAGLIE, R. ; CARRANZA, F.A.jr ; NEWMAN, M.G. and PATTISON, G.A. : Scanning electron microscopy of the gingival wall of deep periodontal pokets in humans. J. Periodont. Res. 17 : 284-293 (1982a).
34. SAGLIE, R. ; NEWMAN, M.G. ; CARRANZA, F.A.jr and PATTISON, G.A. : Bacterial invasion of gingiva in advanced periodontitis in humans. J. Periodont. 53 : 217-222 (1982b).
35. SAGLIE, R. ; CARRANZA, F.A.jr and NEWMAN, M.G. : The presence of bacteria within the oral epithelium in periodontal disease. I. A scanning and transmission electron microscopic study. J. Periodont. 56 :

618-624 (1985).
36. SAGLIE, F.R. ; SMITH, C.T. ; NEWMAN, M.G. ; CARRANZA, F.A.jr., PERTUISET, J.H., CHENG, L. ; AVIL, E. and NISENGAARD, R.J. : The presence of bacteria in the oral epithelium in periodontal disease. II. Immunohistochemical identification of bacteria. J. Periodont. 57 : 492-500 (1986).
37. SAGLIE, F.R. ; PERTUISET, J.H. ; SMITH, M.T. ; NESTOR, M.G. ; CARRANZA F.A.jr. ; NEWMAN, M.G. ; REZENDE, M.T. and NISENGAARD, R.J. : The presence of bacteria in the oral epithelium in periodontal disease. J. Periodont. 58 : 417-422 (1987).
38. SALLAY, K. ; LISTGARTEN, M. ; SANAVI, F. ; RING, I. and NOWOTNY, A. : Bacterial invasion of oral tissues of immunosuppressed rats. Inf. Immunity. 43 : 1091-1094 (1984).
39. SCHAFFER, E.M. : Biopsy studies on necrotizing ulcerative gingivitis. J. Periodont. 24 : 22-25 (1953).
40. SOCRANSKY, S.S. : Relationship of bacteria to the etiology of periodontal disease. J. Dent. Res. 49 : 203-222 (1970).
41. TAKARADA, H. ; CATTONI, M. ; SUGIMOTO, A. and ROSE, G.G. Ultrastructural studies of human gingiva. J. Periodont. 45 : 155-169 (1974).
42. TAKEUCHI, H. ; SUMITANI, M. ; TSUBAKIMOTO, K. and TSUTSUI, M. : Oral microorganisms in the gingiva of individuals with periodontal disease. J. Dent Res. 53 : 132-136 (1974).
43. TURNER, J.G. and DREW, A.H. : An experiemntal inquiry into the bacteriology of pyorrhea. Proc. Royal Soc. Med. 12 : 104-118 (1918).
44. UITTO, V.J. ; TRYGGVASON, K. and SORSA, T. Collagenolytic enzymes in periodontal disases. Proc. Finn. Dent. Soc. 83 : 119-129 (1987).
45. ZAMBON, J.J. : Actinobacillus actinomycetemcomitans in human periodontal disease. J. Clin. Periodont. 12 : 1-20 (1985).

8. Author's Adress :

Robert Frank, Faculté de Chirurgie Dentaire, Université Louis Pasteur
4 Rue Kirschleger, 67000 Strasbourg, France.

Periodontology Today. Int. Congr., Zürich 1988, pp. 160–168 (Karger, Basel 1988)

The Pathogenicity of Haemophilus (Actinobacillus) actinomycetemcomitans
A New Concept

Hans R. Preus

Depts. of Microbiology and Periodontology, Dental Faculty, University of Oslo, Oslo, Norway

Haemophilus (Actinobacillus) actinomycetemcomitans (Ha; although there has been a discussion about the name of this bacterium, studies on the DNA (23) and ribosomal RNA (21) suggest it to be phylogenetically more closely related to the Haemophilus than Actinobacillus family) is a G-, facultative, capnophilic, coccobacillary rod suggested by several authors to play a key role in the development of rapidly destructive periodontal diseases in humans (32,49). Other authors (20) question the role Ha is suggested to play in these diseases. Its habitat in man is not yet established, but it has been considered as being part of the human resident flora (42) of the cavum oris and the upper respiratory system (18,33,49). It is a fastidious organism and constitutes low percentages of the the periodontal flora except in connection with periodontitis. Ha, or elevated serum antibody titers against the bacterium, is found in association with prepubertal periodontitis (25,43), localized juvenile periodontitis (LJP) (31, 50) and adult periodontitis (41), especially in refractory cases (32). 90% of patients with LJP show elevated serum antibody titers against the bacterium (5). It is considered to carry the ability to penetrate epithelium, and it has been recognized in periodontal connective tissues (4). Ha produces several enzymes as well as toxious and noxious products (49). It has also the ability to adhere to glass and agar surfaces in vitro. This characteristic could be mediated by fimbriae (28).

Several observations may indicate Ha to be of exogenous origin in man. First, it is only found in 10 - 15% of humans without LJP (49). Second, it is possible to eliminate the bacterium from the oral environment by the use of bacteriostatic antibiotics, such as tetracycline (19,27,34). An inhabitant of the oral resident flora would hardly be permanently eradicated from its habitat by a bacteriostatic antibiotic. Ha is also rejected by the mature bacterial flora of dental plaque in general (3), and by Streptococcus sanguis and Streptococcus mitis in particular (13,48).

During the last decade we have studied two siblings with

Papillon - Lefèvre syndrome (PLS) (24,27). From the periodontal pockets of these children we isolated several strains of Ha. We also isolated Ha from the PLS family pet dog, and restriction endonuclease mapping suggested that the dog and child strains of Ha was from the same clone, indicating that a transmission had occurred between the dog and the children (29). The finding of Ha in a dog reflects that periodontal pathogens may be found in species within the human environment and might be transmitted between them. There is no evidence that Ha is a normal inhabitant of the dog microflora, but the dogs PMNs are resistant to Ha leukotoxin (39). Also, Zambon et al. (50) have shown that there is a higher frequency of Ha carriers within the family of a LJP patient than in the general population, indicating that Ha is transmitted between family members as well. On the other hand, such transmission can hardly be a common feature since there is a congestion of the bacteria within certain families. These findings might indicate that the bacterium is transmitted to humans with non - mature or non-stable oral microfloras only. Thus a transmission of the bacterium could be expected most frequently to take place in children and juveniles during eruption and shedding of teeth. These periods comprise the ages when prepubertal - and juvenile periodontitis start, and would also theoretically explain why 1st molars and incisors are most frequently affected by the disease. The notion that a transmission of Ha occurs casually and in particular situations and/or in short periods of life may also explain why the diseases it may induce are infrequent.

Despite the recognition of some periodontal diseases as possibly induced by specific and exogenously derived bacteria, it has not been possible to fulfill the postulated requirements of Koch for identifying the etiological agents in this family of infections (36). A main reason for this is that suspected bacteria, have been isolated from diseased as well as healthy sites in humans (49,52). It has also been difficult to explain how Ha, with its postulated high pathogenic potential may reside in healthy sites when other sites in the same mouth are subject to periodontal breakdown and infected with the very same bacterium.

A suggested characteristic of periodontitis is that it shows an intermittant disease activity, characterized by bursts of destruction (37). Several hypotheses, based on studies of local bacteriology and host responses (10), have been put forward to explain these phenomena, but it seems that more questions than answers have accumulated.

A new aspect was introduced when we recently observed that Ha cultured from patients with rapidly destructive periodontitis was infected with several groups of bacteriophages (25,26) In 6 such patients 18 sites with radiographic evidence of recent bone loss, 5 deep periodontal pockets with no such evidence of recent bone loss, and 13 healthy control sites were screened for the presence of Ha and its bacteriophages. Phage activity was exclusively found in the 18 diseased sites that had shown evidence of recent bone loss. In the 5 deep periodontal pockets with no radiographic evidence of recent bone loss, plaque samples showed Ha but no phage activity. None of the 13 healthy control sites showed phage activity although 6 of these sites produced the bacterium. When studying the PLS patient over a period of 7 months, we observed that her only inactive site, which had harbored noninfected Ha became active again concomitantly with the occurrence of Ha phages. These findings suggested an association between bacteriophage infection of Ha and active periodontal destruction.

A possible explanation might be sought in the biological activity of bacteriophages as such. Bacteriophages normally possess both temperate and virulent characteristics. In vitro studies have shown that it is partly the concentration ratio between bacteria and phages, and partly the origin of the recombinant phage-DNA that decide which of the characteristics is to be expressed (35). Most genes in a prophage are kept in an inactive state by the product of the repressor gene, which is frequently the only prophage gene that is expressed. With some phage species genes other than the repressor gene are also expressed. In such cases the prophage genes may express what we recognize as host (bacterial) enzymes, toxins or metabolites. In some diseases phages have been assigned similar roles in the pathogenesis. The production of diphtheria toxin is coded for by a phage genome, and Corynebacterium diphtheria will only cause disease when it is infected with its specific virion. Another classic example of phage infection is scarlatina, in which β-hemolytic streptococci must acquire a specific phage before they can produce erythrogenic toxin. Other examples of toxigenic species of bacteria associated with bacteriophages are Streptococcus pyogenes, Staphylococcus aureus, Clostridium botulinum and Vibrio cholerae (6,7,16,40,47).

There are few reports on phages infecting oral bacteria. A prophage (Aa Φ 17) has been induced in Ha FDC 651 (38), which originated from a patient with LJP. Plaque organisms such as Veillonella (44), Streptococcus mutans PK1 (12) and Actinomyces viscosus (46) have also been observed infected with phage. Electron microscopic investigations have demonstrated phage-like particles in dental plaque (2,11,17), but the role of phages in oral infectious diseases is not known.

In LJP patients 55% of the Ha isolates produce leukotoxin, whereas leukotoxin-producing isolates are rarely recovered from periodontally healthy subjects (51). Furthermore, serum anti-leukotoxin antibodies are present in 94% of LJP patients but only in 19% of healthy reference subjects (45). In spite of this antibody production, it is suggested that leukotoxinproducing strains are generally present in LJP. The possibility cannot be excluded that certain Ha phages code for the production of leukotoxin or other bioactive substances in their hosts even though this could not be demonstrated for Aa Φ 17. C. diphtheria can loose its phage in vivo, and consequently abolish the production of diphtheria toxin. Antibody produced *in vivo* against *C. diphtheria* phage will prevent infection of new bacterial hosts. One may speculate that a similar mechanism might operate in *Ha*, implying that e.g. leukotoxin production may cease when sufficient antibody towards the phage has been produced. Loss of leukotoxin production would arrest periodontal breakdown if this toxin is a major virulence factor in periodontal destruction.

Bacterial products promoting invasion of host tissues may also be a prerequisite of periodontal disease (1). It has been suggested that several of the suspected pathogens in subgingival dental plaque, including *Ha* are able to invade periodontal tissues (1,4). The invading property of the bacteria could be due to phage promoted presence, or abscence, of fimbriae or phage coded production of enzymes necessary for the invasive activity. The genetic background for invasive properties of a bacterium may also be carried by plasmids. Clinical strains of *Ha* has recently been shown to carry 3 plasmids (30). In nature plasmids may be transferred to other bacteria by several mechanisms, for instance transduction. It is thus a possibility that phages may operate in subgingival dental plaque, transferring such genes from one bacterial strain to another.

Whether or not toxin or enzyme production is affected by phage infection, temperate and/or lytic phages in bacteria colonizing periodontal sites may eventually lead to lysis of bacterial cells. This would expose the periodontium to high concentrations of phages, endotoxins, exotoxins and enzymes originating from the lysed bacteria. It has been shown that synthesis of toxin is plasmid-mediated in *Salmonella typhimurium*, *E. coli*, and *Shigella dysenteriae* and that their toxin release is related to lysis of cells by phage (8,9,15,22). This bacterial lysis may also provide large amounts of mitogens capable of producing a polyclonal immunologic response in the periodontium. All these possibilities may separately, or in combination, theoretically promote the rapid destruction of periodontal tissues sometimes observed in humans.

It has been suggested that "burned - out" sites in LJP occur as a result of the emergence of inhibitory bacteria that decrease and control the numbers of *Ha* (14). Another possibility is that the decrease in bacterial numbers is related to phages eliminating susceptible *Ha* from periodontal sites, leaving lysogens and/or a few phage-resistant, or less virulent, non-infected strains of the bacterium at the site.

Being aware of the restrictions due to the low number of test persons examined in our studies, I still find it fruitful to present some working hypotheses that theoretically might explain the nature of rapid periodontal breakdown in man:

* Bursts of destructive periodontitis might occur when prophages from a lysogen in the periodontal pocket are induced and might even be potentiated by the concomitant presence of sensitive strains.
* Lysogeny may increase the pathogenic potential of *Ha*. Phage

infection may also cause lysis of the bacterium, exposing the periodontium to high concentrations of phages and potent antigens and mitogens eliciting immunologically mediated periodontal destruction.

* The periodontally diseased site may remain in remission until the next, if any, local buildup of a periopathogenic phage - bacterium relationship occurs.

In principle, the hypotheses are based on the biological activity of bacteriophages and are not necessarily restricted to Ha-associated periodontitis. The described situation might thus occur in any rapidly destructive periodontitis associated with any bacterium infected with phages.

References.

1. ALLENSPACH-PTRZILKA, G.E. and GUGGENHEIM, G.B.: Bacterial invasion of the periodontium; an important factor in the pathogenesis of periodontitis? J. Clin. Periodontol. 10: 609 - 617 (1983).
2. BRADY, J.M.; GRAY, W.A. and CALDWELL, M.A.: The electron microscopy of bacteriophage-like particles in dental plaque. J. Dent. Res. 56: 991 - 993 (1977).
3. CHRISTERSSON, L.A.; SLOTS, J.; ZAMBON, J.J. and Genco, R.J.: Transmission and colonization of Actinobacillus actinomycetemcomitans in localized juvenile periodontitis patients. J. Periodontol. 56: 127 - 131 (1985).
4. CHRISTERSSON, L.A.; ALBINI, B.; ZAMBON, J.J.; SLOTS, J. and GENCO, R.J.: Demonstration of Actinobacillus actinomycetemcomitans in gingiva of localized juvenile periodontitis lesions. AADR 62th general session, Cincinnati, abstr. 255 (1983).
5. EBERSOLE, J.L.; TAUBMAN, M.A.; SMITH, D.J.; GENCO, R.J. and FREY, D.E.: Human immune responses to oral microorganisms. I. Association of localized juvenile periodontitis (LJP) with serum antibody responses to Actinobacillus actinomycetemcomitans. Clin. Exp. Immunol. 47: 43 - 52 (1982).
6. EKLUND, M.W,; POYSKY, F.T. and REED, S.M.: Bacteriophage and toxigenicity of Clostridium botulinum type D. Nature (New Biol) 235: 16 - 17 (1972).
7. EKLUND, M.W.; POYSKY, F.T.; REED, S.M. and SMITH, C.A.: Bacteriophage and toxigenicity of Clostridium botulinum type C. Science 172: 480 - 482 (1971).

8. GEMSKI, P.; O'BRIEN, A.D. and WOHLHIETER, J.A.: Cellular release of heatlabile enterotoxin of Escherichia coli by bacteriophage induction. Infect. Immun. 19: 1076 - 1082 (1978)

9. GYLES, C.L.; PALCHAUDHURI, S. and MAAS W.K.: Naturally occuring plasmid carrying genes for enterotoxin production and drug resistance. Science 198: 198 - 199 (1977)

10. HAFFAJEE, A.D.; SOCRANSKY, S.S. and EBERSOLE, J.L.: Survival analysi of periodontal sites before and after periodontal therapy. J. Clin. Periodontol. 12: 553 - 567 (1985).

11. HALHOUL, N. and COLVIN, J.R.: Virus-like particles in association with a microorganism from human gingival plaque. Arch. Oral. Biol. 20: 833 - 836 (1975).

12. HIGUCHI, M.; RHEE, G.H.; ARAYA, S. and HIGUCHI, M.: Bacteriophage deoxyribonucleic acid-induced mutation of Streptococcus mutans. Infect. Immun. 15: 938 - 944 (1977).

13. HILLMAN, J.D. and SOCRANSKY, S.S.: Bacterial interference of Actinobacillus. IADR 59th general session, Chicago. Abstr. 1174 (1981).

14. HILLMAN, J.D. and SOKRANSKY, S.S.: Bacterial interference in the oral ecology of Actinibacillus actinomycetemcomitans and its relationship to human periodontosis. Arch. Oral. Biol. 27: 75 - 77 (1982).

15. HOUSTON, C.W.; KOO, F.C. and PETERSON, J.W.: Characterization of Salmonella toxin released by mitomycin C-treated cells. Infect. Immun. 32: 916 - 926 (1981).

16. JOHNSON, L.P.; SCHLIEVERT, P.M. and WATSON, D.W.: Transfer of group A streptococcal pyrogenic exotoxin production to nontoxigenic strains of lysogenic conversion. Infect. Immun. 28: 254 - 257 (1980).

17. KEREBEL, B.; CLERGEAU - GUERITHAULT, S. and FORLOT, P.: Etude ultrastructurale de plaques microbiennes dentaires chez des sujets indemnes de carie. Ann. Microbiol. 126: 203 - 229 (1975).

18. KILIAN, M. and SCHIØTT, C.R.: Haemophili and related bacteria in the human oral cavity. Arch. Oral. Biol. 20: 791 - 796 (1975).

19. LINDHE, J.: Treatment of localized juvenile periodontitis; In GENCO and MERGENHAGEN, Host Parasite Interactions in Periodontal Disease. pp. 399 - 410 (Am. Soc. Microbiol. Washington DC 1982)

20. MOORE, W.E.C.: Microbiology of periodontal disease. J. Periodont. Res. 22: 335 - 341 (1987)

21. PASTER, B.J.; DEWHIRST, F.E. and OLSEN, I.: The phylogeny of Actinobacillus, Haemophilus and Pasteurella by 16S rRNA sequencing. IADR/AADR Montreal; March 9 - 13, 1988.

22. PETERSON, J.W.; HOUSTON, C.W. and KOO, F.C.: Influence of cultural conditions on mitomycin C - mediated bacteriophage induction and release of Salmonella toxin. Infect. Immun. 32: 232 - 242 (1981).

23.POTTS, T.R.; ZAMBON, J.J. and GENCO, R.J.: Proposal for reassignment of *Actinobacillus actinomycetemcomitans* to the genus *Haemophilus* nom. rev. as *Haemophilus actinomycetemcomitans*. Int. J. Sys. Bact. 35: 337 - 341 (1985).

24.PREUS, H.R. and GJERMO, P.: Clinical management of prepubertal periodontitis in two siblings with Papillon - Lefèvre syndrome. J. Clin. Periodontol. 14: 156 - 160. (1987)

25.PREUS, H.R.; OLSEN, I. and NAMORK, E.: Association between bacteriophage infected *Actinobacillus actinomycetemcomitans* and rapid periodontal destruction. J. Clin. Periodontol. 14: 245 - 247 (1987).

26.PREUS, H.R.; OLSEN, I. and NAMORK, E.: The presence of phageinfected *Actinobacillus actinomycetemcomitans* in localized juvenile periodontitis patients. J. Clin. Periodontol. 14: 605 - 609 (1987).

27.PREUS, H.R. Rapidly destructive periodontitis of Papillon-Lefèvre syndrome. Laboratory and clinical observations. J. Clin. Periodontol. in press,No 10 (1988).

28.PREUS, H.R.; NAMORK, E. and OLSEN, I.: Fimbriation of *Actinobacillus actinomycetemcomitans*. Oral Microbiol. Immunol. submitted.

29.PREUS, H.R. and OLSEN, I.: Possible transmittance of *A. actinomycetemcomitans* from a dog to a child with rapidly destructive periodontitis. J. Per. Res. in press (1988).

30.Preus, H.R. and OLSVIK, Ø.: Plasmids in strains of *Actinobacillus actinomycetemcomitans* isolated from patients with rapidly destructive periodontitis. Lancet. submitted (1988).

31.SLOTS, J. and GENCO, R.J.: Microbial pathogenicity. Black-pigmented *Bacteroides* species, *Capnocytophaga* species, and *Actinobacllus actinomycetemcomitans* in human periodontal disease: virulence factors in colonization, survival, and tissue destruction. J. Dent. Res. 63: 412 - 421 (1984).

32.SLOTS, J.: Bacterial specificity in adult periodontitis. A summary of recent work. J. Clin. Periodontol. 13: 912 - 917 (1986)

33.SLOTS, J.; REYNOLDS, H.S. and GENCO, R.J.: *Actinobacillus actinomycetemcomitans* in human periodontal disease: a crossectional microbiological investigation. Infect. Immun. 29: 1013 - 1020 (1980).

34.SLOTS, J. and ROSLING, B.G.: Suppression of the periodontopathic microflora in localized juvenile periodontitis by systemic tetracycline. J. Clin. Periodontol. 10: 465 - 486 (1983).

35.SNYDER, L.A.; FREIFELDER, D. and HARTL, D.L. General Gene tics. chapt.4. (Jones and Bartlet publ. Boston 1985)

36.SOCRANSKY, S.S.: Criteria for the infectious agents in dental caries and periodontal disease. J. Clin. Periodontol. 6: 16 - 21 (1979).

37. SOCRANSKY, S.S.; HAFFAJEE, A.D.; GOODSON, J.M. and LINDHE, J.: New concepts of destructive periodontal disease. J. Clin. Periodontol. 11: 21 - 32 (1984).

38. STEVENS, R.H.; HAMMOND, B.F. and Lai, C.H.: Characterization of an inducible bacteriophage from a leukotoxic strain of Actinobacillus actinomycetemcomitans. Infect. Immun. 35: 343 - 349 (1982).

39. TAICHMAN, N.S.; TSAI, C.C.; SHENKER, B.J. and BÖERINGER, H.: Neutrophil interactions with oral bacteria as a pathogenic mechanism in periodontal diseases; in WAISSMANN, Advances in inflammation Research. pp. 113 - 142 (Raven Press, New York 1984).

40. TAKEYA, K. and SHIMODORI, S.: "Prophage - typing" of El Tor vibrios. J. Bacteriol. 85: 957 - 958 (1963).

41. TANNER, A.C.; HAFFER, C.; BRATTHALL, G.T. VISCONTI, R.A. and SOCRANSKY, S.S.: A study of the bacteria associated with advancing periodontitis in man. J. Clin. Periodontol. 6: 278 - 307 (1979).

42. THEILADE, E.: The non-specific theory in microbial etiology of inflammatory periodontal diseases. J. Clin. Periodontol. 13: 905 - 911 (1986).

43. TINANOFF, N.; TANZER, J.M.; KORNMAN, K.S. MADERAZO, E.G.: Treatment of the periodontal component of Papillon-Lefèvre syndrome. J. Clin. Periodontol. 13: 6 - 10 (1986).

44. TOTSUKA, M.: Studies on veillonella-phages isolated from washings of human oral cavity. Bull. Tokyo. Med. Dent. Univ. 23: 261 - 273 (1976).

45. TSAI, C.C.; MCARTHUR, W.P.; BAEHNI, P.C.; EVIAN, C. et al.: Serum neutralizing activity against Actinobacillus actinomycetemcomitans leukotoxin in juvenile periodontitis. J. Clin. Periodontol. 8: 338 - 348 (1981).

46. TYLENDA, C.A.; CALVERT, C.; KOLENBRANDER, P.E. and TYLENDA, A.: Isolation of Actinomyces bacteriophage from human dental plaque. Infect. Immun. 49: 1 - 6 (1985).

47. VAN DE VIJVER, J.C.M.; VAN ES-BOON, M. and MICHEL, M.F. Lysogenic conversion in Staphylococcus aureus to leukocidin production. Infect. Immun. 10: 318 - 319 (1972).

48. YAMAMOTO, Y.; MASHIMO, P.A.; REYNOLDS, H. and GENCO, R.J.: Antagonistic relations between an oral streptococcal strain and Gram-negative microorganisms. Abstr. Ann. Meet. Am. Soc. Microbiol. Abstr. D41 (1981)

49. ZAMBON, J.J.: Actinobacillus actinomycetemcomitans in human periodontal disease. J. Clin. Periodontol. 12: 1 - 20. (1985)

50. ZAMBON, J.J.; CHRISTERSSON, L.A. and SLOTS, J.: Actinobacillus actinomycetemcomitans in human periodontal disease. Prevalence in patient groups and distribution of biotypes and serotypes within families. J. Periodontol. 54: 707 - 711 (1983).

51. ZAMBON, J.J.; DELUCA, C.; SLOTS, J. and GENCO, R.J. Studies on leukotoxin from *Actinobacillus actinomycetemcomitans* using the premyelocytic HL-60 cell line. Infect. Immun. 40: 205 - 212 (1983).
52. AASS, A.M.; PREUS, H.R. and OLSEN, I.: Association between oral Aa and periodontal bone loss in teenagers. NOF, Scandinavian Division of IADR, Copenhagen. Abstr. No. 22 (1987).

Address:
Hans R Preus, Dept of Microbiology, Dental Faculty,
POB 1052 Blindern, 0316 Oslo 3, Norway

Periodontology Today. Int. Congr., Zürich 1988, pp. 169–177 (Karger, Basel 1988)

Serum Antibodies to Periodontopathic Microorganisms: Specific Induction

Jeffrey L. Ebersole and Stanley C. Holt

Department of Periodontics, The University of Texas Health Science Center at San Antonio, Texas, USA

Introduction

Elevated serum antibodies to suspected periodontal pathogens has been an important factor for associating these specific microorganisms with periodontal disease (1-4). Results in these reports show that the antibodies detected do indeed react with the bacteria; however, there are little data available which demonstrate that these antibodies were elicited by the specific microorganisms cultured from the oral microbiota (5). This circumstantial evidence supports the contention that the antibodies are induced by a specific antigenic stimulus; however, there are numerous reports of polyclonal B cell activators (PBA) in many oral microorganisms (6) and these PBAs may provide nonspecific signals eliciting the antibody in the absence of specific induction. In this report we describe observations which advocate specific antibody induction by selected periodontopathogens in the subgingival microbiota, and show that the majority of data available are inconsistent with a primary function for PBA's in this host-parasite interaction.

Materials and Methods

Patient Samples

Serum was collected for cross-sectional studies from patients at UTHSCSA, at Forsyth Dental Center (FDC) and the Center for Research in Oral Biology, University of Washington, as well as from 22 patients (FDC) at 2-4 month intervals during a monitoring period of 1-5 years (7). Classification of patients as localized juvenile periodontitis (LJP), advanced destructive periodontitis (ADP), adult periodontitis (AP) and normal has been described previously (5).

Microorganisms and Outer Envelope Antigens (OEA)

Actinobacillus actinomycetemcomitans Y4 (FDC), ATCC 29523 and ATCC 33834, *Bacteroides gingivalis* ATCC 33277, W50

(FDC), A7A21 (SUNY at Buffalo (SUNYAB), and 3079.03 (UTHSCSA/ monkey strain), Bacteroides intermedius ATCC 25611, ATCC 25261, and GOR (SUNYAB), Actinomyces viscosus ATCC 15987, Fusobacterium nucleatum ATCC 25586, Eikenella corrodens ATCC 23834, and Wolinella recta ATCC 33238 were cultured and harvested for antigens (8).

OEA were prepared from the various bacterial species using French pressure cell disruption, ultracentrifugation and Sarkosyl solubilization (11). The cell envelope of the bacteria were separated into Sarkosyl-soluble (S-s) and insoluble (S-i) material. The S-s fraction represents the inner membrane and some extracted outer membrane, while the S-s fraction represents the outer membrane. OEA were separated by SDS-PAGE using exponential gels (10-20%) in a discontinuous buffer system and electroblotted to nitrocellulose sheets. Nonspecific binding was eliminated by blocking with 4% BLOTTO. Isotype/subclass specific Ig reagents were used to probe the separated OEA, and developed by a biotin-avidin-horseradish peroxidase system.

Antibody Determinations

Levels & Quantitation. Serum IgG, IgM and IgG subclass antibody levels were determined using an ELISA with formalinized bacteria (1). Monoclonal antibodies to human IgG1, IgG2, IgG3 and IgG4 (Behring Diagnostics) were used to develop the subclass system. Specificity of the monoclonal antibodies was assessed using purified human IgG subclass paraproteins.

A reference human serum standard was used for determining levels of specific antibody and included in all assays. Quantitation of the isotype antibodies was performed by comparing the optical densities of absolute amounts of isolated Ig bound to the microtiter plates and the identical Ig isotypes bound to the bacteria as antibody molecules. Using the identical developing reagents we could then relate an OD value to an amount of Ig bound to the bacteria (9).

Avidity & Specificity. The relative avidity of the antibody population to a particular antigen was assessed by examining the ability of chaotropic ions to dissociate antigen-antibody complexes. The serum was reacted with the antigen covalently bound to the microtiter plates (10). The complexes are then treated with concentrations of $(NH)_4SCN$ between 0.5 and 5M, and that concentration dissociating 50% of the activity is used as the Avidity Index (AI).

The specificity of the antibody was analyzed by cross-adsorptions of human sera with the various microorganisms as described previously (8). The sera were selected based upon elevated IgG reactivity to one of the serotypes of each bacterial species.

Results

Specificity of Serum Antibody. Human sera were adsorbed with the bacteria to examine the specificity of the antibody responses. As seen in Table I the microorganisms were far more efficient in removing homologous antibody activity than the heterologous strains within the species. Adsorption of the sera with F. nucleatum and A. viscosus removed <8% of the activity to each of the antigens.

Table I. Specificity of serum IgG antibody to various periodontopathic microorganisms.

Microorganism (Antigen)	Test Antigen Adsorption	Antibody Activity % Removed* (range)
Aa Y4 (b)	Aa Y4 (b)	89 (81-93)
	Aa 29523 (a)	64 (59-67)
	Aa 33834 (c)	59 (-)
Bg 33277	Bg 33277	88 (84-93)
	Bg W50	72 (67-74)
	Bg A7A21	56 (53-59)
Bi 25611	Bi 25611	95 (92-96)
	Bi 25261	75 (72-77)
	Bi GOR	78 (74-80)

*Percent of antibody removed when compared to unadsorbed serum

Distribution of Antibody Isotype and Subclass Responses. Table II depicts the levels of IgG and IgM antibodies in various periodontitis patients and normal subjects to A. actinomycetemcomitans, B. gingivalis, and B. intermedius. Generally, while both isotypes of antibodies were detected to each organism, there were significant differences in Ig levels in the various disease categories towards the individual bacteria.

Table II. Serum antibodies to oral bacteria.

Disease Category	Microorganism	Serum Antibody Level (ng/ml) IgG	IgM
LJP	Aa Y4 (b)	1830*[a]	61[c]
	Bg 33277	185[a,b]	37[c]
	Bi 25611	360[a,b]	31[c]
ADP	Aa Y4 (b)	265[d]	53[e,f]
	Bg 33277	298[d]	116[e]
	Bi 25611	593[d]	99[f]
AP	Aa Y4 (b)	141[g]	42[h,i]
	Bg 33277	284[g]	85[h]
	Bi 25611	244[g]	73[i]
N	Aa Y4 (b)	70[j]	16
	Bg 33277	28[j]	19
	Bi 25611	272[j]	30

* Mean ± S.E.M. of 25 LJP, 25 ADP, 25 AP and 15 N.
[a,b,d,e,g,h,j] pairs significantly different at $p<0.01$.
[c,f,i] pairs significantly different at $p<0.05$.

Similarly, the results shown in Table III demonstrate the variability in elevated IgG subclass responses to the three microorganisms.

Table III. Distribution of serum IgG subclass antibodies to oral bacteria in periodontitis patients.

Bacteria	Disease Category	Frequency of Elevated Antibody (%)# IgG1	IgG2	IgG3	IgG4
Aa Y4	LJP	51*	81*	68	74
Bg 33277	ADP	24	11*	18	20
	AP	27	21	10*	23
Bi 25611	ADP	3*	26*	11	7

#Elevated levels were determined in serum samples from 65 LJP, 67 ADP and 84 AP patients. Those levels > $\overline{X}$ + 2 S.D. of 82 normal subjects were considered to be elevated.
*Significantly different (p<0.05) than other subclass responses.

Response to Outer Envelope Antigens. The relationship between the amount of antibody to whole cell versus OEA response is seen in Table IV. Note that from 60-200% of the IgG antibody to the intact bacteria is directed towards the OEA. This suggests that some enrichment of the antigens to which the host responds is accomplished in the OEA preparations and is consistent with an active host response to a bacterial infection.

Table IV. Serum IgG antibody to OEA and bacteria.

Microorganism	IgG Antibody (ng/ml) Intact Bacteria@	OEA	%+	Corr. Coef.	p<
Aa Y4 (b)	465 ± 128*	1103 ± 226	237	0.771	0.01
Bg 33277	296 ± 156	183 ± 39	62	0.857	0.01
Bi 25611	297 ± 29	304 ± 61	102	0.714	0.02
Ec 23834	188 ± 55	195 ± 13	104	0.643	0.05
Wr 33238	356 ± 22	433 ± 97	122	0.600	0.05

@Plates were coated with 3-10 ug/well and 3 ug/well of protein for the intact bacteria and OEA, respectively.
+Percentage of antibody to bacteria accounted for by response to S-i ('outer membrane') of OEA.
*Mean ± S.E.M. of 6 samples for each microorganism.
#Spearman Rank Correlation Coefficient comparing intact bacteria to OEA responses for each microorganism.

Antigen Specificity of Response to A. actinomycetemcomitans. Immunoblotting was utilized to examine the specificity of the antibody response to Aa OEA. The OEA were separated (SDS-PAGE) and the antigens were transferred and detected on the blots by probing for IgG, IgA, IgM, and all four subclasses of IgG. A representative serum from an Aa infected periodontal disease patient is presented in figure 1. As can be seen, there are unique antigenic moieties that are primarily detected by restricted isotypes and/or subclasses (Aab120, 95, 75/80). In contrast, certain of the antigens or antigen-complexes exhibit a generalized response pattern across the isotype and subclasses (Aab68/70, 48/50). This observation was consistently found throughout the approximately 50 patients examined.

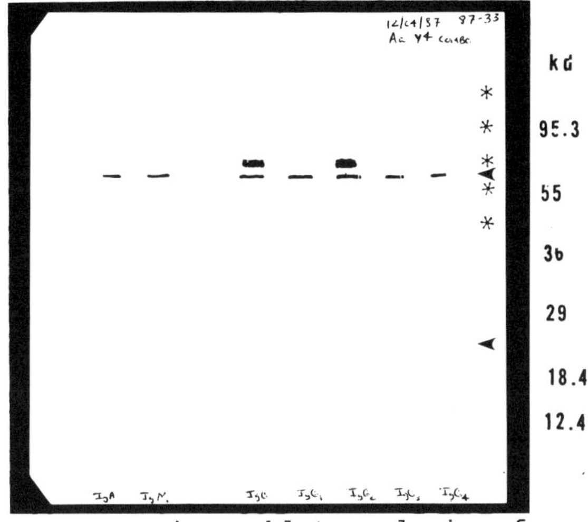

Fig. 1. Western immunoblot analysis of serum antibody specificities to A. actinomycetemcomitans OEA. Lanes were probed for antibody of specific isotype and subclass as labeled. Molecular weight markers are labeled and the arrows indicate the position of goat marker antibodies. Antigens described in the text are signified by the asterisks.

Avidity of Human Antibody Responses. In order to measure the strength of binding, or avidity of the various antibodies to selected test bacteria, we determined an "Avidity Index" (AI). These AIs were also compared to values from serum obtained from nonhuman primates (NhP) that were actively immunized with Aa or Bg. Table IV shows that those sera from periodontitis patients had significantly higher AIs than sera from normal subjects and at least with respect to Bg, the indices were within the range of the immunized NhP.

Table V. Avidity indices of human serum antibodies to periodontopathic bacteria.

Microorganism	Species	Category	Avidity Index
Aa Y4 (b)	Human	Periodontitis	1.42*
	Human	Normal	1.08*
	NhP	Immune	2.33
Bg 33277	Human	Periodontitis	3.09#
	Human	Normal	1.53#
Bg 3079.03	NhP	Immune	3.27

*,# Matched symbols were significantly different at $p<0.05$ and $p<0.025$, respectively, for 4 and 5 periodontitis sera using a Mann-Whitney-U test.

Longitudinal Studies of Serum Antibody Specificities in Periodontitis Patients. Twenty-two periodontitis (4 LJP, 5 ADP, 13 AP) patients were followed clinically, microbiologically and immunologically for a period of up to 5 years. During this interval there were 44 episodes of active disease

(12) with a range of 0.4-2.2 episodes per year and 14/22 patients had multiple episodes. Upon identification of an active disease episode the patient was treated (12). Nine of the 14 patients exhibited a maintenance of or increase in serum IgG antibody to the same microorganism during each active episode (Table VI). The remaining 5 patients showed a significant increase in serum IgG antibody to different bacteria associated with active disease.

Table VI. Longitudinal changes in serum IgG antibodies to periodontal disease-associated microorganisms.

Initial Elevated Response	Elevated During Active Disease	No. of Patients
Aa (b)*, Ec373	Aa (b), Ec373	2
Aa (b)	Aa (b)	3
Bg	Bg	2
Bg, Bi	Bg, Bi	2
Bg	Bi	1
Fn	Bg	1
Bg	Bg, Wr	1
Bi	Ec373	1
Wr	Wr, Bg	1

* Aa (b) = *A. actinomycetemcomitans* Y4, Ec373 = *E. corrodens* 373, Bg = *B. gingivalis* 33277, Bi = *B. intermedius* 25611, Fn = *F. nucleatum*, and Wr = *W. recta*.

Discussion

This report has attempted to distinguish between the production of systemic antibody following induction by specific antigens or bacteria, and the ability of polyclonal B cell activation to account for experimental data showing systemic antibodies to periodontal-disease associated bacteria. Previous studies have shown some correlations between the elevated systemic antibody and the detection of the homologous bacteria in the subgingival flora (5,13,14). In addition, cross-sectional studies generally show an agreement between the percentage of infected patients and the percentage of patients with elevated antibodies to the particular microorganisms (4,15) in different types of periodontitis. This evidence supports the concept that the elevated serum antibodies are elicited by a specific antigenic stimulus; however, there is generally little information available that unequivocally demonstrates the presence of the agent that has elicited these antibodies.

The data presented in this report further support previous observations that the elevated serum antibodies in periodontitis patients to specific microorganisms are the result of specific stimulation of the immune system by these microorganisms. The data are at variance with the presence of polyclonal B cell activators as primary agents in the antibody responses observed. We summarize our observations which support a direct antigen-antibody response in periodontitis with the following points:

1) Antibodies in the human serum not only react with individual bacteria, but in many cases appear to recognize unique antigens among the of *A. actinomycetemcomitans*, *B. gingivalis* and *B. intermedius* (Table 1). Two ubiquitous oral microorganisms, *F. nucleatum* and *A. viscosus*, which contain PBA's cannot remove this antibody. *It is difficult to explain the presence of antibody responses to antigens that are unique among members of the same species, which are elicited by PBA's or which have major cross-reactive moieties in more distantly related bacteria.* If PBA's are primary constituents of the immune response, it would seem more likely to find antibody responses to a few antigens with significant cross-reactions among the oral bacteria.

2) The distribution of IgG and IgM antibody isotype levels (Table II) and elevations in IgG subclasses (Table III) vary among individual patients and disease categories to different microorganisms. If the antibody responses in the patients were primarily associated with PBA's, similar amounts (i.e. either high or low levels) of antibody reactive with the bacteria would be expected. *The present observations do not support a mechanism by which polyclonal activation in a nonspecific manner could account for the immune response variability in the patients. The data is consistent with a specific induction of the antibody.*

3) A major antibody response to the microorganisms is directed to the S-i portion (Table IV) and the S-s portion (data not shown) of the OEA. While the response to S-i and S-s are not mutually exclusive antibody responses, immunoblotting has identified some unique antigen specificities in these preparations for each microorganism. Thus, a summation of the antibody levels showed that with all microorganisms, the OEA were enriched for antigens to which the hosts responded. If PBA's are important in inducing a nonspecific response in the disease, reactivity to a variety of cell antigens would be expected and the major responses would be directed towards substances containing cross-reactive epitopes among numerous microorganisms. *The fact that the primary response was specific and directed towards OEA is consistent with classic host responses to bacterial infections.*

4) The detailed antigenic specificity of the host antibody response varied among *A. actinomycetemcomitans* responsive patients and demonstrated restricted Ig isotypes and subclasses (Figure 1). PBA induction of a systemic response to the bacteria should be manifest by similar antigen response patterns among the isotypes/subclasses. In addition, PBA's are generally associated with the induction of primarily IgM responses. *The uniqueness of the response pattern and the breadth of reactivity among the isotypes is inconsistent with a polyclonal activation as the common factor in the patients and is readily explainable by specific elicitation of the antibody.*

5) The avidity of the host antibody response to the intact bacteria is high and is within the range of actively immunized non-human primate antibody (Table V), which supports an active mature immune response to specific infection with *A. actinomycetemcomitans*. Generally, polyclonally activated antibody is of relatively low avidity.

6) Between 200 and 300 different bacterial species colonize the subgingival plaque. Longitudinal studies have shown that elevations in systemic antibody are distinctive and usually limited to one or a few microorganisms (Table IV). In addition, multiple phases of active disease are associated with continuing elevations to the same microorganism, or an acquisition of an elevated response to a new bacterial species. These results are consistent with specific responses to specific infections, and it would appear that multiple episodes in two-thirds of the patients are associated with the same microorganism. The presence and activity of PBA in the plaque should induce responses to numerous bacterial antigens, and random changes in the responses could be expected. This is not the case.

Acknowledgements

This work was supported by U.S.P.H.S. grants DE-07809 and DE-04881 and NIDR contract DE-52558. We thank Dr. A.D. Haffajee and S.S. Socransky (Forsyth Dental Center) for collection of clinical results from some of the patients used in this report and Dr. R.C. Page (University of Washington) for supplying some of the serum samples used in the analyses. We would like to thank M.J. Steffen, M.N. Sandoval and C. Herrera for expert technical assistance in the performance of the assays. We also thank E. Irizarry and S. Ross for assistance in preparation of the manuscript.

References

1. EBERSOLE, J.L.; TAUBMAN, M.A.; SMITH, D.J.; GENCO, R.J., and FREY, D.E.: Human immune responses to oral microorganisms. I. Association of localized juvenile periodontitis (LJP) with serum antibody responses to *Actinobacillus actinomycetemcomitans*. Clin. Exp. Immunol. 47: 43-52 (1982).
2. GENCO, R.J.; SLOTS, J.; MOUTON, C., and MURRAY, P.: Systemic immune responses to oral anaerobic organisms; in LAMBE, GENCO, and MAYBERRY-CARSON, Anaerobic bacteria: selected topics; pp. 277-293 (Plenum Publishing Corp., New York 1980).
3. NAITO, Y.; OKUDA, K., and TAKAZOE, I.: Immunoglobulin G response to subgingival gram-negative bacteria in human subjects. Infect. Immun. 45:47-51 (1984).
4. TEW, J.G.; MARSHALL, D.R.; MOORE, W.E.; BEST, A.M.; PALCANIS, K.G., and RANNEY, R.R.: Serum antibody reactive with predominant organisms in the subgingival flora of young adults with generalized severe periodontitis. Infect. Immun. 48: 303-311 (1985).

5. EBERSOLE, J.L.; TAUBMAN, M.A.; SMITH, D.J.; FREY, D.E.; HAFFAJEE, A.D., and SOCRANSKY, S.S.: Human serum antibody responses to oral microorganisms. IV. Correlation with homologous infection. Oral Microbiol. Immunol. 2:53-59 (1987).
6. BICK, P.H.; CARPENTER, A.B.; HOLDEMAN, L.V.; MILLER, G.A.; RANNEY, R.R.; PALCANIS, K.G., and TEW, J.G.: Polyclonal B-cell activation induced by extracts of gram-negative bacteria isolated from periodontally diseased sites. Infect. Immun. 34:43-49 (1981).
7. EBERSOLE, J.L.; TAUBMAN, M.A.; SMITH, D.J., and HAFFAJEE, A.D.: Effect of subgingival scaling on systemic antibody responses to oral microorganisms. Infect. Immun. 48:534-539 (1985).
8. EBERSOLE, J.L.; TAUBMAN, M.A.; SMITH, D.J., and FREY, D.E.: Human immune responses to oral microorganisms; Patterns of systemic antibody levels to Bacteroides species. Infect. Immun. 51:507-513 (1986).
9. EBERSOLE, J.L.; FREY, D.E.; TAUBMAN, M.A., and SMITH, D.J.: Human serum antibody responses to oral microorganisms. V. Quantitative relationships between IgG antibody levels in periodontal disease. Clin. Exp. Immunol. (submitted).
10. PULLEN, G.R.; FITZGERALD, M.G., and HOSKING, C.S.: Antibody avidity determination by ELISA using thiocyanate elution. J. Immunol. Methods 86:83-87 (1986).
11. RAPP, V.J.; MUNSON, R.J., and ROSS, R.F.: Outer membrane protein profiles of Haemophilus pleuropneumoniae. Infect. Immun. 52:414-420 (1986).
12. HAFFAJEE, A.D.; SOCRANKSY, S.S., and GOODSON, J.M.: Comparison of different data analyses for detecting changes in attachment level J. Clin. Periodontol. 10:298-310 (1983).
13. EBERSOLE, J.L.; FREY, D.E.; TAUBMAN, M.A.; HAFFAJEE, A.D., and SOCRANSKY, S.S.: Dynamics of systemic antibody responses in periodontal disease. J. Perio. Res. 22:184-186 (1987).
14. WILLIAMS, B.L.; EBERSOLE, J.L.; SPEKTOR, M.D., and PAGE, R.C.: Assessment of serum antibody patterns and analysis of subgingival microflora of members of a family with a high prevalence of early-onset periodontitis. Infect. Immun. 49:742-750 (1985).
15. ZAMBON, J.J.: Actinobacillus actinomycetemcomitans in human periodontal disease. J. Clin. Periodontol. 12:1-20, (1985).

Author's Address

Jeffrey L. Ebersole, Ph.D., Department of Periodontics, School of Dentistry, The University of Texas Health Science Center at San Antonio, 7703 Floyd Curl Dr., San Antonio, TX 78284-7894 (USA).

Periodontology Today. Int. Congr., Zürich 1988, pp. 178–186 (Karger, Basel 1988)

Immunosuppression: An Etiopathogenic Mechanism[1]

Bruce J. Shenker

Department of Pathology, University of Pennsylvania School of Dental Medicine, Philadelphia, PA, USA

Introduction

The nature and contribution of the immune system to the pathogenesis of periodontal infection are poorly understood. A vast literature supports the view that the immune system plays a role in limiting bacterial infection in the gingival region (referenced in 1). Therefore, it is not surprising that there is evidence suggesting that immunologic dysfunction may contribute to susceptibility and progression of periodontal disease (reviewed in 1). Additionally, there are several mechanisms by which periodontal pathogens may evade or directly perturb the host's immune response. It is in this context that we have initiated studies to evaluate putative periodontal pathogens for their ability to alter human lymphocyte responsiveness (reviewed in 1).

We have determined that several microorganisms produce factors capable of depressing human lymphocyte responsiveness (Table I). There is a wide range of potency (i.e., orders of magnitude) among the immunoinhibitory species and it is interesting to note that each of the active organisms appear to function through different mechanisms. For example, *Treponema denticola* inhibits lymphocyte responsiveness by affecting monocytes. Monocytes, in turn, produce substances such as prostaglandins and hydrogen peroxide which have been shown to inhibit a wide range of lymphocyte responses both *in vitro* and *in vivo*. On the other hand, *Centipeda periodontii* selectively kills monocytes and lymphocytes (preferentially B cells) (2). Cytotoxicity involves metabolic alterations (possibly inhibition of protein synthesis) rather than cytolysis as a consequence of damage to the plasma membrane. To date, the immunosuppressive agent derived from *Actinobacillus*

[1]Supported by USPHS DE06014, DE00170 and DE07118.

TABLE I. Suspected periodontal pathogens tested for immunosuppressive potential.

Organism	ID_{50}*
Actinobacillus actinomycetemcomitans	0.03
Oral Treponemes:	
T. denticola	0.50
T. vincentii	-
T. socranskii	50.00
Centipeda periodontii	40.00
Fusobacterium nucleatum	0.75
Veilonella parvula	70.00
Veilonella atypica	100.00
Veilonella dispar	150.00
Capnocytophaga sputigena	-
Capnocytophaga ochracea	40.00
Haemophilus aphrophilus	-
Leptotrichia buccalis	-
Bacteroides spp.:	
B. assacharolyticus	2.00
B. intermedius	6.00
B. melaninogenicus	7.50
B. gingivalis	-
B. loeschii	10.00
B. endodontalis	2.00

*Dose of crude sonic extract (μg protein/ml) required to cause 50% inhibition of Con A activation of human lymphocytes. (-) denotes no effect at concentrations tested.

actinomycetemcomitans (Aa) has been most extensively studied. The purpose of this paper is to present our recent observations concerning the immunosuppressive properties of Aa and relate these findings to an etiologic role in the pathogenesis of periodontal disease.

Aa is a gram-negative, capnophilic bacterium, closely linked to the etiology of localized juvenile periodontitis [4; (LJP)]. Although the mechanism by which Aa might contribute to the development of periodontal disease is not clear, it is known that this organism produces several biologically active mediators. Among these are a leukotoxin capable of killing human neutrophils and monocytes and an immunosuppressive factor [1,3); (ISF)]. As described below, the Aa ISF appears to function via the activation of T-suppressor cells.

Methods

Human lymphocytes were isolated from heparinized blood of healthy donors by bouyant density centrifugation according to methods previously described (2). Following isolation, lymphocytes were suspended to 2 x 10^6 cells/ml in RPMI 1640 containing 2% human AB serum and antibiotics. Lymphocyte cultures were established (with and without ISF); mitogenic and antigenic responses were assessed by ^{3}H-TdR incorporation following a 4 or 6 day incubation, respectively (2). Immunoglobulin production was assessed by measuring IgG and IgM in 8 day culture supernatants by ELISA (1). ISF was prepared from Aa strain 652 and partially purified by ion exchange chromatography as previously described (1).

T-suppressor cells were generated and assayed in a two stage assay system. First, freshly isolated lymphocytes (2 x 10^6) were placed in 1 ml cultures containing medium (control), 10 μg concanavalin A (Con A) or ISF. Following a 48 hr incubation, the nonadherent cells were recovered, washed and X-irradiated (1500 rads). In some instances cells were then treated with monoclonal antibodies against subsets of T-cells (OKT 4 and OKT 8, Orthodiagnostics, Raritan, NJ) and complement. The cells were suspended to 1 x 10^5 cells/ml and suppressor cell activity evaluated by placing these cells into a secondary assay system. The suppressor cells were tested for their ability to inhibit the responsiveness of autologous cells; phytohemagglutinin (PHA; 0.8 μg)-induced ^{3}H-thymidine incorporation was measured following a 3 day incubation in round bottomed microculture plates.

Enumeration of T-suppressor cells was performed by establishing cultures as described above. Following the indicated incubation period, the cells were recovered and the total number of cells enumerated by counting in a Coulter counter. The number of T-helper and T-suppressor cells was determined by rosette formation with insolubilized monoclonal antibodies (Quantigen Assay; BioRad, Richmond, CA).

Results and Discussion

The ISF is a heat-labile protein with a molecular weight of 50,000 daltons. As shown in figure 1, it causes dose-dependent inhibition of lymphocyte responsiveness. Inhibition of lymphocyte protein, RNA and DNA synthesis as well as lymphokine and immunoglobulin production is seen in response to either mitogen or antigen stimulation (1). The ISF has no effect on lymphocyte viability. A series of kinetic experiments were carried out to determine the conditions that result in maximal suppression. The results indicate that the ISF interacts rapidly and irreversibly with lymphocytes; furthermore, the inhibitory agent has to be present 90 min prior to the addition of stimulus. It was surprising, however, to find that suppression was not manifested until 72 hr after initiation of cell culture; responsiveness continued to decline at 96 and 120 hr (1). These conflicting findings between the early requirement for ISF and the delayed observance of suppression suggested that these effects were dependent upon activation of a suppressor cell population. As described below, we have been able to demonstrate that the Aa ISF activates T-suppressor cells both in vitro and in vivo.

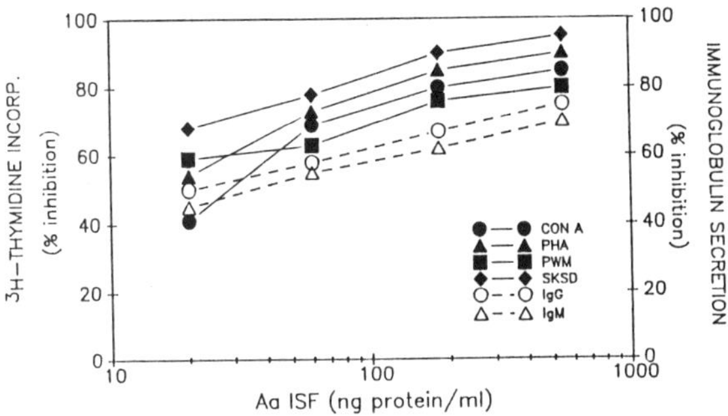

Fig.1. ISF inhibition of mitogen and antigen induced proliferation and Ig production. Abbreviations: concanavalin A (Con A), phtyohemagglutinin (PHA), pokeweed mitogen (PWM) and streptokinase/streptodornase. (SKSD)

We first demonstrated that the ISF activates T-suppressor cells by employing a co-culture assay system. In this assay, lymphocytes are first incubated for 48 hr in the presence of medium (control), Con A (a known activator of T-suppressor cells) or Aa-ISF. After incubation, lymphocytes were washed, irradiated and then tested for their ability to alter the PHA-responsiveness of fresh autologous cells in a second (indicator) culture system. As shown in figure 2A, cells initially exposed to different concentrations of Aa ISF, and Con A to a lesser degree, significantly inhibited autologous cell proliferation. The role of T-suppressor cells was more directly confirmed by depleting the lymphocyte cultures of suppressor cells with anti-T-suppressor cell monoclonal antibodies (OKT8) and complement. These depleted cultures were then added to the second culture system as before. As shown in figure 2B, lymphoid suspensions depleted of suppressor cells were no longer able to inhibit the PHA responsiveness of fresh autologous cells. As a control, lymphocytes were treated with an anti-T-helper cell (OKT 4) monoclonal antibody; the cells remaining after this treatment retained their inhibitory properties. In addition to activating T- suppressor cells, the ISF induces T-suppressor cell proliferation (figure 3). Enumeration of T-helper and T-suppressor cells at 24 hr intervals following exposure to ISF indicates that the number of T-suppressor cells increases

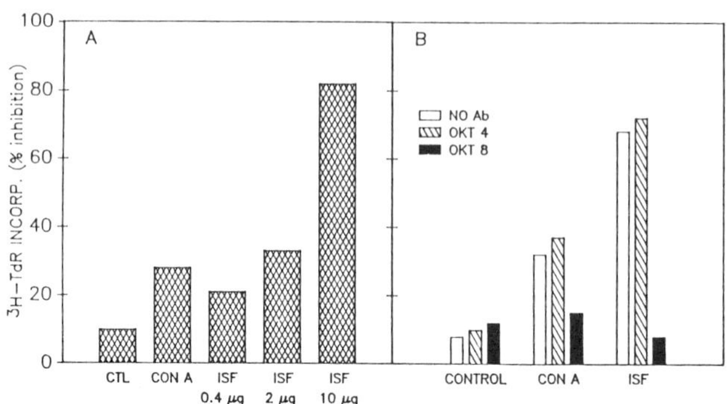

Fig.2. Activation of T-suppressor cells by ISF. Panel A shows the dose-dependent activation of suppressor cells by Aa ISF. Panel B shows the effects of cell depletion by either OKT4 or OKT8 antibody; cells were exposed to 10μg ISF/ml.

between 4 and 6 days. The absolute number of T-helper cells was not altered, hence, the T-helper/ T-suppressor ratios also decreased in these cultures.

In addition to its in vitro activity, the Aa-ISF acts in vivo as well. Rats given IP injections of the inhibitory agent exhibited depressed splenocyte and blood lymphocyte responsiveness (both B and T cell). These animals also showed an increase in the number of functional suppressor cells in the spleen. Using an in vivo correlate of the T-suppressor assay (Table II), spleen cells from ISF treated animals, but not from control animals, inhibited in vitro proliferation of splenocytes obtained from untreated syngeneic animals.

Taken together, these findings strongly implicate T-suppressor cells in the inhibition of lymphocyte responsiveness by Aa-ISF. However, we should point out that this mechanism may not account for the entire immunosuppressive abil-

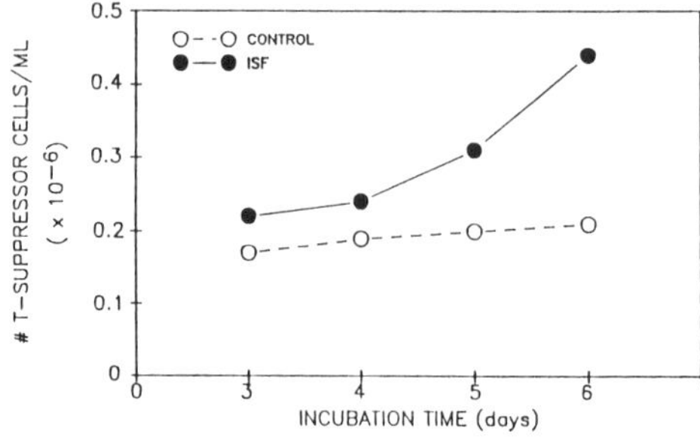

Fig. 3. ISF induced proliferation of T-suppressor cells. Human lymphocytes were incubated with either medium (control) or 2μg ISF/ml and evaluated as described.

TABLE II. *In vivo* activation of suppressor lymphocytes by Aa.

Culture conditions	^{3}H-Thymidine Incorporation* cpm	% inhibition
Responder cells (R) alone	7540	0
R + cells from control animals**	9599	0
R + cells from ISF-treated animals**	3620	52

*Tritiated thymidine incorporation in response to Con A.
**Lymphocytes were harvested from rat spleens 24 hr after ip injection of PBS (control) or ISF. Cells were x-irradiated (1500 rads) prior to placement in culture.

ity of Aa. For example, the Aa leukotoxin can also depress lymphocyte responsiveness (1). Toxin-mediated suppression was the result of: 1) killing and hence depletion of monocytes which are required for lymphocyte responsiveness and 2) direct, but non-lethal, effects on lymphocytes. Similarly, the ISF may function via more than one mode of action. Recent advances in the purification (to homogeneity) of the ISF as well as the generation of monoclonal antibodies will allow us to further address these questions.

Numerous studies suggest a strong association between Aa infection and the etiology of LJP (reviewed in 4). Although the immunologic mechanism(s) involved in periodontal disease, in general, and LJP, in particular, is not clearly defined, there is substantial evidence that impaired host defense mechanisms may contribute to the disease process. Aa, in particular, may be able to upset anti-bacterial defense mechanisms in the gingival crevice. In this regard, we have recently initiated a longitudinal clinical study[2] on the pathogenesis of LJP. The aim of this study is to follow healthy siblings in LJP families in the expectation that they will get LJP. During this study we are measuring clinical, microbiological and immunological parameters and documenting changes as these individuals convert to disease status. Repetitive assessments (every 3 months) are performed on these subjects in order to get accurate baseline data on their immunologic competence. By doing this before, during and after the onset of disease, we shall be in the position to document the earliest changes associated with the pathogenesis of LJP. This will also allow us to relate levels of immunologic responsiveness with the onset of infection. Although we have only recently initiated these studies, we have had one at risk subject "breakdown" or convert to disease status. As shown in figure 4, just prior to the onset

[2]Periodontal Diseases Research Center, Univ. of Penn.

of disease (between visits 1 and 2), this patient showed signs of immunologic abnormalities including a low T-helper/ T-suppressor cell ratio which was accompanied by decreased mitogen and antigen responsiveness. Thereafter, these parameters returned to "normal" levels. It should be pointed out that at the time we detected these depressed responses, Dr. Jorgen Slots was also able to isolate Aa from the gingival crevice[3]. Although preliminary, these observations tend to provide indirect support for a role for immunologic dysfunction in the pathogenesis of LJP. Hence, Aa may conceivably be capable of causing immunologic dysfunction (local and/or systemic) in patients who harbor the organism.

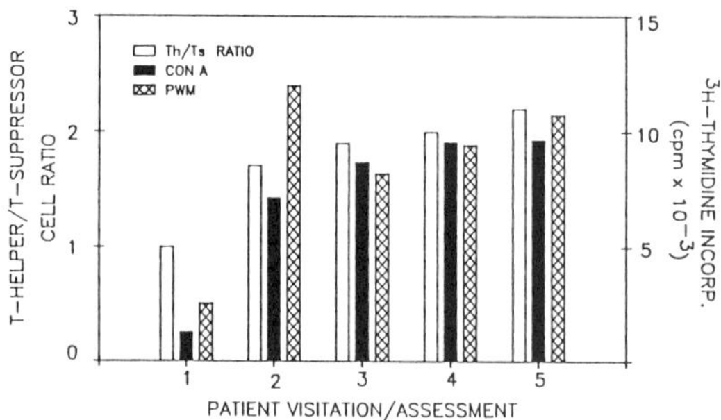

Fig.4. Immunologic competence during onset of LJP. The patient was evaluated for T-helper (Th)/ T-suppressor (Ts) cell ratio as well as mitogen responsiveness at 3 month intervals. The subject developed LJP between visits 1 and 2.

There has been some reluctance, however, to accepting the possibility that immunologic dysfunctions play an etiologic role in periodontal disease. The basis for this hesitancy is that some patients exhibit high antibody titers and sensitized T-cells to suspected periodontal pathogens. The contradictory findings of immune dysfunction and elevated antibody titers (or T cell responsiveness) are not uncommon in infectious disease. For example, acquired immunodeficiency syndrome (AIDS) patients simultaneously display gross signs of immunodeficiency while also eliciting an immune response to the causative agent, human immunodeficiency virus. Similarly, periodontal patients may also be afflicted with immunologic abnormalities (but on a smaller or local scale than the more severely ill AIDS patients) and yet generate an immune response to oral pathogens. Such abnormalities might permit an immune response to develop, but it may be depressed in magnitude or delayed in onset. Alternatively, the response may be against wrong or irrelevant antigens; this

[3]J. Slots, Abstract, Int'l Assoc. Dent. Res., 1988

would not benefit the host in any appreciable way.

Therefore, any working model for the pathogenesis of periodontal disease must take into account several conflicting clinical findings. The first involves reports of both active as well as depressed immune responses in apparently similar patient populations. This may be the result of mis-groupings of patients exhibiting similar clinical manifestations but at different stages of disease progression. Alternatively, these findings may represent heterogeneity amongst the patient population whose conditions are due to different etiologic or pathogenetic events. The second paradox relates to reports of persistent infection in the face of an active immune response. This contradiction is more difficult to account for. One possible model that may help resolve these antithetical observations and incorporate current knowledge regarding the immunomodulatory properties of oral pathogens is presented below.

In this model we propose that the development of disease depends heavily upon the outcome of the initial interaction or contact of pathogen(s) with the host's defense systems. If this interaction leads to a "productive" and rapid immune response, then the organism should be contained and ultimately eliminated without the production of disease. However, if this interaction fails to produce an "appropriate" response (qualitatively or quantitatively) then the microorganism would be free to colonize and persist in the gingival crevice and perhaps even invade the periodontal tissue. Failure of the host's response may be due to several factors: 1) inability to recognize the pathogen as a result of genetic and/ or environmental factors; 2) subversion and/or evasion of the immune response by the microbe itself. As described, several suspected oral pathogens produce immunoinhibitory factors; if these agents act _in vivo_, they could impede the development of humoral and/or cell mediated immune responses. As a result, the host would be left immunologically compromised (particularly at the local level) and infection by the initiating organism as well as by secondary or succeeding microorganisms could proceed. Consequently, disease or tissue injury would occur initially as a result of insult by the microbes themselves. In this regard, several bacterial factors (enzymes, toxins, etc) have been described which could conceivably cause tissue injury. Since many periodontal patients eventually develop a detectable humoral and/or cellular immune response to infection, the immunosuppressive state must be a relatively short-lived phenomenon. Regardless of its intensity, a "delayed" immune response may be unable to control infection. This failure may occur because sufficient time has elapsed to allow high numbers of organisms (antigenic overload) to populate the crevice. A delay in the onset of the immune response could also result in antibody production in the presence of antigen excess; such relationships between antigen and antibody concentration could result in activation of immunopathologic-mediated pathways of tissue injury. Under these conditions the immune system would then play a destructive role in the progression of disease.

Despite recent advances in our understanding of periodontal disease, the role of the immune system in these inflammatory disorders remains poorly defined. Recent studies strongly suggest a role for altered host defenses as a possible underlying mechanism. If this hypothesis is valid, the immune response so often documented in cross-sectional clinical studies of established disease only represents a single moment in the duration of an evolving disease. It is likely that such studies could miss temporary or transient depressions in immunologic reactivity. The duration and extent of this delay may be critical to the establishment of infection and disease. Therefore, we propose that one of the determinants contributing to the etiology of periodontal disease is the time interval from first exposure to the pathogen to the production and delivery of "sufficient" amounts of functional antibodies and possibly T cells to sites of infection. Additionally, individual susceptibility to disease may be related to sensitivity to the effects of microbial virulence factors such as the immunoinhibitory agents. In summary, we see the immune system as playing a dynamic role in the pathogenesis of periodontal disease; one that changes with the course of the disease. Such dynamics may also help account for the cyclical or episodic nature of periodontal disease progression.

References

1. SHENKER, B.J.: Immunologic dysfunction in the pathogenesis of periodontal disease. J. Clin. Periodontol. 14: 489-98 (1987).
2. SHENKER, B.J., BERTHOLD, P., DOUGHERTY, P. and PORTER, K.: Immunosuppressive effects of Centipeda periodontii: selective cytotoxicity for lymphocytes and monocytes. Infect. Immun. 55: 2332-40 (1987).
3. TAICHMAN, N.S., DEAN, R.T. and SANDERSON, C.J.: Biochemical and morphological characterization of killing of human monocytes by a leukotoxin derived from Actinobacillus actinomycetemcomitans. Infect. Immun. 28: 258-68 (1980).
4. ZAMBON, J.: Actinobacillus actinomycetemcomitans in human periodontal disease. J. Clin. Periodontol. 12:1-20 (1985).

Bruce J. Shenker, Ph.D., Department of Pathology, University of Pennsylvania School of Dental Medicine, 4010 Locust Street, Philadelphia, PA 19104-6002 (USA)

Periodontology Today. Int. Congr., Zürich 1988, pp. 187–195 (Karger, Basel 1988)

What Can in vitro Lymphocyte Data Tell Us about the Pathogenesis of Periodontal Diseases?

Denis F. Mangan

Departement of Dental Research, University of Rochester, Rochester, New York, USA

Immunity and Immunopathology

Excessive or inappropriate reactions to an antigen cause a spectrum of clinical symptoms ranging in severity from mild, brief inflammation to asphyxia and death. These hypersensitivity reactions occur only after prior exposure to the antigen and are mediated by immunoglobulins (Igs) or by direct damage by activated lymphocytes and macrophage.

The immune response, whether protective or harmful, involves complex interactions between cells (lymphocytes and macrophage) and soluble factors (Igs and lymphokines). Because of this complexity, the immune system must be experimentally dissected in order to understand the role of each component in the immune response. In vivo dissection of the immune system occurs in "experiments of nature" in which one or more specific components of the immune system is lacking in the host. A classic example of this is the nude mouse or rat, which lacks mature T cells yet has normal B cell function (25).

Much information on lymphocyte biology has accrued from dissecting the immune system in vitro. In vitro methods limit complexity by defining and controlling variable parameters. Lymphocytes which are stimulated in vitro with an antigen undergo enhanced cell growth, and Ig and lymphokine secretion. These responses are considered to represent the events which occur when lymphocytes encounter antigen in vivo. Lymphocytes from animals sensitized to an antigen are activated upon subsequent exposure to that antigen in tissue culture, whereas lymphocytes from control, non-sensitized animals remain unactivated when cultured with the antigen. A similar in vitro scenario occurs with human lymphocytes shortly after infection or vaccination.

Methodology for in vitro lymphocyte studies

The basic strategy for in vitro lymphocyte experiments is shown in the FIGURE. Human lymphocytes are obtained from peripheral blood or inflamed gingival tissue, whereas rodent lymphocytes are usually obtained from the spleen or lymph nodes since blood is difficult to obtain in sufficient quantities. Solid tissues are minced and digested with collagenase to release lymphocytes from the connective tissue. Single cell suspensions are then centrifuged on a density gradient (e.g. Ficoll-Hypaque™) which separates mononuclear cells (lymphocytes + monocytes) from contaminating RBCs, neutrophils, or epithelial cells. Monocytes/macrophage are reported to suppress activation of lymphocyte by bacterial components (12) and therefore are removed by adherence to plastic, glass, or Sephadex™ beads prior to culturing the lymphocytes. Lymphocytes are cultured without further manipulation, or are separated into B and T cell-rich populations in order to study regulatory effects by the two subsets (2). Lymphocytes are typically cultured in RPMI 1640 tissue culture media containing 10-20% autologous or fetal bovine serum. The test stimulant is added to the cultures, and the cultures are incubated for an appropriate length of time (typically 3-9 da.) to obtain the desired activation response. Lymphocyte functions routinely assayed in vitro include blastogenesis (DNA synthesis), lymphokine secretion, cytotoxicity, and Ig production.

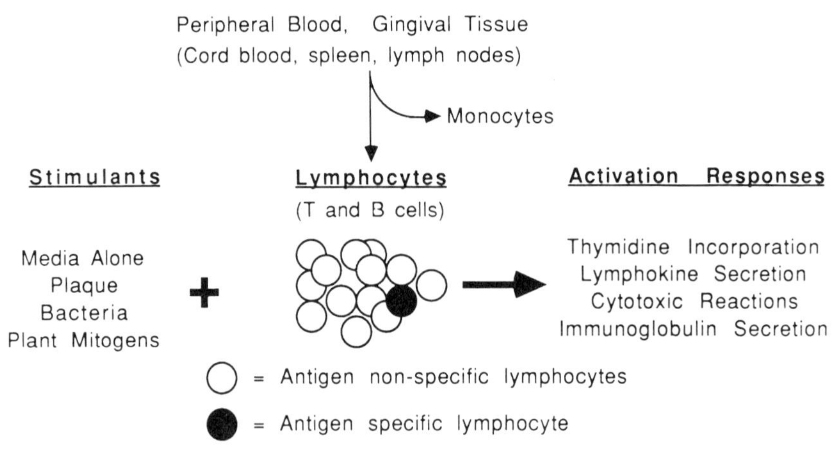

FIGURE. Basic strategy for in vitro lymphocyte studies.

In vitro lymphocyte data and periodontal disease

In general, four approaches are used to evaluate the role of the immune system in periodontitis: 1) compare and contrast healthy controls and patients with varying types and severity of periodontal disease, 2) compare periodontitis patients before and after therapy, 3) measure responses from healthy subjects undergoing experimental gingivitis, and 4) examine plaque-induced stimulation and regulation of lymphocytes from healthy subjects. In vitro lymphocyte responses from these studies suggest that lymphocytes are stimulated as well as suppressed by subgingival plaque.

Blastogenesis

When antigen-specific B and T cells are cultured with the homologous antigen in vitro, antigen interacts with receptors on the surface of the lymphocytes causing the cells to undergo blastogenesis (i.e. an increase in size, "blast formation", and synthesis of DNA). Antigen-specific lymphocytes cultured with unrelated antigens remain quiescent. Blastogenesis also occurs when lymphocytes are cultured with mitogens which non-specifically activate multiple clones of lymphocytes. The incorporation of radio-labeled (^{3}H-)thymidine, a DNA constituent, is commonly used as a measurement of the quantity of newly synthesized DNA and thus a measurement of lymphocyte stimulation. Blastogenesis itself is probably not a pathogenic response in vivo, but does indicate lymphocyte activation which may be associated with tissue destruction in vivo (see Brandtzaeg, this volume).

Early studies suggested that blastogenic responses induced by plaque bacteria correlated with the incidence and severity of periodontal diseases (6; for review see 16). However, subsequent reports clearly indicated that plaque bacteria induce equivalent blastogenic responses from orally healthy subjects and periodontitis patients (4, 8, 22). Thus, both healthy and diseased individuals appear to be sensitized to plaque bacteria antigens. Since hypersensitivity reactions occur after the host has been sensitized, these findings suggest that healthy individuals somehow suppress harmful immune responses.

Several reports indicated that plaque has suppressive effects on the host immune system. Patients undergoing rigorous oral hygiene to remove subgingival plaque demonstrate enhanced blastogenic responses after therapy (1, 10). Furthermore, in experimental gingivitis studies, subjects with fast-accumulating plaque have decreased blastogenic responses compared with subjects with slow-accumulating plaque (18). These reports support in vitro studies using lymphocytes from healthy donors which clearly showed a bell-shaped, blastogenic response curve to plaque, plaque bacteria, or bacterial components.

Supraoptimal concentrations of stimulant in the cultures cause a sharp decrease in blastogenesis.

Plaque bacteria contain potent B and T cell mitogens capable of stimulating unsensitized umbilical cord blood lymphocytes and spleen cells from germ-free mice (23). Nonspecific stimulation makes it extremely difficult to assess antigen-specific activation in vitro. Thus, blastogenesis is not a useful diagnostic or prognostic indicator of periodontal disease, although the data from these studies do provide valuable information on immunostimulation and regulation by plaque bacteria.

There is one blastogenesis assay which seems to hold promise as a diagnostic tool. Lymphocytes from periodontitis patients consistently have lower blastogenic responses than do lymphocytes from healthy controls when cultured in media alone, without deliberate stimulation with plant or bacterial macromolecules (19). The blastogenesis is reported to be due to autologous mixed lymphocyte reactions (AMLR) in which T cells are activated by autologous HLA-DR positive non-T cells in the cultures (19). Low AMLR reactions represent a putative defect in immunoregulation which is speculated to have deleterious effects on the immune response in the periodontium (19).

Lymphokine production

Lymphokines are soluble, biologically active proteins produced by activated B and T lymphocytes. These proteins are involved in 1) regulation and growth of B and T lymphocytes, macrophage, and fibroblasts (e.g. interleukin [IL]-2, IL-4), 2) migration of phagocytes and lymphocytes (e.g. macrophage inhibitory factor), and 3) tissue damage and bone resorption (e.g. lymphotoxin, IL-1). Lymphokine production is therefore extremely relevant to the immunopathogenesis of periodontal diseases.

Lymphokine production induced by plaque bacteria is increased in lymphocytes from periodontitis patients compared to those of orally healthy controls (7). The amount of lymphokines produced is reported to correlate more closely with disease severity than does blastogenesis, suggesting a dissociation between these measures of lymphocyte activation. O'Neill et al. (15) isolated lymphocytes from gingival tissues and noted that the amount of cytotoxicity and lymphotoxin production is directly related to the degree of inflammation and severity of disease. Interestingly, the blood lymphocytes from these patients did not secrete lymphokines above control levels, which supports the concept of a local immune response in the gingival tissue.

Ig production

Chronically inflamed periodontitis lesions are densely infiltrated with B cells and plasma cells. Recent studies in our lab (5) indicate that activated B cells are chemokinetically attracted into filters soaked with plaque bacterial extracts, whereas T cells fail to migrate into these filters. These results suggest that plaque bacteria may contribute to the accumulation of B cells within periodontitis lesions.

Many species of bacteria isolated from subgingival plaque stimulate B cell proliferation and Ig production in vitro. The quantity of Ig produced, the large number of B cells activated, and the capacity of the bacteria to stimulate splenocytes from nude rodents (lacking mature T cells) suggest stimulation is nonspecific (i.e. polyclonal B cell activation, PBA). Moreover, adsorption of culture supernates with the stimulating bacteria has little effect on the total Ig or the antibody titers to serologically unrelated oral bacteria (13). Immunoregulation studies indicate that bacteria-induced PBA in vitro is suppressed by macrophage (12) and is regulated by T cells (2). Smith et al. (20) found that young adults with severe periodontitis are hyperresponsive to PBA mitogens in oral and non-oral bacterial extracts compared to age-matched controls. These results support the hypothesis that B cell hyperactivity is involved in the pathogenesis of severe periodontitis.

Igs mediate tissue damage via 1) IgE-mediated immediate type hypersensitivity, 2) antibody-dependent cellular cytoxicity (ADCC), or 3) immune complex formation. Although mast cells are present in the gingiva, the role of IgE in periodontitis has not been convincingly demonstrated in vivo or in vitro. Lopatin et al. (9) clearly showed that ADCC is possible in the gingiva and that antibodies to bacterial macromolecules bound to the surface of host cells mediate ADCC reactions. Furthermore, PBA activation of lymphocytes induces the production of autoimmune antibodies which might react with periodontal tissues and cause ADCC reactions (14). Whether subgingival plaque bacteria which contain PBA factors stimulate such autoimmune antibodies remains to be determined. There is little evidence for immune complex deposition in inflamed periodontal tissues (16). Although bacterial antigens and functional antibody-secreting plasma cells are present in the lesions, PBA is likely to result in the production of (relatively) low affinity antibodies which do not form stable immune complexes capable of inducing complement activation (16).

LJP patients frequently have enhanced levels of antibodies which react with *A. actinomycetemcomitans* (*AA*) (see Ebersole, this volume). A recent report (24) indicated that enhanced titers of antibodies to *AA* are produced in vitro when sensitized lymphocytes are co-stimulated with *AA* and *Fusobacterium nucleatum (FN)*, a polyclonal B cell activator. *AA* or *FN* alone induced only low levels of anti-*AA* antibodies. Therefore, enhanced Ig responses to specific oral antigens may result from the adjuvant effects of PBA factors in plaque bacteria.

Interpretation of in vitro lymphocyte data

Many experimental factors can alter lymphocyte responses in vitro. Suzuki et al. (21) showed the importance of in vitro culture conditions on blastogenesis of lymphocytes from normal controls and periodontitis patients. There was considerable variation in responses among the individuals regardless of disease status, although all subjects responded to the plaque bacteria. The optimal response occurred in cultures which were incubated for 5-8 days, in conical-shaped wells, and contained >2 x 10^6 cells/well (the cell concentration commonly used by many laboratories). Thus, a "low-responder" can be converted into a "high-responder" simply by changing the in vitro conditions.

Lymphocytes extracted from peripheral blood or inflamed gingival tissue may respond dissimilarly when cultured in vitro. O'Neill and Woodson (15) reported that blood lymphocytes fail to produce chemotactic lymphokines or undergo blastogenesis above unstimulated, baseline levels when stimulated with plaque, *Bacteroides gingivalis*, or *Actinomyces viscosus* whether or not the donors had healthy gingiva, gingivitis, or periodontitis. In contrast, gingival lymphocytes from patients with gingivitis and periodontitis (but not from healthy tissue) produced significantly higher levels of lymphokines and blastogenesis when cultured with the same stimulants. The reason for the differences in responses between blood and gingival lymphocytes is not clear. Peripheral blood and gingival tissue contain different ratios of B-to-T cells and T helper-to-T suppressor cells. This suggests a substantial difference in T cell regulation and B cell activity in the in vitro cultures (3). Moreover, immunocompetent cells are released into the circulation in highest numbers 7-14 days after sensitization (11). The point at which blood is drawn from an individual may be before or after specifically sensitized cells are released into the circulation. This may explain why there is variability in blastogenesis between individuals and between the responses from one donor on a day-to-day basis.

Host-related factors, such as age, genetic background, and health status, regulate immune responses in vitro. In syphilis and leprosy, overwhelming infection leads to anergy, tolerance or immunosuppression rather than sensitization. Therefore, disease can occur without corresponding lymphocyte responsiveness in vitro (for review, see Ref. 16).

The stimulant also plays a critical role in lymphocyte activation. As mentioned, bacteria contain a variety of antigens and polyclonal T and B cell activating factors. Lymphocyte activation in vitro cannot easily be ascribed to specific or non-specific stimulation (see 16). Patters et al. (17) noted that lymphocytes from both healthy donors and patients respond to *A. viscosus* and fail to respond to *Streptococcus sanguis*. Thus, regardless of the disease status, some bacteria fail to induce blastogenesis in vitro.

Finally, each lymphocyte activation response is regulated independently from other responses. For example, lymphocytes from patients with severe periodontitis are weakly blastogenic yet secrete increased amounts of lymphokines and are more cytotoxic compared with lymphocytes from healthy controls (7).

Therefore, only particular in vitro responses may be elevated or depressed during periodontal diseases.

Conclusion

In vitro studies show that plaque bacteria specifically and nonspecifically stimulate as well as suppress lymphocyte activation. Activated lymphocytes in the periodontium (periodontitis), synovium (arthritis), or mucosa of the bowel (inflammatory bowel disease) are associated with inflammation and tissue damage. Cytotoxic cells and lymphokines, Igs, and cell-mediated hypersensitivity reactions appear to play a role in pathogenesis of periodontal disease. The in vitro reactions do not correlate well with disease (with the possible exception of AMLR) due to in vitro experimental variables, host factors, and use of inappropriate assays. However, in vitro lymphocyte studies are necessary to dissect the immune responses to plaque bacteria. Improved in vitro models are clearly needed which more accurately resemble the in vivo environment while being carefully standardized to give reproducible and meaningful results. Multiple measures of lymphocyte activation should be used to obtain a more global view of the immune response. Modern techniques in cell biology and molecular biology will greatly aid the study of periodontal diseases. With new techniques at hand, in vitro lymphocyte studies will continue to provide valuable information on the pathogenesis of periodontal diseases.

References

1. BAKER, J.J.; WRIGHT, W.E.; CHAN, S.P., and OPPENHEIM, J.J.: Longitudinal effects of clinical therapy and the edentulous state on the transformation of lymphocytes from patients with severe periodontitis. Clin. Exp. Immunol. 34: 199-205 (1978).
2. CARPENTER, A.B.; SULLY, E.C.; RANNEY, R.R., and BICK, P.H.: T-cell regulation of polyclonal B-cell activation induced by extracts of oral bacteria associated with periodontal diseases. Infect. Immun. 43: 326-336 (1984).
3. COLE, K.L.; SEYMOUR, G.J., and POWELL, R.N.: Phenotypic and functional analysis of T cells extracted from chronically inflamed human periodontal tissues. J. Periodontol. 58: 569-573 (1987).
4. DONALDSON, S.L.; RANNEY, R.R.; BURMEISTER, J.A., and TEW, J.G.: Blastogenic responses by lymphocytes from periodontally healthy populations induced by periodontitis-associated bacteria. J. Periodontol. 53: 743-751 (1982).

5. GHORABA, N.; KRIGER, P.S., and MANGAN, D.F.: Activated B-lymphocytes migrate into filters containing *Fusobacterium nucleatum*. J. Dent. Res. 66: 188 (1987).
6. IVANYI, I., and LEHNER, T.: Stimulation of lymphocyte transformation by bacterial antigens in patients with periodontal disease. Archs. Oral Biol. 15: 1089-1096 (1970).
7. IVANYI, I.; WILTON, J.M.A., and LEHNER, T.: Cell-mediated immunity in periodontal disease; cytotoxicity, migration inhibition and lymphocyte transformation studies. Immunol. 22: 141-145 (1972).
8. KIGER, R.D.; WRIGHT, W.H., and CREAMER, H.R.: The significance of lymphocyte transformation responses to various microbial stimulants. J. Periodontol. 45: 780-785 (1974).
9. LOPATIN, D.E., and BLACKBURN, E.: Sensitization with *Fusobacterium nucleatum* targets antibody-dependent cellular cytotoxicity to mammalian cells. Infect. Immun. 52: 650-6546 (1986).
10. LOPATIN, D.E.; SMITH, F.N.; SYED, S.A., and MORRISON, E.C.: The effect of periodontal therapy on lymphocyte blastogenesis to plaque associated microorganisms. J. Periodont. Res. 18: 93-102 (1983).
11. MALLISON, S.M.; SZAKAL, A.K.; RANNEY, R.R., and TEW, J.G.: Antibody synthesis specific for nonoral antigens in inflamed gingiva. Infect. Immun. 56: 823-830 (1988).
12. MANGAN, D.F.; WON, T., and LOPATIN, D.E.: Nonspecific induction of immunoglobulin M antibodies to periodontal disease-associated microorganisms after polyclonal human B-lymphocyte activation by *Fusobacterium nucleatum*. Infect. Immun. 41: 1038-1045 (1983).
13. MANGAN, D.F.; WON, T., and LOPATIN, D.E.: Monocyte suppression of *Fusobacterium nucleatum*-induced human polyclonal B-lymphocyte activation. Infect. Immun. 46: 332-339 (1984).
14. MOLLER, E.; STROM, H., and AL-BALAGHII, S.: Role of polyclonal activation in specific immune responses. Scand. J. Immunol. 12: 177-182 (1980).
15. O'NEILL, P.A., and WOODSON, D.L.: Lymphokine production by human gingival lymphocytes. J. Periodont. Res. 21: 338-350 (1986).
16. PAGE, R.C., and SCHROEDER, H.E.: Periodontitis in humans; in Periodontitis in man and other animals, pp. 5-57 (Karger, New York 1982).
17. PATTERS, M.R.; CHEN, P.; MCKENNA, J., and GENCO, R.J.: Lymphoproliferative responses to oral bacteria in humans with varying severities of periodontal disease. Infect. Immun. 28: 777-784 (1980).
18. PATTERS, M.R.; SEDRANSK, N., and GENCO, R.J.: The Lymphoproliferative response during human experimental gingivitis. J. Periodont. Res. 14: 269-278 (1979).

19. SEYMOUR, G.J.; BOYATZIS, S., and POWELL, N.: The autologous mixed lymphocyte reaction (AMLR) as a possible indicator of immunoregulation in chronic inflammatory periodontal disease. J. Clin. Periodontol. 13: 639-645 (1986).
20. SMITH, S.; BICK, P.H.; MILLER, G.A.; RANNEY, R.R.; RICE, P.L.; LALOR, J.H., and TEW, J.G.: Polyclonal B-cell activation: severe periodontal disease in young adults. Clin. Immunol. Immunopathol. 16: 354-366 (1980).
21. SUZUKI, J.B.; SIMS, T.J., and PAGE, R.C.: Effect of factors other than pathologic status on responsiveness of peripheral blood mononuclear cells from patients with chronic periodontitis. J. Periodontol. 54: 408-419 (1983).
22. SUZUKI, J.B.; SIMS, T.J., and PAGE, R.C.: Blastogenic responsiveness of human lymphoid cells to mitogens and to homogenates of periodontal pocket bacteria. J. Periodont. Res. 19: 352-365 (1984).
23. TEW, J.G.; RANNEY, R.R., and DONALDSON, S.L.: Blastogenic responsiveness in periodontally healthy subjects. Evidence for mitogenic activity in oral bacteria. J. Periodont. Res. 17: 466-468 (1982).
24. TEW, J.G.; THOMAS, S.S., and RANNEY, R.R.: *Fusobacterium nucleatum*-mediated immunomodulation of the in vitro secondary antibody response to tetanus toxoid and *Actinobacillus actinomycetemcomitans*. J. Periodont. Res. 22: 506-512 (1987).
25. YOSHIE, H.; TAUBMAN, M.A.; EBERSOLE, J.L.; SMITH, D.J.; and OLSON, C.L.: Periodontal bone loss and immune characteristics of congenitally athymic and thymus cell-reconstituted athymic rats. Infect. Immun. 50: 403-408 (1985).

Dennis F. Mangan, PhD, Department of Dental Research, University of Rochester, Rochester, NY 14642 (USA)

Periodontology Today. Int. Congr., Zürich 1988, pp. 196–208 (Karger, Basel 1988)

Role of the Immune System – Dangers of a Nonholistic Approach in Explaining Health and Disease

Per Brandtzaeg

Laboratory for Immunohistochemistry and Immunopathology (LIIPAT), Institute of Pathology, University of Oslo, The National Hospital, Rikshospitalet, Oslo, Norway

Inflammation - a Two-edged Sword

After the pioneering studies of Waerhaug (36) in the early 1950s, it has become widely accepted that periodontal disease (PD) is caused by bacteria of dental plaque. Variants of this disorder may thus be viewed as different host responses to more or less poorly defined foreign material. Progressive PD shows features of both acute (exudative) and chronic (proliferative) inflammation. In a nutshell it fits with Sobin's (27) elegant description of inflammatory reactions in general:

"Inflammation is meant to be good
That's the way it would be if it would
Remain in proportion
Avoid all distortion
Resolve at the time that is should.

Inflammation may last and turn chronic
Situation that is most ironic
Instead of defending
Result is offending
Protractive destructive demonic."

The leukocyte population present in inflamed gingivae is quite similar to that usually found in reactive lymph nodes with a predominance of activated B cells and CD4-positive (T4) putative helper T lymphocytes. The protective effects of B- and T-cell responses in organized lymphoid tissues are obvious, and these tissues usually survive with well-preserved function. However, similar immune responses in connective tissues like the gingiva, skin and synovia, often result in a state of hypersensitivity which clinically appears injurious. In lymphoid tissues the various immunologically active cells are apparently organized adequately for elimination of antigens and immune complexes without the induction of excessive tissue damage. The follicular dendritic cells, for example, which retain immune complexes in germinal centres, seem to be protected against the cytolytic effect of in situ terminal complement activation by concomitant binding of S-protein or vitronectin (15). So what is mainly protective for the host in one tissue, may be quite damaging in another.

An additional important difference is that lymphoid organs are chiefly engaged in defence against exogenous infections, in which the immunogenic agent is introduced from the outside environment. With the possible but unproven exception of juvenile periodontitis (JP), PD is non-infectious in the sense that it is not communicable. Rosebury (22) appropriately suggested more than 35 years ago that PD, instead, should be called an "infective disease" because it is caused by the indigenous or commensal oral bacteria. As in other endogenous microbial diseases, the development of PD depends on significant preceeding circumstances in addition to the infective agent. Some of these predisposing factors are undoubtedly determined by a variable host response (2); but in relation to PD the most obvious preceeding circumstances are the teeth with their hard surfaces which allow prolonged retention and accumulation of indigenous bacteria. A non-pathogenic dental plaque, in the sense of not causing gingivitis, has never been observed (31).

Immune Response, Immune Reaction and Hypersensitivity

Immune response refers to the morphological alterations and biological activities induced by stimulation of acquired immunity (figure 1). It depends on macrophages, antigen-presenting dendritic cells expressing class II determinants (HLA-DR, -DQ and -DP) of the major histocompatibility complex (MHC) as genetically determined restriction elements, and CD4-positive (T4) helper lymphocytes. Regulation of the response probably also involves CD8-positive (T8) suppressor cells. All of these cell categories are present in the gingiva (25) so an immune response to plaque antigens can undoubtedly be mounted locally.

A long-lasting, secondary type of immune response gives rise to differentiation to effector cells and release of biologically active substances aiming at neutralization and elimination of antigen. Such immunological effector mechanisms, and the non-specific biological amplification often triggered by them, are collectively referred to as immune reactions (figure 1). Acquired immunity is thus based on specific immune responses but is expressed by immune reactions. The effector cells of the B-cell system are the immunoglobulin(Ig)-producing plasma cells which abound in the established gingival lesion (2-5,9). Progressive PD is therefore a typical B-cell lesion (26), but the early stabil

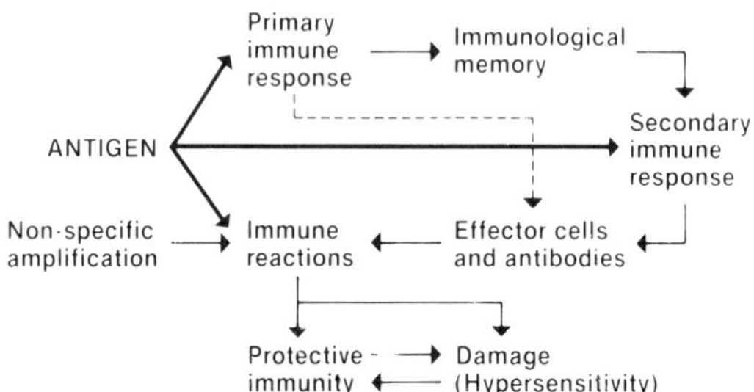

Fig. 1. Schematic representation of the relationships between immune response, immune reaction, protection and hypersensitivity.

lesion may nevertheless be dominated by T-cells (25). Although immune reactions are initially directed specifically against antigen(s), they often induce extensive non-specific events which may be considered variations on the theme of inflammation. When the result is judged to be damaging, the underlying immune reactions are referred to as immunopathology and the clinical effect is called hypersensitivity (figure 1).

For didactic reasons, the hypersensitivity mechanisms were categorized into four types (figure 2) by Coombs and Gell in the 1960s (21). These types do not necessarily occur isolated but one type may be dominating in a particular immunopathological lesion. It should also be emphasized that hypersensitivity is principally an expression of protective immune reactions which, however, become tissue-damaging mainly when immune elimination for some reason is hampered (figure 1). This may be due to continuous supply of antigen (e.g., chronic virus infection, autoimmunity, dental plaque) or an inefficient (e.g., low-affinity antibodies) or exaggerated (e.g., atopic IgE) immune response, probably often genetically determined. The hypersensitivity mechanisms involved in PD have not been defined, although circumstantial evidence points to Types 2 and 3 and probably also Type 4, the latter especially in the early lesion (25,26). A high degree of complexity can be expected. It may be of some comfort that our immunological knowledge is just as meagre with regard to most other chronic inflammatory diseases.

Immunogenicity, Mitogenicity and Tolerogenicity of Plaque

Plaque bacteria produce a variety of toxins and enzymes which may be directly involved as virulence factors in the pathogenesis of PD (17,19). However, there is no reason to

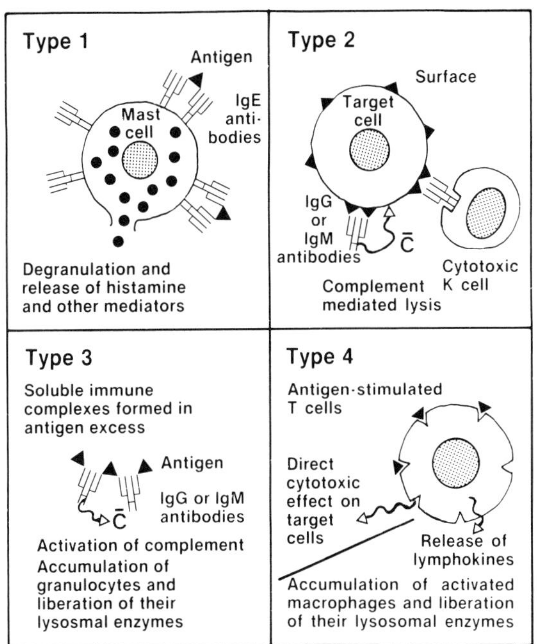

<u>Fig. 2</u>. Schematic representation of Type 1 (immediate, atopic or anaphylactic), Type 2 (cytotoxic or lytic), Type 3 (immune complex-mediated) and Type 4 (T cell-mediated) hypersensitivity mechanisms.

doubt that also immunopathological mechanisms are engaged. Numerous studies have reported that antibodies to plaque bacteria are present in serum (33) and these antibodies, which are mainly of the IgG class, will by extravascular distribution be available to react with corresponding antigens in the gingival area (9). Such a local immune reaction may increase the influx of irrelevant antigens as part of an immunopathological development (10). The initial gingival lesion is probably an ideal situation for the development of an "Auer phenomenon"; that is, aggravation of mild inflammation by local accumulation of serum antibodies combined with (systemical or) topical supply of the corresponding antigen(s) (4).

There is, moreover, direct evidence for local production of antibodies to plaque components in the gingiva (9,24,29). Nevertheless, based on experimental topical immunization with a purified immunogen, the fraction of "non-specific" plasma cells in the lesion can be expected to be larger than 60% (3,4); and this fraction will increase according to the number of immunogenic antigens involved (35). The "non-specific" local plasma cells are to a large extent producing antibodies to immunogens encountered elsewhere in the body (4); their development in the lesion is apparently a result of polyclonal B-cell activation. This may be induced by non-specific immunoregulatory signals released during the local specific response (4). In addition, several plaque components are mitogenic and can function as polyclonal B-cell activators (25). At present, therefore, it is impossible to define to what extent the immunologically active cells in the periodontal lesion are actually directed against plaque antigens.

The complexity increases by the fact that components of plaque bacteria have been shown to cause suppression of both T- and B-cell activities *in vitro* (25). The mechanisms are poorly defined; but it is known that antigen exposure of the intestinal mucosa of experimental animals under certain conditions may have a tolerogenic effect, perhaps by induction of suppressor T8 cells (18). There is some indirect evidence that hyporesponsiveness of T cells may be associated with susceptibility to PD (30), and a decreased T4- to T8-cell ratio has been observed in established PD lesions of adults (25). However, it remains to be determined whether the low-responder patients have been partially tolerized to plaque antigens as a secondary event or show a poor immune response due to incompatible genetic restriction. This distinction likewise cannot be made with regard to the suggested possibility that a poor serum antibody response to *Actinobacillus (Haemophilus) actinomycetemcomitans* contributes to the severity of JP (14).

Interactions between Dental Plaque and the Secretory Immune System

Most immunological studies of PD have been performed on circulating lymphocytes and serum antibodies; but the periodontium should in fact be viewed as a watershed between the systemic and secretory immune systems (figure 3). The balance of evidence indicates that secretory IgA antibodies in saliva can inhibit bacterial colonization on the teeth (6,7), although IgA-specific proteases of plaque bacteria may counteract this effect (19). Accumulation of dental plaque has in most studies been shown to induce enhanced production of salivary IgA (7). The stimulatory effect of plaque on the secretory immune system may be afforded both by increased amounts of swallowed bacteria (stimulating migratory B cells in tonsils and Peyer's patches) and by increased absorption of immunogens through the gingiva. Thus, elevated levels of parotid IgA antibodies to *A. actinomycetemcomitans* were often seen in subjects whose gingival crevices harboured this microorganism (28).

Much therefore remains to be learned about the assumed

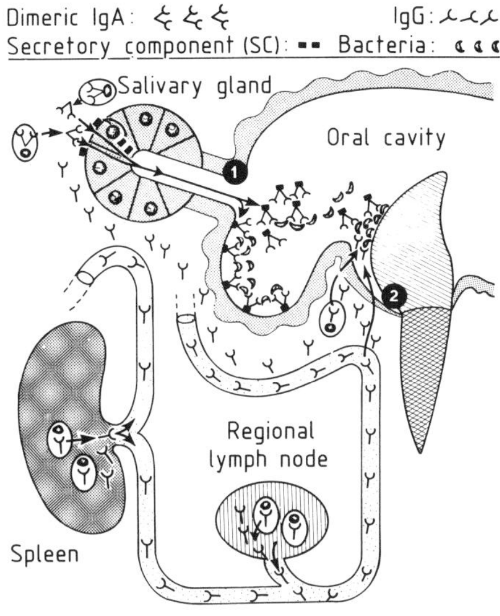

Fig. 3. Schematic representation of the two principal Ig systems influencing the oral microbiota. 1. The secretory IgA system: Dimeric IgA produced by plasma cells in major and minor salivary glands is transported to the oral cavity by complexing with the epithelial receptor (SC). Secretory IgA is incorporated in the mucus layer covering the soft surfaces and it is assumed to mediate protection by limiting colonization of microorganisms on epithelial cells and by inhibiting influx of soluble antigens. Secretory IgA antibodies also influence colonization of bacteria on the teeth. 2. The IgG system: Most IgG reaches the oral cavity by passive diffusion through the gingival crevicular epithelium. This IgG is mainly derived from serum and originates in lymph nodes and spleen. A small fraction is, in addition, produced by local plasma cells when the gingiva is inflamed. Reproduced with permission from Ref. 6).

protective effects of host responses within the secretory immune system on the development of PD. This seems particularly important in view of the recent finding that the two major potentially periodontopathic microorganisms, Bacteroides gingivalis and A. actinomycetemcomitans (31), may invade the gingiva from the oral side in relation to lesions of advanced adult PD and JP, respectively (23).

Interactions between Dental Plaque and the Systemic Immune System

The immunogenicity, mitogenicity and tolerogenicity of plaque bacteria discussed above, have been studied mainly with peripheral blood lymphocytes in vitro; to what extent the findings obtained may be extrapolated to the in vivo situation in the gingival area is uncertain. Conversely, demonstration of serum antibodies has direct gingival relevance as they are extravascularly distributed (9), and at least 80% of the IgG in gigival fluid from patients with PD seems to be serum-derived (3).

Most of the increased serum levels of plaque-directed antibodies found in the patients (33) may actually be explained by gingival production. Thus, the highest levels in adult PD and JP are against *B. gingivalis* and *A. actinomycetemcomitans*, respectively, which are prominent in the corresponding plaques (12,31) and invade the respective lesions (23). Furthermore, the antibody levels drop when plaque is removed (11,34). It therefore appears that the systemic antibody response reflects the degree of gingival exposure to particular microorganisms. Although interesting, this information does not necessarily elucidate the degree of protection or hypersensitivity ensuing the actual immune response; and it cannot be excluded that a considerable and variable fraction of the antibodies are produced in tonsils, lymph nodes and spleen (figure 3) because increased amounts of oral bacteria are probably swallowed and more plaque antigens may enter lymph and blood in PD patients than in subjects with a healthy gingiva.

Immunopathological Interpretations According to Availability of Immunological Methods

Our initial observation of Ig-producing plasma cells in gingival lesions in the mid-1960s (8), stimulated an interest in PD-related humoral immunity which peaked around 1970. The reason for a shift to an enormous interest in cell-mediated immunity (figure 4) could be ascribed to the development of methods for studying lymphoid cells in vitro (16). Transformation of peripheral blood lymphocytes in response to plaque components was erroneously taken to suggest that PD is mainly a Type 4 hypersensitivity lesion (figure 2); the predominance of Ig-producing plasma cells in the established lesion was more or less neglected. In the beginning of the 1980s, when convenient techniques for measuring antibodies became available (33), the emphasis was again placed on humoral immunity as an important aspect of PD (figure 4). These trends show how limited methodological competence may jeopardize a holistic biological approach. This is of course not unique in relation to PD, but it is certainly a danger young researchers should

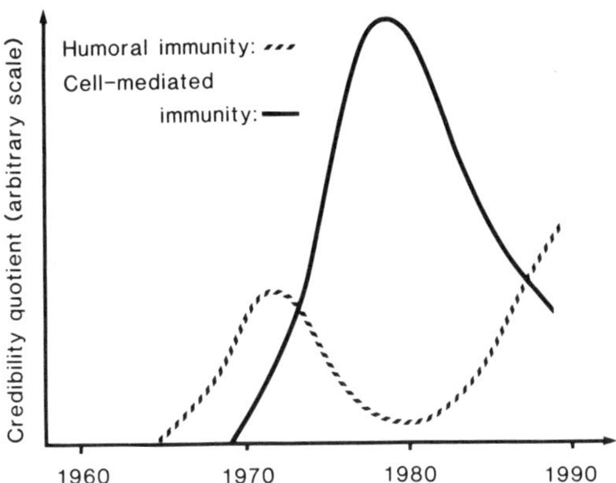

Fig. 4. Trends in immunopathological research on periodontal disease since 1965.

be aware of.

The Overwhelming Complexity of the Immune System

The complexity of the immune system makes it necessary to select defined aspects for studies of the relationship between protective and tissue-damaging mechanisms. But the honest scientist should not forget that the findings obtained are of little value unless they are fitted into a holistic approach. Some workers have attempted this in relation to PD (figure 5). The result is necessarily perplexing and based on numerous questionable extrapolations because specific information is still limited. It has to be admitted that the detailed immunological mechanisms operating in the gingiva remain obscure, and nothing is known about how MHC class II-related genetic restriction influences an individual's immune response to pathogenetic antigens. Again, this is not unique to PD. Thus, the immunopathology of the apparently much simpler coeliac disease is still unsolved despite the fact that gluten peptides have been identified as etiological factors and much is known about the immune response-related genetic aspects of this disorder.

Dissection of the Immune System by Immunodeficiency or Immunosuppression

As "experiments of Nature", immunodeficiencies have served to enhance tremendously our understanding of the immune

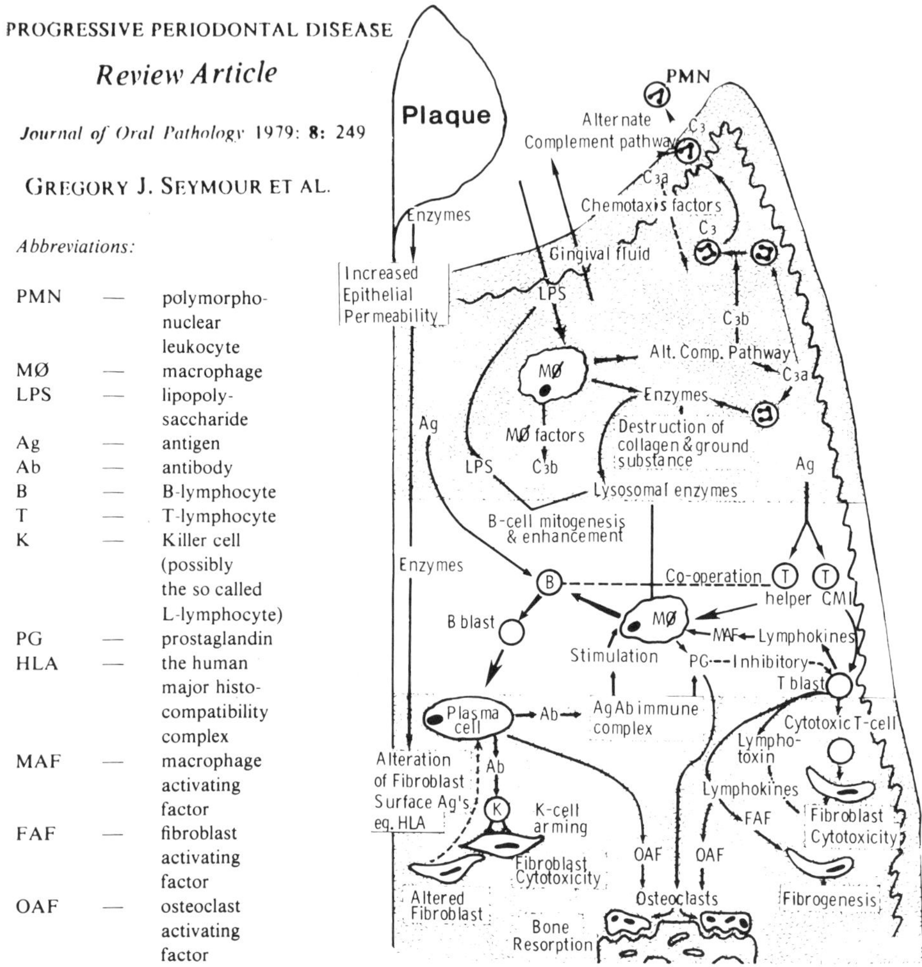

Fig. 5. Hypothetical concept of interactions between immunopathological mechanisms in progressive periodontal disease. Reproduced with permission from Ref. 26.

system in general. In relation to PD, however, studies of immunodeficiency are difficult to interpret because of the superimposed variable effects of general health status, antibiotic treatment, mouth breathing due to nasal congestion, oral hygiene status and professional dental care. Nevertheless, observations in patients with various humoral immune defects have indicated less severe PD than in matched controls (20), which may suggest that antibodies contribute to gingival

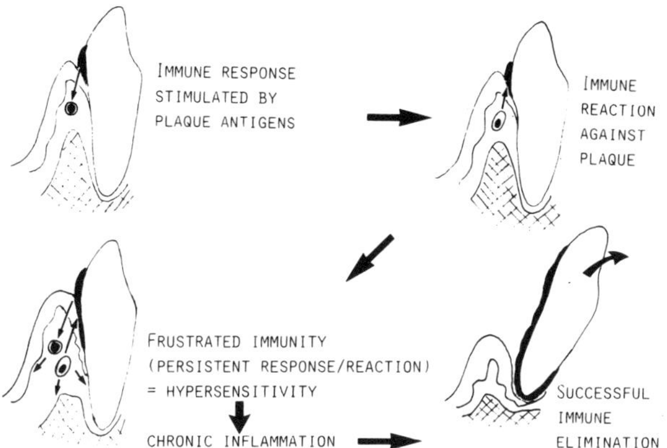

Fig. 6. A simplistic immunopathological concept of progressive periodontal disease.

inflammation. Similar conclusions have been made from studies of patients treated with immunosuppressive drugs (1,32). The interpretation is again difficult, however, because most such drugs do not affect selectively immunocompetent cells but are in addition antiphlogistic. Conversely, rapidly progressive PD has been observed in patients with the acquired immunodeficiency syndrome (AIDS), suggesting that gingival defence deteriorates when regulatory T4 cells are destroyed by the AIDS virus (37). We have observed almost complete lack of T4 cells in the inflamed periodontium of such a patient (13).

A Simplistic Concept of Progressive Periodontal Disease

Both observations in AIDS patients (37) and in experimental animals (25) have indicated that an intact immune system has an important protective role in the periodontium. However, when plaque is allowed to accumulate on the teeth, the periodontium apparently becomes an area in immunological conflict. Immune mechanisms most likely contribute significantly to the prevention of microbial spread to deeper and distant tissues but antigen elimination, which is the ultimate goal of the immune system, cannot be achieved as long as plaque persists. Such "frustrated immunity" may be settled either by mechanical (and antibiotic) plaque removal or by tooth loss - which in fact may be viewed as successful immune elimination (figure 6). Superimposed on this simplistic immunopathological concept of PD, come the individual patterns of disease progression, which may be explained both by microbial and immunological variables. We will never reach full understanding of these variables without a holistic approach. Acceptance of a high level of complexity, however, should not detract from further studies of the host-parasite relationship in the gingival area.

References

1. BEEN, V. and ENGEL, D.: The effects of immunosuppressive drugs on periodontal inflammation in human renal allograft patients. J. Periodontol. 53: 245-248 (1982).
2. BRANDTZAEG, P.: Local factors of resistance in the gingival area. J. Periodont. Res. 1: 19-42 (1966).
3. BRANDTZAEG, P.: Local formation and transport of immunoglobulins related to the oral cavity; in MacPHEE, Host resistance to commensal bacteria; pp. 116-150 (Churchill-Livingstone, London 1972).
4. BRANDTZAEG, P.: Immunology of inflammatory periodontal lesions. Internat. dent. J. 23: 438-454, 1973.
5. BRANDTZAEG, P.: Immunoglobulin systems of oral mucosa and saliva; in DOLBY. Oral mucosa in health and disease; pp. 137-213 (Blackwell Scientific Publications, Oxford 1975).
6. BRANDTZAEG, P.: The oral secretory immune system with special emphasis on its relation to dental caries. Proc. Finn. dent. Soc. 79: 71-84 (1983).
7. BRANDTZAEG, P.: Salivary immunoglobulins; in TENOVUO, Human saliva: clinical chemistry and microbiology; Chapter 5, in press (CRC Press, Boca Raton, Florida 1988).
8. BRANDTZAEG, P. and KRAUS, F.W.: Autoimmunity and periodontal disease. Odont. Tidskr. (Scand. J. dent. Res.) 73: 281-393 (1965).
9. BRANDTZAEG, P. and TOLO, K.: Immunoglobulin systems of the gingiva; in LEHNER, The borderline between caries and periodontal disease; pp. 145-189 (Academic Press, London 1977).
10. BRANDTZAEG, P. and TOLO, K.: Influence of parenteral immunization in rabbits on the penetrability of oral mucosa for macromolecules. Advanc. exp. Med. Biol. 107: 227-232 (1978).
11. EBERSOLE, J.L., FREY, D.E., TAUBMAN, M.A., HAFFAJEE, A.D., and SOCRANSKY, S.S.: Dynamics of systemic antibody responses in periodontal disease. J. periodont. Res. 22: 184-186 (1987).
12. EBERSOLE, J.L., TAUBMAN, M.A., SMITH, D.J., and SOCRANSKY, S.S.: Humoral immune responses and diagnosis of human periodontal disease. J. periodont. Res. 17: 478-480 (1982).
13. GERNER, N.W., HURLEN, B., DOBLOUG, J., and BRANDTZAEG, P.: Endodontic treatment and immunopathology of periapical granuloma in an AIDS patient. Endodont. Traumatol. In press (1988).

14. GUNSOLLEY, J.C., BURMEISTER, J.A., TEW, J.G., BEST, A.M., and RANNEY, R.R.: Relationship of serum antibody to attachment level patterns in young adults with juvenile periodontitis or generalized severe periodontitis. J. Periodontol. 58: 314-320 (1987).
15. HALSTENSEN, T.S., MOLLNES, T.E., GARRED, P., and BRANDTZAEG, P.: Distribution of vitronectin and terminal complement complex (TCC) on follicular dendritic cells (FDC) in human lymphoid tissue. Abstracts 9th International Conference on Lymphatic Tissues and Germinal Centres in Immune Reactions; A17 (Oslo, Norway 1987).
16. LEHNER, T.: Cell-mediated immune responses in oral disease: A review. J. oral. Path. 1: 39-58 (1972).
17. LISTGARTEN, M.A.: Nature of periodontal diseases: Pathogenic mechanisms. J. periodont. Res. 22: 172-178 (1987).
18. MOWAT, A. McI.: The regulation of immune responses to dietary protein antigens. Immunol. Today 8: 93-98 (1987).
19. REINHOLDT, J. and KILIAN, M.: Interference of IgA protease with the effect of secretory IgA on adherence of oral streptococci to saliva-coated hydroxyapatite. J. dent. Res. 66: 492-497 (1987).
20. ROBERTSON, P.B., MACKLER, B.F., WRIGHT, T.E., and LEVY, B.M.: Periodontal status of patients with abnormalities of the immune system. II. Observations over a 2-year period. J. Periodontol. 51: 70-73 (1980).
21. ROITT, I.: Essential immunology; 4th ed., pp. 217-252 (Blackwell, Oxford 1980).
22. ROSEBURY, T.: Etiology factors in periodontal disease. Oral Surg., oral Med., oral Pathol. 5: 473-482 (1952).
23. SAGLIE, F.R., SMITH, C.T., NEWMAN, M.G., CARRANZA, F.A., PERTUISET, J.H., CHENG, L., AUIL, E. and NISENGARD, R.J.: The presence of bacteria in the oral epithelium in periodontal disease. II. Immunohistochemical identification of bacteria. J. Periodontol. 57: 492-500 (1986).
24. SCHONFELD, S.E. and KAGAN, J.M.: Specificity of gingival plasma cells for bacterial somatic antigens. J. periodont. Res. 17: 60-69 (1982).
25. SEYMOUR, G.J.: Possible mechanisms involved in the immunoregulation of chronic inflammatory periodontal disease. J. dent. Res. 66: 2-9 (1987).
26. SEYMOUR, G.J., POWELL, R.N., and DAVIES, W.I.R.: The immunopathogenesis of progressive chronic inflammatory periodontal disease. J. oral Path. 8: 249-265 (1979).
27. SOBIN, L.H.: A pathology primer in verse; pp. 5-7 (H.K. Lewis, London 1978).
28. SMITH, D.J., EBERSOLE, J.L., TAUBMAN, M.A., and GADALLA, L.: Salivary IgA antibody to Actinobacillus actinomycetemcomitans in a young adult population. J. periodont. Res. 20: 8-11 (1985).
29. SMITH, D.J., GADALLA, L.M., EBERSOLE, J.L., and TAUBMAN, M.A.: Gingival crevicular fluid antibody to oral microorganisms. III. Association of gingival homogenate and

gingival crevicular fluid antibody levels. J. periodont. Res. 20: 357-367 (1985).

30. STASHENKO, P., RESMINI, L.M., HAFFAJEE, A.D., and SOCRANSKY, S.S.: T cell responses of periodontal disease patients and healthy subjects to oral microorganisms. J. periodont. Res. 18: 587-600 (1983).

31. THEILADE, E.: The non-specific theory in microbial etiology of inflammatory periodontal diseases. J. clin. Periodontol. 13: 905-911 (1986).

32. TOLLEFSEN, T., STRØMME KOPPANG, H., and MESSELT, E.: Immunosuppression and periodontal disease in man. Histological and ultrastructural observations. J. periodont. Res. 17: 329-344 (1982).

33. TOLO, K. and BRANDTZAEG, P.: Relation between periodontal disease activity and serum antibody titres to oral bacteria; in GENCO and MERGENHAGEN, Host-parasite interactions in periodontal diseases; pp. 270-282 (Amer. Soc. Microbiol., Washington 1982).

34. TOLO, K., SCHENCK, K., and JOHANSEN, J.R.: Activity of human serum immunoglobulins to seven anaerobic oral bacteria before and after periodontal treatment. J. periodont. Res. 17: 481-483 (1982).

35. VOS-CLOETENS, C. de, MINSART-BALERIAUX, V., and URBAIN-VANSANTEN, G.: Possible relationships between antibodies and non-specific immunoglobulins simultaneously induced after antigenic stimulation. Immunology 20: 955-962 (1971).

36. WAERHAUG, J.: The gingival pocket. Anatomy, pathology, deepening and elimination. Odont. Tidskr. (Scand. J. dent. Res.) 60 (Suppl. 1): 1-186 (1952).

37. WINKLER, J.R. and MURRAY, P.A.: Periodontal disease. A potential intraoral expression of AIDS may be rapidly progressive periodontitis. Calif. dent. Assoc. J. 15: 20-24 (1987).

Dr. P. Brandtzaeg, Laboratory for Immunohistochemistry and Immunopathology, The National Hospital Rikshospitalet, 0027 Oslo 1, Norway

Periodontology Today. Int. Congr., Zürich 1988, pp. 209–217 (Karger, Basel 1988)

Mechanisms and Consequences of Neutrophil Interaction with the Subgingival Microbiota

T. E. Van Dyke, R. L. Duncan, C. W. Cutler, J. R. Kalmar und R. R. Arnold

Department of Periodontology and Dental Research Center, Emory University, Atlanta, Georgia, USA

INTRODUCTION

Periodontal diseases are inflammatory lesions of the gingival and periodontal tissue which affect most of the human adult population to some degree and may cause sufficient destruction of the periodontium to result in the loss of teeth (1,2). Histologically, periodontal diseases resemble an acute inflammatory response, characterized by a polymorphonuclear leukocyte infiltrate. The neutrophils migrate from the gingival tissue into the gingival crevice. This migration is in response to chemotactic substances elaborated by bacteria or by complement derived chemotactic factors. Once in the gingival crevice, the neutrophils are capable of interacting with crevicular microorganisms, which are generally considered to be the etiological agents in these diseases. Factors which influence migration of neutrophils and the subsequent interaction between neutrophils and crevicular microorganisms may play a key role in the outcome of the disease.

The importance of the neutrophil in host defense against periodontal disease microorganisms is emphasized by the relationship between periodontitis and impaired neutrophil function. For example, neutrophil chemotactic and bactericidal defects are frequently found in patients with localized juvenile periodontitis (3,4). Because of the importance of the neutrophil in host defense against periodontal pathogens, an understanding of the effect that biologically active products from periodontal pathogens may have on the neutrophil is important to understanding these diseases.

Although more than 260 distinct types and species of bacteria have been isolated from sites of periodontal disease, several lines of evidence suggest that certain microorganisms are more relevant to periodontal diseases than others (5). Recent studies have demonstrated a correlation between an increase in the proportion of Gram-negative anaerobic organisms in the subgingival microflora and an increasing severity of periodontal disease (5,6,7). Of particular interest are the Gram-negative organisms, Actinobacillus actinomycetemcomitans (associated with juvenile periodontitis) and Bacteroides gingivalis (associated with adult periodontitis).

The most outstanding characteristic of these microorganisms is the presence of lipopolysaccharides (LPS), which are major components of the outer membrane of Gram-negative bacteria. LPS consists of a lipid component (Lipid A) attached to a core polysaccharide and a polysaccharide side chain of varying length. LPS modulates a plethora of biological activities both in vivo and in vitro. Several lines of evidence using enteric bacteria suggest that lipid A is the part of the LPS molecule responsible for these biological activities. First, lipid A obtained from LPS following mild acid hydrolysis retains the biological activities associated with the intact LPS molecule (8). Second, the cationic protein polymixin B, which binds to the lipid A region of the LPS molecule, blocks the biological activity of LPS (9). Third, synthetic lipid A has been demonstrated to manifest the biological activities of intact native LPS (10).

In vitro, LPS can initiate B lymphocyte proliferation (11, 12), immunoglobulin production (13,14), complement activation, coagulation, affect T-lymphocyte responses (15, 16), and activate macrophages to become tumoricidal (17, 18) and release colony stimulating factor (19, 20), interleukin 1 (21), prostaglandins (22), and interferon (23, 24). Perhaps one of the more important observations with respect to possible host-bacterial interactions in periodontal diseases is the recent observation that LPS can modulate certain neutrophil functions (25). It should be emphasized, however, that the LPS used in these experiments were derived from well characterized, non-periodontal pathogens. Although striking similarities exist among the lipid A structures of LPS of the Enterobacteriaceae (26), recent evidence suggest that the lipid A structure of Bacteroides may differ in several respects from enterobacterial lipid A (27,28). Unlike enterobacterial lipid A, the fatty acid residues of Bacteroides lipid A are isobranched with five distinct 3-hydroxy fatty acids. Furthermore, 3-hydroxytetradecanoic acid is not a predominate fatty acid component of Bacteroides lipid A (28). These rather significant differences between the LPS structure of Bacteroides lipid A and the more thoroughly studied, biologically active, enterobacterial lipid A raise questions regarding the biological activity of B. gingivalis LPS. In this regard, it is noteworthy that highly purified Bacteroides LPS has been reported to be less active than the LPS of Enterobacteriaceae in the 10-day-old chick embryo lethality assay, the Limulus amoebocyte lysate assay, and Schwartzman reaction (29). Under certain conditions, Bacteroides LPS has also been reported to be less active than enterobacterial LPS in bone resorption assays (30) and mitogenic assays (31). Thus, it is tempting to speculate that in adult periodontitis, Bacteroides LPS may suppress normal neutrophil functions locally, creating a bacterial- induced neutrophil defect, which in turn leads to disease. This possibility is consistent with the observation that, in contrast to the inflammatory properties normally induce by the in vivo administration of LPS, LPS can also have anti-inflammatory properties. For example, LPS inhibits the reversed passive Arthus reactions in rabbit skin (32), and inhibits a variety of immunologically induced inflammatory responses in guinea pigs, including the active Arthus reaction. Verghese and Snyderman (33) demonstrated that a single dose of LPS inhibits the response in mice to intraperitoneal injections of either complement activating substances or nonspecific stimulants such as pokeweed mitogen. While some of these effects have been explained, in part, by induction of hypotension or leukopenia by LPS, it is noteworthy, with respect to this investigation, that the anti-inflammatory response induced by LPS is also partially caused by a modification of neutrophil responses to C5a. Therefore, of particular interest with respect to periodontal diseases, is the effect that B. gingivalis LPS may have on neutrophil functions relevant to host defense. These include chemotaxis in response to a chemical gradient, cell surface receptor mediated attachment, engulfment, killing and superoxide anion generation.

METHODS and MATERIALS

Subjects

All patients have been obtained from the patient population of Emory University School of Dentistry, Emory Dental Research Center, Emory Clinic and affiliated hospitals. Informed consent was obtained from all subjects or, in the case of minors, from their parents or legal guardians. A complete medical history and battery of clinical laboratory tests including SMA-22, prothrombin time and urinalysis was completed on all patients. Health questionnaires were administered to patient and controls on each each day of neutrophil function testing which elicited information regarding tobacco use, drug and alcohol consumption, illnesses and blood loss; and for females, additional information regarding birth control medication, menstruation and pregnancy was gathered.

The adult periodontitis group was defined as patients who exhibited generalized severe alveolar bone loss with multiple vertical osseous defects. The control group consisted of healthy individuals from laboratory and dental school populations who had no radiographic evidence of bone loss or evidence of periodontal disease other than mild gingivitis. Patients and controls were age and sex matched for most experiments.

Isolation of LPS

Microorganisms: Two clinical isolates of B. gingivalis (CDC designated A7436 and A7438) were used in this investigation. They were maintained by serial passage in Schaedler broth in an atmosphere of 10% H_2, 5% CO_2, 85% N_2 at 35° C. These isolates were characterized in the laboratory of Dr. V.R. Dowell Jr., Director of the Anaerobic Bacteria Branch of the Centers for Disease Control (CDC).

Endotoxin preparations: The LPS was extracted from the Bacteroides by hot phenol-water extraction (34). The phenol-water extracted LPS was then further purified on CsCl isopycnic density gradients as described previously (35). Individual fractions were dialyzed to remove CsCl and those fractions containing peak endotoxic activity (densities of 1.42-1.52 gm/cm^2), as determined by murine splenocyte proliferation and Limulus anaeobocyte clotting, were pooled and and lyophlyzed. Prior to each experiment LPS was resuspended in saline to the concentrations indicated and sonicated briefly to disperse the LPS.

Isolation of Neutrophils and Neutrophil Functional Assays

Chemotaxis: Neutrophils were isolated as previously described (36). The chemotaxis assay, as it is routinely performed in our laboratory, has been described in detail elsewhere (36). In summary, neutrophils were suspended in an assay medium consisting of Gey's Balanced Salt Solution (GBSS) supplemented with 2% bovine serum albumin (BSA), at a concentration of 2.5×10^6 cells/ml. The cell suspension was placed in the upper compartment of a modified Boyden chamber separated by a 5 μ-pore micropore filter (Sartorius membrane filter, GmbH, Gottingen, FRG). The lower compartment contained the synthetic chemotactic peptide N-formylmethionylleucylphenylalanine (FMLP) or C5a. Chemotaxis was evaluated by counting the number of neutrophils that accumulate on the distal surface of the filter after a 60 minute incubation. Ten high power fields (400x) were counted for each of triplicate filters. Statistical differences between 0.01-10μg LPS and GBSS were determined by analysis of variance.

Bactericidal Activity: The phagocytosis and killing assay used in our laboratory was an adaptation of the method of van Furth *et al.* (37). Briefly, isolated neutrophils were suspended in sterile Gey's Balanced Salt Solution with 0.1% gelatin at a concentration of 1×10^7 cells/ml. The indicator organism, Staphylococcus epidermidus, was grown in Trypticase-Soy Broth, washed in PBS and the concentration adjusted to an optical density of 0.6 at 540nM. The organisms were centrifuged, resuspended in 5ml of 1:10 dilution of pooled human serum for opsonization for 30 minutes at 37°C. After 2 washes in PBS, the organisms are suspended in GBSS at 4×10^8 cells/ml. The reaction mixture consists of 0.5ml of neutrophil suspension and 0.5ml of preopsonized S. epidermidus suspension in Falcon 2003 tubes. The mixture was gently inverted for

30 minutes at 37°C on an Ames aliquot tilt table. The reaction is stopped by the addition of 3ml of cold GBSS and centrifuged at 4°C at 400 x g for 5 minutes. The pellet is resuspended in 0.2ml of a 20 U/ml solution of lysostaphin (Sigma) in phosphate buffered saline (PBS) to lyse non-phagocytosed bacteria including those attached to the surface of the neutrophils. The cells were repelleted, washed 2 x with PBS and resuspended in 300μl of PBS. The suspension was diluted to 1.5ml with distilled water to lyse the neutrophils at appropriate time intervals. The resulting bacterial suspension was serially diluted and plated in trypticase soy agar using a spiral plater. After 24 hours at 37°C, the colony forming units were counted and the kinetic data were used to quantify bactericidal activity. Statistical differences between 0.01-10μg LPS and GBSS in the bactericidal activity assay was determined by analysis of variance.

Superoxide Generation: Superoxide (O_2^-) generation was evaluated using opsonized zymosan or 1mM FMLP as a stimulant as described by Cohen *et al.* (38). Neutrophils were isolated from venous blood by Ficoll-Hypaque centrifugation and superoxide release was quantified by measurement of cytochrome C reduction using a colorimetric assay. Briefly, 2.5 x 10^6 cell/ml was preincubated with LPS (1-100 μg/ml) or GBSS for 30 minutes at 37°C. Cytochrome C (0.08mm) was added to the cells in the cuvettes [the reference cuvette also contained superoxide dismutase (50 mg/ml)] and colorimetric changes recorded at 500nm using Cary spectrophotometer. After the tracing had stabilized, 1μ of FMLP or 1 mg/ml opsonized Zymosan was added as a stimulus. Superoxide production was recorded at a rate function, i.e. ng cytochrome C reduced per unit time.

B.gingivalis Resistance to Phagocytosis by Normal Human Neutrophils

In order to evaluate phogocytosis of B. gingivalis (CDC isolate A7436) by normal human neutrophils, the bacteria were grown to exponential phase (O.D.=0.15 at 660nm) in Schaedler broth in an anaerobic (5% CO_2, 5% H_2, 90% N_2) environment overnight, centrifuged and resuspended in 10 μl/ml, 4′,6-diamidino-2-phenylindole (DAPI, a fluorescent DNA-specific dye). Actinobacillus actinomycetemcomitans (A.a) prepared under similar conditions, served as positive control (2). The cells were then washed 3 times in normal saline to remove growth media, metabolic end products and wash out excess DAPI. At an O.D. of 0.15, the bacterial population is approximately 10^8 CFU/ml. This concentration and a 1:10 dilution in saline was used for phagocytosis by normal human neutrophils enriched by Ficoll-Hypaque centrifugation and suspended to a concentration of 10^7 cells/ml. For opsonization, 100μl of B. gingivalis were combined with 32μl patient serum or control serum and 1.6μl of 500 mg/ml propidium iodide (a fluorescent DNA-binding dye which is excluded by viable cells), and incubated for 15 minutes at 37°C. Then 208μl neutrophil suspension were added and incubated for 15 minutes and 60 minutes. At 15 and 60 minutes, 10μl of bacterial/neutrophil suspension was removed and examined by fluorescent microscopy using narrow band excitation. Ten fields were observed from each slide. Bacteria appearing blue were counted as viable and red bacteria as non-viable. Neutrophils with propidium iodide-stained red nuclei were also recorded as non-viable.

RESULTS

Chemotaxis- To assess the effect of B. gingivalis LPS on normal neutrophil chemotaxis to FMLP, normal peripheral blood neutrophils were suspended in buffer containing 10 μg/ml B. gingivalis LPS or 10 μg/ml E. coli LPS in the Boyden chamber assay. Care was taken to insure equal concentrations of LPS in both compartments of the Boyden chamber to avoid creating an LPS gradient in the system. Optimal FMLP concentration (10^{-8}M) was used. The results suggest that E. coli LPS enhances the neutrophil chemotactic response to FMLP whereas B. gingivalis LPS markedly suppressed the chemotactic response to FMLP (Table I).

A Checkerboard experiment was performed to evaluate the chemotactic activity of E. coli LPS(Table II). Top refers to the upper compartment of the Boyden Chamber where cells are placed. Bottom refers to the lower compartment where the chemotactic factor is placed. The concentration of E. coli LPS in each compartment is indicated. Empty boxes represent reverse gradient and are not evaluated. Note that cell motility increases with increasing concentration of LPS. However, the presence of a gradient does not result in an increase in mobility. Therefore, E. coli LPS is chemokinetic for human neutrophils, but not chemotactic. There was no toxic activity for neutrophils at any concentration tested, as determined by Trypan blue dye exclusion. In similar experiments with B. gingivalis LPS, no neutrophil mobility was detected under any conditions. There was, likewise, no toxicity.

TABLE I

Effect of E. coli and B. gingivalis LPS on Neutrophil Chemotaxis to FMLP (10^{-8})

	Additions		
	None	10 μg/ml E. coli LPS	10 μg/ml B. gingivalis LPS
Chemotaxis (Cells/HPF)	73.7 ± 2.7	91.6 ± 10.2	19.5 ± 0.5

TABLE II

CHECKERBOARD EXPERIMENT FOR CHEMOTACTIC ACTIVITY OF E. coli LPS

	TOP			
	PBS	1 μg/ml	10 μg/ml	100 μg/ml
PBS	5.1 ± 1.7			
1 μg/ml	10.5 ± 1.2	11.7 ± 1.7		
10 μg/ml	13.2 ± 5.3	12.6 ± 2.2	13.2 ± 2.6	
100 μg/ml	16.0 ± 1.8	11.6 ± 2.5	12.7 ± 2.9	13.0 ± 2.6

Phagocytosis and Bactericidal Activity: Two types of experiments were performed: 1) the effect of B. gingivalis LPS on neutrophil bactericidal activity of an non-related indicator organisms and 2) phagocytosis and killing of opsonized B. gingivalis by normal neutrophils. Bactericidal activity of normal human neutrophils was inhibited in a dose dependent manner with increasing concentrations of B. gingivalis LPS. As demonstrated in Figure 1, at the concentration of 10 μg/ml killing of S. epidermidis by neutrophils is completely inhibited.

In a separate set of experiments, the interaction of B. gingivalis with normal neutrophils was assessed. Without serum opsonization, no phagocytosis of DAPI-labelled B. gingivalis by normal human neutrophils was observed, both at 15 minutes and 60 minutes. Opsonization using serum from normal health subjects also failed to augment phagocytosis. Opsonization of B. gingivalis with serum from an adult periodontitis (A.P.) patient revealed limited phagocytosis with only 7% of the neutrophils ingesting very few organisms (Table III). The AP sera that was tested contained high titer antibody to B. gingivalis (ELISA). A.a, another Gram-negative periodontal pathogen opsonized with high titer LJP serum, served as a positive control in these assays. In contrast to the limited phagocytosis seen with B. gingivalis, when A.a labelled with DAPI are used, about 60% of the neutrophils had ingested over 15 bacterial cells per neutrophil. (Table III).

TABLE III

Phagocytosis of Bacteroides gingivalis

Opsonization	% of phagocytosis[a]	Bacteria/Neutrophil
A.P. Sera	7.3 ± 1.5	0.074 ± .021[b]
Control Sera	1.05 ± .05	0.005 ± .007[b]
PBS	0	0
LJP Sera	56.2 ± 4.2	16.9 ± 4.5[c]

[a] -percentage of neutrophils containing bacteria
[b] -B.g./neutrophil
[c] -A.a./neutrophil

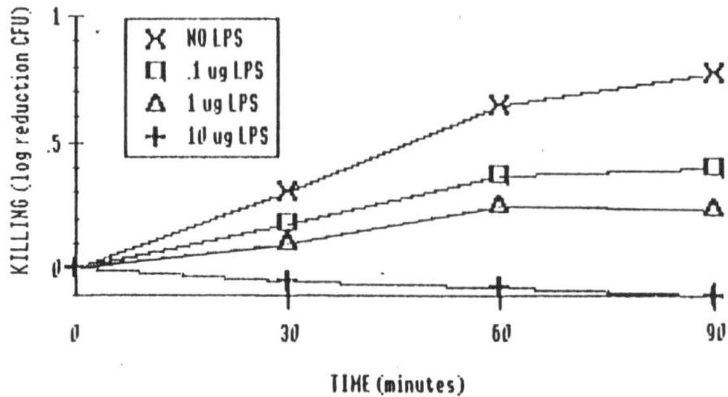

Figure 1- Bactericidal Activity of normal neutrophils to S. epidermidis, expressed as reduction in colony forming units (CFU), after preincubation with B. gingivalis LPS.

Superoxide- As with other experiments, the effect of B. gingivalis LPS was compared to E. coli LPS in the superoxide assay. In this case, the effect of E. coli LPS was biphasic, being inhibitory at high concentrations but enhancing the response at lower concentrations (Figure 2). In contrast to E. coli LPS, B. gingivalis LPS had no effect on the rate of O_2^- production by normal neutrophils. Further experiments were performed to assess the response of neutrophils from adult periodontitis patients infected with B. gingivalis. Under those circumstances, the A.P. neutrophils exhibited a a biphasic response to B. gingivalis LPS similar to that of E. coli (Figure 3). Hence, in uninfected individuals there is no effect of B. gingivalis LPS on superoxide generation, whereas, in B. gingivalis infected individuals, B. gingivalis LPS markedly inhibits superoxide generation at high doses and enhances superoxide generation a low doses.

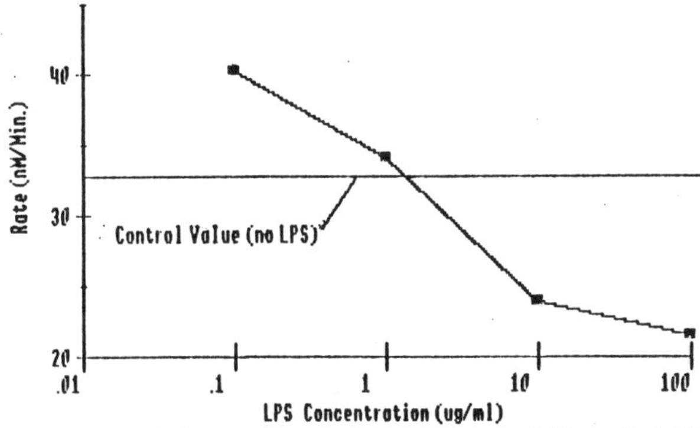

Figure 2- The effect of increasing concentrations of E. coli LPS on the rate of superoxide generation (nM cytochrome C reduced per minute).

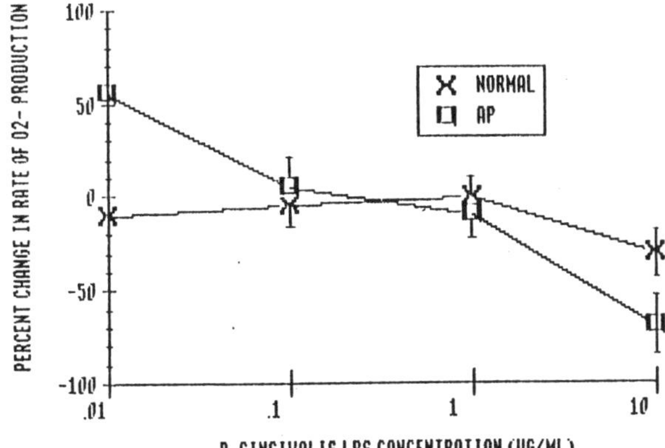

Figure 3- The change in rate of superoxide generation expressed as percent change from control (no LPS), for B. gingivalis LPS. Normal human neutrophils from non-infected individuals are compared to neutrophils from AP patients infected with B. gingivalis.

DISCUSSION

In these studies we demonstrate that lipopolysaccaride (LPS) from B. gingivalis has potent inhibitory effects upon host response by direct inhibition of neutrophil function. This is in contrast to LPS from enteric organisms that generally enhance neutrophil function. Specifically, B. gingivalis LPS markedly inhibits neutrophil motility, both directed (chemotaxis) and random (chemokinesis). Bactericidal activity of a non-related indicator organism is completely inhibited at high doses of LPS and the B. gingivalis organism itself is resistent to phagocytosis.

The effect of LPS on neutrophil superoxide generation is of interest. E. coli LPS modifies the O_2^- response of the neutrophil to stimulus (FMLP or opsonized zymosan) in a biphasic manner, enhancing the response at low dose and inhibiting at high dose. B. gingivalis LPS had no effect on normal neutrophils at any concentration tested. It was of interest, therefore, to elucidate the effect of B. gingivalis LPS on neutrophils of AP patients who were infected with B. gingivalis. B. gingivalis infection was confirmed by culture of periodontal pockets and serum antibody titer (ELISA). Neutrophils from AP patients exhibited the same response to B. gingivalis and E. coli LPS, that of biphasic enhancement or inhibition. These data suggest that prior exposure of the host to the LPS is necessary to respond to the LPS in vitro.

There are reports in the literature of Bacteroides inhibition of phagocytosis and killing of indicator organisms (38,39). In order to further investigate these phenomenon, we performed experiments to evaluate the effect of B. gingivalis LPS on phagocytosis and killing of a non-related indicator organism (S. epidermidis) and to evaluate the direct interaction of neutrophils with B. gingivalis LPS on phagocytosis and killing experiments in which B. gingivalis was the indicator organism.

In contrast to previous reports, our data indicated that there was no effect of B. gingivalis LPS on phagocytosis of S. epidermidis (data not shown). However, B. gingivalis LPS inhibited killing of S. epidermis by normal neutrophils in a dose dependent manner, such that at 10 $\mu g/\mu l$ LPS there was no reduction in C.F.U. (Figure I).

Of greater significance is the interaction of B. gingivalis and neutrophils when the phagocytosis of B. gingivalis by normal neutrophils is directly evaluated. Previous work in our laboratories related to the phagocytosis and killing of A.a. by LJP neutrophils revealed that normal neutrophils will phagocytose and kill opsonized A.a. rapidly and efficiently (2, see Table III). Using this interaction as a positive control, the phagocytosis and killing of opsonized B. gingivalis by neutrophils in the same assay was evaluated. In contrast to the rapid uptake of A.a. by neutrophils (16.9 A.a./neutrophil, about 60% of neutrophils contain bacteria), B. gingivalis was markedly resistant to phagocytosis (0.07 B. gingivalis/neutrophils, <8% of neutrophils contain bacteria).

The data presented strongly suggest that there are many diverse effects of LPS upon phagocytic cell function. Of particular note is the fact that all LPS are not alike; each exhibiting properties unique to its' structure. The implication is, therefore, that the LPS from each periodontal organism is capable of direct inhibition of the host via unique molecular properties.

Of further significance, are the properties of B. gingivalis. The mechanism of the avoidance of neutrophil phagocytosis is unknown. However, the known properties of B. gingivalis suggest possible mechanisms, such as fibriae, capsule, LPS or degradation of opsonizing antibody. Overall, the pathogenic potential of B. gingivalis appears enormous and the further elucidation of host cell-B. gingivalis interaction will aid in the understanding of the pathogenesis of microbial infection.

REFERENCES

1. Ranney, R.R., Debski, B.F. and Tew, J.G. Pediatr. Dent. 3:89 (1981).
2. Socransky, S.S. J. Periodontol. 48:497 (1977).
3. Cianciola, L.J., Genco, R.J., Patters, M.R., McKenna, J., van Oss, C.J. Nature (London), 256:445 (1977).
4. Kalmar, J.R., Arnold, R.R. and Van Dyke, T.E. J. Period. Res. 22:179-181 (1987).
5. Moore, W.E.C., Ranney, R.R. and Holdeman, L.V. American Soci. Micro.
6. Slots, J. J. Clin. Periodontal. 6:351 (1979).
7. White, D. and Mayrand, D. J. Periodontal. Res. 16:259 (1981).
8. Galanose, C., Luderitz, O. Reitschel, E. and Westphal, O. Int. Rev. Biochem. 14:239.
9. Morrison, D.C. and Jacobs, D.M. Immunochemistry 13:813 (1976).
10. Kotani, S., Takada, H, Tsujimoto, M., Ogawa, T., Harada, K., Mori, Y., Kawasake, A., Tanaka, A., Nagao, S., Tetsuo, S., Shoichi, K., Imuto, M., Yoshimura, H., Yamamoto, M. and Shimamoto, T. Infect. Immun 45:293 (1984).
11. Gerg, I., Kruyer, J. and Spiesel, S.F. J. Immunol. 108:1088 (1972)
12. Anderson, J., Moller, G. and Sjoberg, O. Cell. Immunol. 4:381 (1972).
13. Ortiz-Ortiz, L. and Jaroslow, B.N. Immunol. 19:387 (1970).
14. Rank, W.R.,Di Pauli, R. and Flugge-Rank, U. Eur. J. Immunol. 2:517 (1972).
15. Scheid, M.P., Hoffmann, M.K., Komuro, K., Hammerling, V., Abbott, J., Boyse, E.A., Cohen, G.H., Hooper, J.A., Schulof, R.S. and Goldstein, A.L. J. Exp. Med. 138:1027 (1973).
16. Schmidake, J.R. and Najarian, J.S. J. Immunol. 114:742 (1975).
17. Ruco, L.P. and Meltzer, M.S. J. Immunol. 120:329 (1978).
18. Ruco, L.P. and Meltzer, M.S. J. Immunol. 121:2935 (1978).
19. Evans, A.C. and Bruce, W.R. Cell Tissue Kinet 7:19 (1974).
20. Cohen, D.W. and Morris, A.L. J. Periodontol. 32:159 (1961).
21. Unanue, E.R., Kiely, J.M. and Calderon, J. Exp. Med. 144:155 (1976).
22. Morley, J. Prostaglandins 8:272 (1974).
23. Smith, T.J. and Wagner, R.R. J. Exp. Med. 125:559 (1967).
24. Finkelstein, M.S., Bausek, G.H. and Merigan, T.C. Science 161:465 (1968).
25. Guthrie, L.A., McPhail, L.C., Henson, P.M. and Johnston, Jr., R.B. J. Exp. Med 160:1656 (1984).
26. Hase, S. and Rietschel, E.T. Eur. J. Biochem. 63:101 (1976).
27. Hofstad, T. and Kristoffeinsen, T. J. Gen. Microbiol 61:15 (1970).
28 Wollenweber, H.W., Rietschel, E.T., Hofstad, T., Weintraub, A. and Lindberg, A.A. J. Bacteriol. 144:898 (1980).
29. Kasper, D.L. J. Infect. Dis. 134:59 (1984).
30. Iino, Y. and Hopps, R.M. Arch. Oral Biol. 29:59 (1984).
31. Donaldson, S.L., Ranney, R.R. and Tew, J.G. Infect. and Immun. 42:487 (1983).
32. Humphrey, J.H. Br. J. Exp. Pathol. 36:268 (1955).
33. Verghese, M.W. and Snyderman, R. J. Immunol. 127:288 (1981).
33. Duncan, Jr., R.L. and Morrison, D.C. J. Immunol. 132:1416 (1984).
34. Westphal, O. and Jann, K,:Bacterial lipopolysaccharides:Extraction with phenol-water and further applications of the procedure; Vol 5 (Academic Press, N.Y.).
35. Van Dyke, T.E., Reilly, A.A., Horoszewicz, H.U., Gagliardi, N. and Genco, R.J. J. Immunol. Meth. 31:271 (1979).
36. Van Furth, R., Van Zwet, T.L. and Leijh, P.C.J.:Handbook of Experimental Immunology, p. 31 (London, Blackwell).
37. Ingham, H.R., Sisson, P.R., Tharagonnet, D., Selkon, J.B. and Codd, A.P. The Lancet ii:1252 (1977).
38. Church, J.A. and Nye, C.A. Ann. Allergy 43:333 (1979).

Dr. T.E. Van Dyke, Department of Periodontology and Dental Research, Emory University, 1462 Clifton N.E., Atlanta, Georgia 30322, USA

Periodontology Today. Int. Congr., Zürich 1988, pp. 218–226 (Karger, Basel 1988)

Mediators of Osteoclast Activation in vitro and their Relevance to Resorption in Periodontal Diseases

John Reynolds

Cell Physiology Department, Strangeways Research Laboratory, Cambridge, UK

1. Introduction

During inflammatory diseases activated leukocytes produce many cytokines which influence not only the behaviour of other leukocytes but also have profound effects on the activities of non-leukocyte cell populations. Cytokines are thus the key mediators of the host response to exogenous antigens, and they include the interleukins, tumour necrosis factors, transforming growth factors and interferons. Interleukin-1 (IL-1), for example, enhances various immune responses and also mediates non-immunological events, including synthesis of acute phase proteins, endogenous pyrogen-induced fever, fibroblast proliferation, muscle breakdown, and metalloproteinase and prostaglandin production by tissue cells. IL-1 is also potent in inducing bone resorption and it is what was hitherto termed osteoclast activating factor (OAF; 5). While most cytokine responses are beneficial to the host, those involving connective tissues are potentially damaging. We proposed that a major cause of tissue breakdown in periodontal diseases is due to the interaction between bacterial antigens and inflammatory cells, resulting in the production of cytokines (23). Unlike gingivitis, periodontitis results in acute and chronic episodes of bone loss (33). Thus the relationship of the production of cytokines to tissue destruction is of great current interest.

2. Physiological Mediators of Bone Resorption In Vitro

Before discussing pathological bone resorption it is first necessary to summarise the presently perceived situation in physiology. In intact bone parathyroid hormone (PTH) and 1,25-dihydroxycholecalciferol (1,25$(OH)_2D_3$) are the most important stimulaters of bone resorption. There is a wealth of literature on their effects *in vitro* (see also Table IA): both hormones can increase osteoclast numbers and increase resorption by the stimulation of existing mature osteoclasts. An intriguing fact that long remained an enigma is that osteoclasts lack receptors for PTH and $1,25(OH)_2D_3$. It was shown recently that when osteoclasts are separated from non-osteoclastic bone cells, PTH and $1,25(OH)_2D_3$ no longer increase resorption (20). The realisation that osteoblasts and not osteoclasts were the target cells for the bone resorbing hormones and prostaglandins suggested that osteoblasts both synthesize bone and, by mediating osteoclast control, co-ordinate its removal.

One mechanism by which osteoblasts can initiate resorption by resident osteoclasts is by mineral exposure. Bone is formed with a thin covering of unmineralized osteoid, which appears to shield the underlying bone from osteoclast attack. Calvarial cells can remove osteoid and thereby permit resorption to commence (2), and this initiating action of calvarial cells is

Table I. Factors that can cause increased bone resorption *in vitro* and may be important *in vivo*.

Factor	Approx. Dose Range (M)
A: Physiological Agents	
$1,25(OH)_2D_3$	10^{-9} - 10^{-11}
Parathyroid Hormone (PTH)	10^{-7} - 10^{-9}
B: Pathological (?) Agents	
Interleukin 1s: IL-1a and IL-1ß	10^{-10} - 10^{-12}
Tumour Necrosis Factors: TNF-a (cachectin):TNF-ß (lymphotoxin)	10^{-7} - 10^{-9}
Transforming Growth Factors: TGF-a; TGF-ß	10^{-9} - 10^{-11}
Epidermal Growth Factor (EGF)	10^{-8} - 10^{-10}
Platelet-Derived Growth Factor (PDGF)	10^{-8} - 10^{-10}
Prostaglandin E_2 (PGE_2)	10^{-6} - 10^{-8}

The data is representative of many studies (see text) on the relative activities of the various bone resorbing factors and is mostly from work with calvariae *in vitro*: there are differences between various test systems and the table is not meant to give a precise definition of all the factors.

enhanced by PTH, and can be mimiced by mammalian collagenase (3). We showed that osteoblasts synthesize latent collagenase and that its production is increased by bone resorbing hormones (11). Osteoblasts were shown to be able to resorb collagen by culturing them on films of type I collagen (41). The balance between metalloproteinases and TIMP (tissue inhibitor of metalloproteinases) production could provide an initiation mechanism for bone resorption that is dependent on resident cells and subject to hormonal regulation (41). Tetracyclines inhibit bone resorption in organ culture (7) and are in use in periodontal diseases: GOMES et al. (7) suggested that they act by inhibiting collagenase as well as by being antibiotics.

Osteoid destruction alone, however, is not sufficient to account for osteoclast stimulation by osteoblasts. Stimulated osteoblasts produce a factor which directly induces mature osteoclasts to resorb (21,22). PERRY (26) demonstrated the production of a factor from PTH-treated mononuclear leukocytes which stimulates cultured bone to resorb: this factor may be related to IL-1 (27) and be made by osteoblasts. Thus there may be several pathways for osteoblasts to signal to osteoclasts.

3. Pathological Mediators of Bone Resorption In Vitro

IL-1.

Work in this author's laboratory first demonstrated that cultured human monocytes produce a non-prostanoid factor which can stimulate bone resorption *in vitro* (8). We suggested that the resorptive activity was due to an IL-1-like factor and later showed that pure pig IL-1a is a potent stimulater of bone resorption (13). Concentrations as low as 25 pM are effective (Table IB), demonstrating that it is an order of magnitude more potent than 1,25$(OH)_2D_3$. THOMSON et al. (39) suggested that IL-1 stimulates bone resorption through a primary action on osteoblasts that is not prostaglandin mediated (see below).

IL-1 is now recognized as a family of polypeptides. In the human two distinct gene products have been cloned and termed IL-1a (pI 5) and IL-1ß (pI 7); these two forms have been found in every species studied to date. The predominant species produced by activated human monocytes is IL-1ß which seems to be more active than IL-1a. Although mononuclear phagocytes were once thought to be a unique source of IL-1 it is clear that a wide variety of cell types can produce it. Monolayer cultures of rabbit periosteal fibroblasts synthesize a factor that stimulates bone resorption and which has IL-1 activity (12), suggesting that periosteal cells may also play a role in bone biology. This fibroblast factor stimulates mouse osteoblasts and rabbit chondrocytes to increase collagenase production. Recently a resorbing factor from human gingival fibroblasts has been described (18), which seems to be IL-1-like.

Transforming Growth Factors (TGF-a and TGF-ß)

TGF-a is a polypeptide mitogen that is 35% homologous with

epidermal growth factor (EGF). Both factors stimulate bone resorption (see Table IB) and increase prostaglandin E_2 (PGE_2) production (16,32,37). TGF-a also inhibits collagen synthesis in cultured calvaria. As a solid tumour product with potent bone resorbing activity TGF-a has been implicated as a factor in the pathogenesis of hypercalcemia of malignancy (16).

TGF-ß belongs to a family of dimeric polypeptide growth factors which act in organisms ranging from drosophila to man. They do not interact with the TGF-a/EGF receptor. TGF-ß has been implicated in embryogenesis and tissue repair and seems to be involved in the control of differentiation and cell growth (4). Although most normal cells and tumours (17) produce TGF-ß, it is particularly abundant in bone (6). TGF-ß is synthesized by osteoblasts (30) and is a potent inducer of bone resorption (37). Interestingly bone resorbing hormones all increase TGF-ß release from organ cultured calvaria (29), either by increasing synthesis or the liberation of TGF-ß from lysing bone matrix.

In normal individuals bone replacement matches bone destruction so that turnover occurs without a change in skeletal mass. Many hypotheses have invoked "coupling" factors to co-ordinate the two events but it now seems likely that this results from a complex interplay of the various local hormones with systemic hormones, and that intercellular mediators are involved in controlling the recruitment, maturation and activation of bone cells. Present data suggest that TGF-ß may be a very important local regulator in skeletal tissue.

<u>The Tumour Necrosis Factors (TNF-a and TNF-ß)</u>

These cytokines, TNF-a and TNF-ß, are products of activated macrophages and lymphocytes respectively. Although having no effect on lymphocytes, the TNFs share many of the actions of IL-1, including those on connective tissues: they can induce bone resorption (1,31,38), although they are not as potent as IL-1 (Table I). The TNFs act on osteoclasts by way of osteoblasts (40) and they also inhibit collagen synthesis (1).

<u>Platelet-derived growth factor (PDGF)</u>

PGDF induces bone resorption via a prostaglandin-mediated pathway since its action is inhibited by indomethacin, a cyclo-oxygenase inhibitor (36, and see below). Its importance is not yet clear, nor how it interacts with other cytokine factors.

<u>Prostaglandins</u>

It has been long-established that prostaglandins can stimulate bone resorption, particularly PGE_2 (reviewed in 10), although relatively high levels are needed <u>in vitro</u> (Table IB). Some actions of cytokines are mediated by prostaglandin-dependent pathways and consequently prostaglandins may have a key role in mediating much pathological resorption. For example, the actions of TNF-a and TGF-ß on resorption <u>in vitro</u> are prevented by indomethacin (32,37). <u>In vivo</u> prostaglandin synthesis inhibitors can reduce periodontitis in dogs (42).

Interferon-gamma (IFN-γ)

IFN-γ prevents IL-1- and TNF-induced bone resorption *in vitro* (9,15) and inhibits prostaglandin-mediated resorption (15). It may act by inhibiting osteoclast formation (35). Presently there is some divergence of opinion as to whether IFN-γ can prevent PTH-induced resorption (9,28).

4. Bone Resorption In Vivo and Periodontal Diseases

We presented evidence (14,23) that pathogens might mediate tissue destruction in periodontal diseases through the ability of bacterial antigens to stimulate cytokine production in circulating monocytes, and perhaps fibroblasts. We envisaged that the cytokines then induce metalloproteinase synthesis in resident gingival cells, resulting in matrix degradation, with the final destructive phase being the loss of alveolar bone. Although some of the cytokines responsible for tissue destruction remain poorly characterized, much circumstantial evidence suggests that the IL-1s are the most important.

We cultured monocytes from patients with severe periodontal destruction to ascertain if they had been pre-activation *in vivo*. We found a wide range in the levels of IL-1 produced, but our findings did indicate that monocytes from patients with *active* disease, particularly those who do not respond to treatment, release IL-1ß spontaneously into the culture medium (24). However, since this investigation was initiated it has become clear that antigen-activated monocytes also produce TNF. An additional complication is that human gingival fibroblasts in culture, and stimulated with lipopolysaccharide (LPS, from *Actinobacillus actinomycetemcomitans*), produce IL-1 (MEIKLE, M.C., personal communication). This finding has implications for the early development of the periodontal lesion because IL-1 can act as a chemoattractant for neutrophils, monocytes and lymphocytes. Hitherto only chemotactic substances derived either from plaque bacteria or resulting from complement activation have been thought important in promoting leukocytosis during the generation of the initial response. Fibroblasts could be acting as an antigen-presenting cell.

We found that both LPS and LTA (lipotechoic acid) from several bacterial strains commonly present in plaque were equally effective in inducing the production of cytokines able to stimulate gingival fibroblasts to synthesize collagenase (14). We have concluded that if a cytokine-mediated mechanism is important in tissue destruction during periodontitis, then the disease may be triggered by a large variety of bacteria, or by combinations. This is at variance with theories which assume that either one or a small number of bacterial strains mediate the onset and progress of the disease. We think that disease is more likely to be initiated in a susceptible individual by a critical number of organisms, comprising a mixture of strains able to exploit the environmental conditions pertaining.

5. Concluding Comments

It is clear that many hormones and cytokines can influence bone resorption and that there is probably a complex synergism (31). Therefore a much more detailed knowledge of the factors involved in modulating the synthesis and actions of cytokines is needed if a better understanding of bone resorption at one sight *in vivo* is to be gained. One major problem is that the number of agents that affect bone resorption is still increasing. Recently a polypeptide with significant homology to PTH has been cloned and which may be important in normal bone physiology as well as in the humoral hypercalcemia of malignancy (34). Also the various cytokines may modulate the synthesis and activity of each other. For example, with vascular cells TNF induces the release of IL-1 (19,25), and TNF and IL-1 can have synergistic effects on bone. Better assays for cytokines are becoming available and studies on periodontal diseases could provide data that would be of value in understanding the destructive events in many inflammatory diseases.

6. Acknowledgements

Work in the author's laboratory is funded by the Medical Research Council (U.K.). Thanks are given to MURRAY MEIKLE and BRIAN THOMSON for helpful discussions of the manuscript.

7. References

1. BERTOLINI, D.R.; NEDWIN, G.E.; BRINGMAN, T.S.; SMITH, D.D., and MUNDY, G.R.: Stimulation of bone resorption and inhibition of bone formation *in vitro* by human tumour necrosis factors. Nature 319: 516-518 (1986).
2. CHAMBERS, T.J., and FULLER,K.: Bone cells predispose bone surfaces to resorption by exposure of mineral to osteoclastic contact. J. Cell Sci. 76: 155-165 (1985).
3. CHAMBERS, T.J.; DARBY,J.A., and FULLER,K.: Mammalian collagenase predisposes bone surfaces to osteoclastic resorption. Cell Tissue Res. 241: 671-675 (1985).
4. CHEIFETZ, S.; WEATHERBEE, J.A.; TSANG,M.L.S.; ANDERSON,J.K.; MOLE, J.E.; LUCAS, R., and MASSAGUE, J.: The transforming growth factor-ß system, a complex pattern of cross-reactive ligands and receptors. Cell 48: 409-415 (1987).
5. DEWHIRST, F.E.; STASHENKO, P.P.; MOLE, J.E., and TSURUMACHI, T.: Purification and partial sequence of human osteoclast-activating factor: identity with interleukin 1ß. J. Immunol. 135: 2562-2568 (1985).
6. ELLINGSWORTH ,L.R.; BRENNAN, J.E.; FOK, K.; ROSEN, D.M.; BENTZ, H.; PIEZ, K.A., and SEYEDIN, S.M.: Antibodies to the N-terminal portion of cartilage-inducing factor A and transforming growth factor B. Immunohistochemical localization and association with differentiating cells.

J. Biol. Chem. 261: 12362-12367 (1986).
7. GOMES, B.C.; GOLUB, L.M., and RAMAMURTHY, N.S.: Tetracyclines inhibit parathyroid hormone-induced bone resorption in organ culture. Experientia 40: 1273-1275 (1984).
8. GOWEN, M.; MEIKLE, M.C., and REYNOLDS,J.J.: Stimulation of bone resorption *in vitro* by a non-prostanoid factor released by human monocytes in culture. Biochim. Biophys. Acta 762: 471-474 (1983).
9. GOWEN, M.; NEDWIN, G.E., and MUNDY, G.R.: Preferential inhibition of cytokine-stimulated bone resorption by recombinant interferon gamma. J. Bone Mineral Res. 1: 469-474 (1986).
10. HARVEY, W., and MEGHJI, S.: Prostaglandins in pathological bone resorption. Agents Actions 19: 73-79 (1986).
11. HEATH, J.K.; ATKINSON, S.J.; MEIKLE, M.C., and REYNOLDS, J.J.: Mouse osteoblasts synthesize collagenase in response to bone resorbing agents. Biochim. Biophys. Acta 802: 151-154 (1984).
12. HEATH, J.K.; SAKLATVALA, J.; MEIKLE, M.C.; ATKINSON, S.J., and REYNOLDS, J.J.: Periosteal fibroblasts synthesize a cytokine that stimulates bone resorption and demonstrates interleukin-1 activity after partial purification. Br. J. Rheum. 24: (Suppl. 1), 136-139 (1985).
13. HEATH, J.K.; SAKLATVALA, J.; MEIKLE, M.C.; ATKINSON, S.J., and REYNOLDS, J.J.: Pig interleukin 1 (catabolin) is a potent stimulator of bone resorption *in vitro*. Calcif. Tissue Int. 37: 95-97 (1985).
14. HEATH, J.K.; ATKINSON, S.J.; HEMBRY, R.M.; REYNOLDS, J.J., and MEIKLE, M.C.: Bacterial antigens induce collagenase and prostaglandin E_2 synthesis in human gingival fibroblasts through a primary effect on circulating mononuclear cells. Infection Immunity 55: 2148-2154 (1987).
15. HOFFMANN, O.; KLAUSHOFER, K.; GLEISPACH, H.; LEIS, H.J.; LUGER, T.; KOLLER, K., and PETERLIK, M.: Gamma interferon inhibits basal and interleukin 1-induced prostaglandin production and bone resorption in neonatal mouse calvaria. Biochem. Biophys. Res. Commun. 143: 38-43 (1987).
16. IBBOTSON, K.J.; TWARDZIK, D.R.; D'SOUSA, S.M.; HARGREAVES, W.R.; TODARO, G.J., and MUNDY, G.R.: Stimulation of bone resorption *in vitro* by synthetic transforming growth factor-alpha. Science 228: 1007-1009 (1985).
17. INSOGNA, K.L.; WEIR, E.C.; WU, T.L.; STEWART, A.F.; BROADUS, A.E.; BURTIS, W.J., and CENTRELLA, M.: Co-purification of transforming growth factor ß-like activity with PTH-like and bone-resorbing activities from a tumor associated with humoral hypercalcemia of malignancy. Endocrinology 120: 2183-2185 (1987).
18. LERNER, U., and HANSTROM, L.: Human gingival fibroblasts secrete non-dialyzable, prostanoid-independent products which stimulate bone resorption *in vitro*. J. Periodont. Res. 22: 284-289 (1987).
19. LIBBY, P.; ORDOVAS, J.M.; AUGER, K.R.; ROBBINS, A.H.; BIRINYI, L.K., and DINARELLO, C.A.: Endotoxin and tumor

necrosis factor induce interleukin-1 gene expression in adult human vascular endothelial cells. Am. J. Pathol. 124: 179-185 (1986).

20. MCSHEEHY, P.M.J., and CHAMBERS, T.J.: Osteoblastic cells mediate osteoclastic responsiveness to parathyroid hormone. Endocrinology 118: 824-828 (1986).

21. MCSHEEHY, P.M.J., and CHAMBERS, T.J.: Osteoblast-like cells in the presence of parathyroid hormone release soluble factor that stimulates osteoclastic bone resorption. Endocrinology 119: 1654-1659 (1986).

22. MCSHEEHY, P.M.J., and CHAMBERS, T.J.: 1,25-dihydroxyvitamin D_3 stimulates rat osteoblastic cells to release a soluble factor that increases osteoclastic bone resorption. J. Clin. Invest. 80: 425-429 (1987).

23. MEIKLE, M.C.; HEATH,J.K., and REYNOLDS,J.J.: Advances in understanding cell interactions in tissue resorption. Relevance to the pathogenesis of periodontal diseases and a new hypothesis. J. Oral Pathol. 15: 239-250 (1986).

24. MEIKLE, M.C.; MCALPINE, C.G.; HEATH,J.K.; NEWMAN,H.N., and REYNOLDS,J.J.: Interleukin-1 production by peripheral blood mononuclear cells from patients with severe periodontitis; in LEHNER and CIMASONI, The Borderland Between Caries and Periodontal Disease III, pp. 283-290 (Editions Medecine et Hygiene, Geneva 1986).

25. NAWROTH, P.P.; BANK, I.; HANDLEY, D.; CASSIMERIS, J.; CHESS, L., and STERN, D.: Tumor necrosis factor/cachectin interacts with endothelial cell receptors to induce release of interleukin 1. J. Exp. Med. 163: 1363-1375 (1986).

26. PERRY, H.M.: Parathyroid hormone-lymphocyte interactions modulate bone resorption. Endocrinology 119: 2333-2339 (1986).

27. PERRY, H.M.; SKOGEN, W.; CHAPPEL, J.C.; WILNER, G.D.; KAHN, A.J., and TEITELBAUM,S.L.: Conditioned medium from osteoblast-like cells mediate parathyroid hormone induced bone resorption. Calcif. Tissue Int. 40: 298-300 (1987).

28. PETERLIK, M.; HOFFMANN, O.; SWETLY, P.; KLAUSHOFER, K., and KOLLER, K.: Recombinant γ-interferon inhibits prostaglandin-mediated and parathyroid hormone-induced bone resorption in cultured neonatal mouse calvaria. FEBS Lett. 185: 287-290 (1985).

29. PFEILSCHIFTER, J., and MUNDY, G.R.: Modulation of type ß transforming growth factor activity in bone cultures by osteotropic hormones. Proc. Natl. Acad. Sci. USA 84: 2024-2028 (1987).

30. ROBEY, P.G.; YOUNG, M.F.; FLANDERS, K.C.; ROCHE, N.S.; KONDAIAH, P.; REDDI, A.H.; TERMINE, J.D.; SPORN, M.B., and ROBERTS, A.B.: Osteoblasts synthesize and respond to transforming growth factor-type ß (TGF-ß) in vitro. J. Cell Biol. 105: 457-463 (1987).

31. STASHENKO, P.; DEWHIRST, F.E.; PEROS, W.J.; KENT, R.L., and AGO, J.M.: Synergistic interactions between interleukin 1, tumor necrosis factor, and lymphotoxin in bone resorption. J. Immunol. 138: 1464-1468 (1987).

32. STERN, P.H.; KRIEGER, N.S.; NISSENSON, R.A.; WILLIAMS, R.D.; WINKLER, M.E.; DERYNCK, R., and STREWLER, G.J.: Human transforming growth factor-alpha stimulates bone resorption in vitro. J. Clin. Invest. 76: 2016-2019 (1985).
33. STERRETT, J.D.: The osteoclast and periodontitis. J. Clin. Periodontol. 13: 258-269 (1986).
34. SUVA, L.J.; WINSLOW, G.A.; WETTENHALL, R.E.H.; HAMMONDS, R.G.; MOSELEY, J.M.; DIEFENBACH-JAGGER, H.; RODDA, C.P.; KEMP, B.E.; RODRIGUEZ, H.; CHEN, E.Y.; HUDSON, P.J.; MARTIN, T.J., and WOOD, W.I.: A parathyroid hormone-related protein implicated in malignant hypercalcemia: cloning and expression. Science 237: 893-896 (1987).
35. TAKAHASHI, N.; MUNDY, G.R., and ROODMAN, G.D.: Recombinant human interferon-γ inhibits formation of human osteoclast-like cells. J. Immunol. 137: 3544-3549 (1986).
36. TASHJIAN, A.H.; HOHMANN, E.L.; ANTONIADES, H.N., and LEVINE, L.: Platelet-derived growth factor stimulates bone resorption via a prostaglandin-mediated mechanism. Endocrinology 111: 118-124 (1982).
37. TASHJIAN, A.H.; VOELKEL, E.F.; LAZZARO, M.; SINGER, F.R.; ROBERTS, A.B.; DERYNCK, R.; WINKLER, M.E., and LEVINE, L.: a and ß human transforming growth factors stimulate prostaglandin production and bone resorption in cultured mouse calvaria. Proc. Natl. Acad. Sci. USA 82: 4535-4538 (1985).
38. TASHJIAN, A.H.; VOELKEL, E.F.; LAZZARO, M.; GOAD, D.; BOSMA, T., and LEVINE, L.: Tumor necrosis factor factor-a (cachectin) stimulates bone resorption in mouse calvaria via a prostaglandin-mediated mechanism. Endocrinology 120: 2029-2036 (1987).
39. THOMSON, B.M.; SAKLATVALA, J., and CHAMBERS, T.J.: Osteoblasts mediate interleukin 1 stimulation of bone resorption by rat osteoclasts. J. Exp. Med. 164: 104-112 (1986).
40. THOMSON, B.M.; MUNDY, G.R., and CHAMBERS, T.J.: Tumor necrosis factors a and ß induce osteoblastic cells to stimulate osteoclastic bone resorption. J. Immunol. 138: 775-779 (1987).
41. THOMSON, B.M.; ATKINSON, S.J.; REYNOLDS, J.J., and MEIKLE, M.C.: Degradation of type I collagen films by mouse osteoblasts is stimulated by 1,25 dihydroxyvitamin D_3 and inhibited by human recombinant TIMP (tissue inhibitor of metalloproteinases). Biochem. Biophys. Res. Commun. 148: 596-602 (1987).
42. WILLIAMS, R.C.; JEFFCOAT, M.K.; HOWELL, T.H.; HALL, C.M.; JOHNSON, H.G.; WECHTER, W.J., and GOLDHABER, P.: Indomethacin or flurbiprofen treatment of periodontitis in beagles: comparison of effect on bone loss. J. Periodont. Res. 22: 403-407 (1987).

8. Author's Address

John J. Reynolds, Cell Physiology Department, Strangeways Research Laboratory, Cambridge CB1 4RN (U.K.)

Periodontology Today. Int. Congr., Zürich 1988, pp. 227–235 (Karger, Basel 1988)

A Critical Assessment of the Burst Hypothesis

Henning Birkedal-Hansen, Marilyn S. Lantz and Ronald B. Cogen

University of Alabama School of Dentistry, University of Alabama at Birmingham, Birmingham, Alabama, USA

Introduction

Data from cross sectional and longitudinal studies indicate that the severity of chronic adult periodontitis increases slowly but continuously with age in a population (1,2,18,22). In the absence of any direct evidence, these observations have evolved into a model which portrays the disease as slowly and continuously progressive within individual subjects and in individual sites. This model adequately accounts for averaged population data but fails to explain the rapid progression of the disease in individual sites observed by some investigators. Results from several studies suggest that a disproportionately large fraction of sites loses probing attachment, often exceeding 2-3 mm, within a relatively short period of time (for review see 4,8). This observation is inconsistent with a slowly, continuously progressive disease model and led the authors to formulate a new concept of disease progression based on bursts of disease activity separated by longer periods of remission or quiescence. In recent publications (4,7,8,11,12,23), the statistical treatment of the data has been expanded in attempts to gather evidence in support of the model. However, concerns have been raised over the interpretation of the underlying data sets on both statistical and biological grounds. In this paper, we have summarized the evidence for and against the burst hypothesis. In addition, we have raised two questions which need to be considered in the discussion of periodontal disease models: (i) does the burst model apply only to a small, unrepresentative disease entity? and (ii) are rapid changes of probing attachment level indicative of loss or gain of connective tissue attachment?

Arguments in favor of the burst model

Goodson et al. (6) examined 22 untreated patients (1155

sites) by repeat monthly probing measurements and reported that 5.7% of sites showed significant probing attachment loss ($p<0.01$) over a one year period when analyzed by sequential linear regression. In order to account for the apparent numerical excess of deteriorating sites over those expected from measurement error alone (1% at the $p=0.01$ level), the authors suggested that the disease progresses by alternating periods of exacerbation and remission. It was proposed that over a given period of time, in this case one year, only a small percentage of sites actually lost attachment. However, the sites in question lost a disproportionate amount of attachment which far exceeded the approximately 0.1 mm per year estimated on a population basis (for review see (24)).

The authors subsequently introduced two new analytical techniques, the running medians method and the tolerance method, designed to discriminate between disease "active" and "inactive" sites (10,11). The first method analyzes running medians of three in a succession of individual measurements at the same site over time in order to dampen the "noise" of attachment level measurements. The tolerance method analyzes the difference between two sets of duplicate site measurements based on the site specific variability. A study of 3,414 sites monitored by repeat bimonthly measurements revealed that sequential linear regression identified almost twice as many "losing" sites (5.1%) as either the running medians (2.6%) or the tolerance method (2.8%)(10,11). The data illustrate how sensitive the results are to the choice of analytical method and to the arbitrary choice of cut-off level to distinguish losing from non-losing sites (trade-off of type I and type II error). These problems notwithstanding, the incidence of probing attachment loss in this data set (11) was similar to that reported in two other studies. In a Swedish population (4101 sites in 64 patients), 3.9% of sites lost more than 2 mm attachment over a 3 year period, and 11.6% lost this much or more in 6 years (16). In a U.S. population (3210 sites in 36 subjects), 3.2% of sites lost more than 2 mm attachment over a 1 year period (16). A more detailed analysis of patterns of probing attachment loss led Socransky et al. (24) to suggest that bursts of disease activity may occur with higher frequency during certain periods of an individual's life and that burst sites "may show no further activity or could be subject to one or more bursts at later time periods."

In an effort to correlate probing attachment loss with radiographic bone loss, Goodson et al. (5) analyzed a subset of sites in 22 patients from the 1982 study (6). Fourteen of 231 sites (6.1%) showed loss of alveolar bone height in excess of 0.48 mm, but none of these sites showed probing attachment loss during the same time period. In most sites, loss of probing attachment preceded loss of bone by 6-8 months. Somewhat surprisingly, virtually all of the lost probing attachment was regained before radiographic bone loss was detected.

With the application of survival functions to (treated and untreated) periodontitis sites, Haffajee et al. (9) introduced a new method of analysis. Sites that lost more than 3 mm (4 x standard deviation) of probing attachment between two successive measurements were considered to have "died." The annual hazard rate, i.e. that fraction of sites that "died" within a year, was in the range of 0.10-0.16. Therapy reduced the annual hazard rate by a factor between 2 and 10. The number of sites that lost more than 3 mm of attachment (10-16%) was substantially higher than that expected from measurement error alone (<< 1%). These observations are consistent with the burst hypothesis but also with other disease models.

Based on curve fitting analysis of the frequency distribution of attachment level measurements in 61 chronic adult periodontitis patients, Haffajee and Socransky (7) and Socransky and Haffajee (23) identified three patterns of attachment loss. Each of these patterns could be accounted for by a single normal distribution or by summation of 2 or 3 independent normal distributions. By comparison with computer simulated distribution functions, the authors determined the range of burst sizes (0.3-3.4 mm attachment loss) that could account for the observed distributions. The data were consistent with a burst hypothesis although not necessarily to the exclusion of other disease models. As emphasized by the authors, however, such simulations are highly arbitrary and reflect the biases of the simulators.

In recent reviews, Goodson (4) and Haffajee and Socransky (8) summarized the arguments in favor of the burst hypothesis. It was a principal conclusion that a disproportionately large fraction of sites showed probing attachment loss which could not be accounted for by measurement error alone. Intraclass correlation among sites within an individual and autocorrelation of errors within sequential measurements were considered but were not found to significantly alter this conclusion. As will be discussed later, much of the concern over the statistical treatment of the data used in support of the burst hypothesis has focused on intraclass correlation and autocorrelation of errors. The argument in favor of the burst model is essentially a statistical one as are most of the counter arguments raised so far. The validity of the conclusion that significant loss of attachment occurs in a higher-than-expected fraction of sites hinges on the estimate of the standard deviation for probing attachment level measurements, the "cut-off" level chosen for significance of loss, and on the level of intraclass correlation and autocorrelation of errors in the data sets.

Arguments against the burst model

The evidence in favor of the burst hypothesis is largely based on analysis of probing attachment level measurements. It is widely recognized that a combination of unfavorable circumstances (large standard deviation, insensitivity to small changes, low incidence of disease) renders probing attachment level measurements unsatisfactory for assessment of disease progression. Variables such as probing force, anatomy of probing sites, probe positioning and state of inflammation contribute to a large standard deviation (0.3 - 1.1 mm)(24) which makes detection of small changes impossible. In essence, the noise overpowers the signal. An additional source of insensitivity of probing attachment level measurements is that the measurements are made in 1 mm increments and therefore fail to accurately detect small changes. Each of these problems can be managed if the disease in question occurs with high frequency but it does not. The incidence of bursts of significant size is often so low that the numbers of "false positives" and "true positives" are of the same order of magnitude.

Statistical concerns. The statistical criticism of the burst model does not necessarily imply that the model is incorrect but that the underlying data may be accounted for entirely by measurement error. The thrust of the argument is that intraclass correlation within sites and autocorrelation of errors result in underestimation of the type I error (assuming change when there is none) and therefore lead to erroneous conclusions. These concerns have been detailed by Morrison and Kowalski (20), Imrey (13), Laster (15) and Ralls and Cohen (21).

Morrison and Kowalski's criticism (20) focused on two issues: (i) the logical inconsistency of testing a burst hypothesis by linear regression analyses of sequential measurements, and (ii) the risk of underestimating the type I error when the measurement errors are autocorrelated. On the basis of computer simulations, the authors concluded that even moderate autocorrelation results in a substantial increase in type I error. Moreover, computer simulated tests showed that when the effects of sequential linear regression and correlated errors were combined "all of the changes detected by Goodson et al. (1982) can be accounted for in the context of a no change model in which the errors are moderately correlated when sequential linear regressions are used to monitor the sites over time." In a detailed review of the statistical and analytical problems associated with clinical periodontal disease trials, Imrey (13) and Laster (15) echoed these concerns and emphasized that both intraclass correlation and autocorrelation of errors lead to underestimation of type I error.

Two major studies of untreated periodontitis patients have shown that sites with significant gain of probing attachment outnumber those with loss (6,16). This observation is not readily accounted for by any disease progression model. Lindhe et al. (16) suggested that the frequent surveillence of the subjects stimulated improved self-performed plaque control and that a high proportion of initially deep sites disposed this group for gain of probing attachment. The biological meaning of probing attachment gain at untreated periodontitis sites, however, remains unclear. In view of data such as these, it is difficult to ignore the statistical concern over possible underestimation of the type I error. It is possible that there was no real change, gain or loss, in either direction.

Ralls and Cohen (21) raised another concern, namely that the dichotomous categorization of sites as "changed" or "unchanged" harbors an inherent danger and suggests that "it is a mistake to assume that a diagnostic criterion results in a new disease reality." Moreover, the authors suggested that "even if chance rates are exceeded, this does not compel acceptance of the burst model over a model of continuous loss with varying rates." The authors also showed that computer simulated sequential measurements can generate patterns of apparent burst-like attachment loss, similar to those presented in the literature, in the absence of any true change.

In the absence of sufficiently sensitive measurement techniques, the debate continues. It is widely accepted that the large standard deviation of probing measurements (0.3 to 1.1 mm; reviewed in (24)) remains an imposing obstacle. It is highly desirable to lower the standard deviation by refinement of probing techniques, and efforts in this area are continuing at several institutions. It is equally important to refine the statistical and analytical techniques to permit a more accurate estimation of the type I error. As a first step, it is necessary to ascertain whether probing attachment level measurements are normally distributed and whether all other conditions for statistical tests and analyses based on the normal distribution are fulfilled. Along with intraclass correlation and autocorrelation of errors, deviation from normality is an additional source of underestimation of type I error. We must learn to manage the statistical and analytical problems created by our complex experimental designs and to compensate for intraclass correlation, autocorrelation and other confounding factors that influence the type I error. If these problems can be managed, it may become possible to resolve the question whether periodontal disease sites actually undergo burst losses of attachment. Unfortunately, the complexity of the issues is not limited to the statistical problems summarized above. Even if we set aside the statistical concerns and assume that all apparent probing attachment level changes are real, there are still other problems associated with the burst hypothesis which merit consideration.

Risk of selecting for a particular disease entity. In order to lower the type I error, the cut-off level between "changed" and "unchanged" sites is often chosen 2-4 standard deviations from the mean (2-3 mm). Even if it is assumed that all sites that fall beyond the cut-off have lost attachment, an error may have been committed by excluding all other losing sites from consideration. If rates of attachment loss are continuously and possibly even normally distributed, it is likely that only the tail end of the distribution has been identified and that the majority of disease sites has been excluded. A related but altogether different concern arises from the possibility that we may have selected for an infrequent, unrepresentative, exacerbating disease entity characterized by loss of 2-3 mm attachment within a few weeks. If so, all sites affected by the disease we refer to as slowly progressive chronic adult periodontitis may have been missed. In addition, Ralls and Cohen (21) pointed out that bursts identified by the running median method may be artifacts because of the discontinuous nature and the large measurement error of attachment level determinations. A "sudden" large change may in fact have occurred gradually over a long period of time but registered only when the cumulated loss exceeded the cut-off value. The assumption that all of the loss occurred in a short period of time may be incorrect.

Probing attachment level change versus destruction of functional periodontium. Another potentially important problem is the relationship of attachment level change to disease progression. Clinical trials have shown probing attachment gains of 1-2 mm after scaling and root planing (14,19). It has also been shown that probe penetration is highly dependent on the resistance of the tissue and may vary by 1.0-1.5 mm depending on the state of inflammation (3,17). We interpret these findings to suggest that, as inflammation subsides and the tissue "firms-up," there is a substantial gain of probing attachment, as defined by the deepest penetration of the probe, but not necessarily a gain of functional connective tissue attachment. Moreover, we suggest that substantial losses and gains of probing attachment may occur only as a consequence of spontaneous exacerbation or resolution of inflammation without any change in functional connective tissue attachment. Probing attachment level changes, therefore, should not be accepted uncritically as absolute evidence of loss (or gain) of functional attachment. If a 1-2 mm probing attachment level change accounted for by inflammation alone is added to a 2-3 mm apparent loss accounted for by measurement error, it is possible to envision substantial probing attachment loss without any true progression of disease. While probing attachment measurements may be "the best estimator of periodontal attachment" currently available (8), it is not clear that they are useful to assess rates of disease progression.

Clarification of the mechanism(s) of progression of functional attachment loss in periodontitis is important both for establishing diagnostic criteria and for developing rational therapeutic strategies. Unfortunately, however, at the current time we may lack appropriate tools to measure loss of functional attachment in a manner that would allow us to sort out the mechanisms of attachment loss at individual sites in human periodontitis. As a consequence, we may need to put on "hold" attempts to resolve the many questions raised by formulation of the "burst" hypothesis until such time as appropriate measurement tools for functional attachment loss are available.

This study was supported by U.S.P.H. grants DE 06028, DE 05817, DE 02670, DE 07256, and DE 08228.

References

1. AXELSON, P. and LINDHE, J. Effect of controlled oral hygiene procedures on caries and periodontal disease in adults. J. Clin. Periodontol. 5: 133-151 (1978).
2. BECKER, W., BERG, L. and BECKER, B. E.: Untreated periodontal disease: a longitudinal study. J. Periodontol. 50: 234-244 (1979).
3. FOWLER, C., GARRETT, S., CRIGGER, M. and EGELBERG, J.: Histologic probe position in treated and untreated human periodontal tissues. J. Clin. Periodontol. 9: 373-385 (1982).
4. GOODSON, J.M.: Clinical measurements of periodontitis. J. Clin. Periodontol. 13: 446-455 (1986).
5. GOODSON, J.M., HAFFAJEE, A.D. and SOCRANSKY, S.S.: The relationship between attachment level loss and alveolar bone loss. J. Clin. Periodontol. 11: 348-359 (1984).
6. GOODSON, J.M., TANNER, A.C.R., HAFFAJEE, A.D., SORNBERGER, G.C. and SOCRANSKY, S.S.: Patterns of progression and regression of advanced destructive periodontal disease. J. Clin. Periodontol. 9: 472-481

(1982).
7. HAFFAJEE, A.D. and SOCRANSKY, S.S.: Frequency distributions of periodontal attachment loss. J. Clin. Periodontol. 13: 625-637 (1986).
8. HAFFAJEE, A.D. and SOCRANSKY, S.S.: Attachment level changes in destructive periodontal diseases. J. Clin. Periodontol. 13: 461-472 (1986).
9. HAFFAJEE, A.D., SOCRANSKY, S.S. and EBERSOLE, J.L.: Survival analysis of periodontal sites before and after periodontal therapy. J. Clin. Periodontol. 12: 553-567 (1985).
10. HAFFAJEE, A.D., SOCRANSKY, S.S. and GOODSON, J.M.: Periodontal disease activity. J. Periodontal Res. 17: 521-522 (1982).
11. HAFFAJEE, A.D., SOCRANSKY, S.S. and GOODSON, J.M.: Comparison of different data analyses for detecting changes in attachment level. J. Clin. Periodontol. 10: 298-310 (1983).
12. HAFFAJEE, A.D., SOCRANSKY, S.S. and LINDHE, J.: Comparison of statistical methods of analysis of data from clinical periodontal trials. J. Clin. Periodontol. 10: 247-256 (1983).
13. IMREY, P.B.: Considerations in the statistical analysis of clinical trials in periodontitis. J. Clin. Periodontol. 13: 517-528 (1986).
14. KNOWLES, J.W., BURGETT, F.G. NISSLE, R.R., SHICK, R.A., MORRISON, E.C. and RAMFJORD, S.P.: Results of periodontal treatment related to pocket depth and attachment level. Eight years. J. Periodontol. 50: 225-233 (1979).
15. LASTER, L.L.: The effect of subsampling sites within patients. J. Periodontal Res. 20: 91-96 (1985).
16. LINDHE, J., HAFFAJEE, A.D. and SOCRANSKY, S.S.: Progression of periodontal disease in adult subjects in the absence of periodontal therapy. J. Clin. Periodontol. 10: 433-442 (1983).
17. LISTGARTEN, M.A.: Periodontal probing: What does it mean? J. Clin. Periodontol. 7: 165-176 (1980).
18. LOE, H., ANERUD, A., BOYSEN, H. and SMITH, M.: The natural history of periodontal disease in man. J. Periodontol. 49: 607-620 (1978).
19. LOESCHE, W.J., SYED, S.A., MORRISON, E.C., KERRY, G.A., HIGGINS, T. and STOLL, J.: Metronidazole in periodontitis. J. Periodontol. 55: 325-335 (1984).
20. MORRISON, E.C. and KOWALSKI, C.J.: Discussion: Clinical measurements of periodontitis. J. Clin. Periodontol. 13: 456-458 (1986).
21. RALLS, S.A. and COHEN, M.E.: Problems in identifying "bursts" of periodontal attachment loss. J. Periodontol. 57: 746-752 (1986).
22. RAMFJORD, S.P., KNOWLES, J.W., NISSLE, R.R., BURGETT, F.G. and SCHICK, R.A.: Results following three

modalities of treatment. J. Periodontol. 46: 522-526 (1975).
23. SOCRANSKY, S.S. and HAFFAJEE, A.D.: Frequency distributions of periodontal attachment loss. J. Clin. Periodontol. 13: 617-624 (1986).
24. SOCRANSKY, S.S., HAFFAJEE, A.D., GOODSON, J.M. and LINDHE, J.: New concepts of destructive periodontal disease. J. Clin. Periodontol. 11: 21-32 (1984).
25. SUOMI, J.D., GREENE, J.C., VERMILLION, J.R., DOYLE, J. CHANG, J.J. and LEATHERWOOD, E.C.: The effect of controlled oral hygiene procedures on the progression of periodontal disease in adults: results after third and final year. J. Periodontol. 42: 152-160 (1971).

Henning Birkedal-Hansen, D.D.S, Dr. Odont., Department of Oral Biology, University of Alabama School of Dentistry, Birmingham, AL 35294 USA

Periodontology Today. Int. Congr., Zürich 1988, pp. 236–243 (Karger, Basel 1988)

Clinical Criteria for Evaluation of Periodontal Therapy

Jan Egelberg

Postgraduate Dental Education Center, Örebro Country Council, Örebro, Sweden

Introduction

Periodontal therapy is generally provided with the purpose of preventing further loss of periodontal attachment. It appears, however, that the appropriate recordings to evaluate the effect of therapy - attachment level measurements - are not commonly used in clinical practice, presumably due to the time consuming nature of these recordings. Instead, clinical signs of the conditions of the gingival tissues seem to be used to monitor the outcome of therapy. These signs are less demanding to record and they may also have the advantage of allowing observations and corrections of undesirable gingival conditions prior to the development of attachment loss.

In the periodontal patient, clinicians often record the presence of dental plaque, probing depths, and bleeding and suppuration on probing at several sites around each tooth. Apart from initial recordings, these scores may be obtained at various intervals during the therapeutic phase and subsequently during the maintenance phase. At a given magnitude of these various scores, the clinician may decide to intervene with therapeutic procedures. The purpose of this intervention, thus, is to prevent further loss of periodontal attachment.

In other words, the clinician is using the clinical signs to predict attachment loss. The predictive values of such signs have been investigated in a limited number of studies (HAFFAJEE ET AL. 1983, BADERSTEN ET AL. 1985b, LANG ET AL. 1986, VANOOTEGHEM ET AL. 1987). The overall findings indicate that the clinical signs have little or moderate predictive value for attachment loss. This may partly be due to the fact that the observation intervals were limited to 2 years or less in these studies.

The present report presents a summary of the results from 2 more recent studies, where longitudinal data over 5 years (BADERSTEN ET AL. 1988) and $3\frac{1}{2}$ years (CLAFFEY ET AL. 1988) are available. Due to the longer observation intervals, these studies permitted evaluation of the diagnostic predictability of scores obtained during the first years of observation relative to attachment loss established at the end of the observation periods.

Subjects and treatment

In the study by BADERSTEN ET AL. (1988) 49 adult patients with severe periodontitis were included. The incisors, cuspids and premolars in either the maxilla or the mandible were studied. The patients were treated with a series of oral hygiene instructions and supra- and subgingival debridement, completed within 9 months after baseline. Periodontal surgery was not performed. Maintenance therapy, which included reinforcement of plaque control, tooth polishing and subgingival debridement of sites demonstrating marked bleeding, suppuration and/or deep probing depth, was given twice yearly.

In the study by CLAFFEY ET AL. (1988) 17 adult patients with advanced periodontitis participated. Both non-molar and molar teeth were studied. The patients received a series of oral hygiene instructions and a single episode of supra- and subgingival debridement. Periodontal surgery was not performed. The maintenance therapy varied among these subjects. Although all patients received oral hygiene reinforcement and tooth polishing 4 times per year throughout the 42 months of observation, subgingival debridement was only performed at these visits during the period between 12-27 months.

Measurements

Recordings of supragingival dental plaque (presence/absence), bleeding and suppuration on probing (presence/absence), probing depth (mm) and probing attachment level (mm) were performed at 6 sites per non-molar tooth and 8-10 sites per molar. In the CLAFFEY study recordings were obtained every 3rd month throughout the 42 months of observation. In the BADERSTEN study scores were taken every 3rd month during the first 24 months of observation and subsequently every 6th month.

Calculation of plaque, bleeding and suppuration frequencies

Accumulated frequencies of the presence of supragingival plaque and bleeding on probing at each individual site were calculated for the following intervals; 3-12, 3-24 and 3-36 months. For example, during the 3-24 month interval 8 examinations had been made. A positive score at 1 of these examinations would give a frequency of 12.5 % (1/8); at 2 examinations 25 % (2/8), etc. This type of frequency scores were calculated for the above variables at indicated intervals. Accumulated frequencies of suppuration on probing were expressed as the number of examinations with suppuration.

Identification of sites with probing attachment loss

Linear regression analysis. The recordings during the 0-42/0-60 month periods provided series of 15/21 probing attachment level measurements for each site for the CLAFFEY and BADERSTEN studies respectively. These data points from each site were subjected to linear analysis of regression (GOODSON ET AL. 1982, HAFFAJEE ET AL. 1983, BADERSTEN ET AL. 1985a). The slope of the regression line for each of these sites was calculated together with the projected probing attachment loss during the 0-42/0-60 month periods (Δy). The probability for each slope being different from a horizontal line was determined using 13/19 degrees of freedom. A minimum projected Δy of 1.5 mm and a probability of $p<0.05$ were required to classify a site as showing probing attachment loss.

End point analysis. In the BADERSTEN study duplicate recordings of probing attachment levels by 2 independant examiners were available at 0 and 60 months. Therefore, probing attachment loss for individual sites during the 0-60 month interval was also determined from analysis of the change from the 0- to the 60-month measurements only. To classify a site as showing probing attachment loss a difference of $\geq$ 1.5 mm was required between the deepest value of the initial pair of recordings obtained by the 2 examiners and the shallowest value of the final pair of probings by these examiners (BADERSTEN ET AL. 1987).

Sites which demonstrated probing attachment loss using both methods and those identified using either regression analysis or end point analysis were included in the determination of diagnostic predictability for the BADERSTEN study.

Determination of diagnostic predictability

The reliability of scores for plaque, bleeding, suppuration, and probing depth in identifying sites with probing attachment loss was evaluated from calculations of diagnostic predictability ratios, in %, as follows.

	Probing attachment loss	
Score	Presence	Absence
positive	a	b
diagnostic predictability	a/(a+b)	

Thus, diagnostic predictability gives the proportion of sites with positive scores that shows loss of probing attachment.

Only sites with initial probing depth $\geq$ 4.0 mm were included (BADERSTEN study, N=1136; CLAFFEY study, N=1480). Calculations were not performed if the sum of a+b was less than 20, due to the uncertainty associated with such small number of sites.

Results

The diagnostic predictability of the various clinical scores recorded after 12, 24 and 36 months to identify sites with probing attachment loss observed after 42 and 60 months respectively is presented in Tables I-V. The results showed that all the investigated scores were associated with probing attachment loss. This association was demonstrated by increased diagnostic predictability along with increased frequency or magnitude of the various scores. Also, the diagnostic predictability improved with increase in length of time for recording of the scores.

Table I. Diagnostic predictability (%) of accumulated plaque frequency scores of increasing magnitude after 12, 24 and 36 months for probing attachment loss at the end of the maintenance period in the study by BADERSTEN ET AL. (60 months) and in the study by CLAFFEY ET AL. (42 months)

Plaque frequency (%)	BADERSTEN ET AL. (1988)			CLAFFEY ET AL. (1988)		
	12	24	36	12	24	36
		months			months	
≥ 25	9	11	12	12	12	11
≥ 50	12	18	18	13	13	12
≥ 75	7	13	28	13	15	13

Comments to table I. For plaque scores, the diagnostic predictability was low and showed no or little increase with heightened plaque frequency or with lengthened observation interval. The highest predictability (28 %) was observed in the BADERSTEN study for plaque frequency ≥ 75 % after 36 months. This means that 28 % of sites with plaque present at 75 % or more of all examinations performed during 36 months from baseline demonstrated probing attachment loss at 60 months.

Table II. Diagnostic predictability (%) of accumulated bleeding frequency scores

Bleeding frequency (%)	BADERSTEN ET AL. (1988)			CLAFFEY ET AL. (1988)		
	12	24	36	12	24	36
		months			months	
≥ 25	10	11	12	11	11	12
≥ 50	11	13	14	13	14	17
≥ 75	13	14	23	15	21	31

Comments to table II. Bleeding frequency ≥ 75 % reached a diagnostic predictability of 31 % after 36 months in the CLAFFEY study. This means that 31 % of the sites that bled upon probing at 75 % or more of all examinations performed during 36 months from baseline demonstrated probing attachment loss at 42 months.

Table III. Diagnostic predictability (%) of accumulated suppuration frequency

Suppuration frequency (no. of exams)	BADERSTEN ET AL. (1988)			CLAFFEY ET AL. (1988)		
	12	24	36	12	24	36
		months			months	
≥ 1	14	14	15	<*	26	28
≥ 2	<	<	20	<	<	<

* less than 20 sites available for calculation

Comments to table III. Suppuration reached a maximum predictability of 28 %. However, suppuration was not a frequent finding. Few sites demonstrated suppuration more than twice during the entire 42/60-month observation intervals.

Table IV. Diagnostic predictability (%) of residual probing depth

Residual probing depth (mm)	BADERSTEN ET AL. (1988)			CLAFFEY ET AL. (1988)		
	12	24	36	12	24	36
		months			months	
≥ 4.0	9	9	10	16	14	18
≥ 5.0	10	13	16	22	24	27
≥ 6.0	12	16	28	26	32	36
≥ 7.0	20	26	37	26	38	45
≥ 8.0	<	<	<	26	39	63
≥ 9.0	<	<	<	21	35	72

Comments to table IV. Diagnostic predictability for sites 7.0 mm or deeper at 36 months were 37 % and 45 % respectively for the 2 studies. In the CLAFFEY study there was sufficient number of sites with residual depths ≥ 8.0 mm and ≥ 9.0 mm available for calculation, providing predictabilities of 63 % and 72 % respectively at 36 months.

Table V. Diagnostic predictability (%) of residual probing depth for sites without/with reduction in depth compared to baseline

Residual probing depth ≥ 7.0 mm	BADERSTEN ET AL. (1988)			CLAFFEY ET AL. (1988)		
	12	24	36	12	24	36
		months			months	
Without reduction	20	26	37	26	38	45
With reduction ≥ 1.0 mm	5	14	<	22	37	17

Comments to table V. Residual probing depth ≥ 7.0 mm showed a decreased predictability for sites with reduced probing depth from baseline compared to sites without reduction in probing depth. In other words, the predictive power of residual probing depth ≥ 7.0 was related to the baseline probing depth of the investigated sites.

Table VI. Diagnostic predictability (%) of increase in probing depth

Increase in probing depth (mm)	BADERSTEN ET AL. (1988) 12	24 months	36	CLAFFEY ET AL. (1988) 12	24 months	36
≥ 0.0	28	24	35	28	28	37
≥ 0.5	31	31	52	36	42	55
≥ 1.0	<	39	<	29	45	61
≥ 1.5	<	<	<	<	45	72

Comments to table VI. Increase in probing depth 1.0 mm or more at 24 months compared to baseline showed a predictability of 39 % and 45 % respectively for the 2 studies. Compared to the other recordings, increase in probing depth showed the highest overall predictability values.

Calculations of diagnostic predictability were performed for a multitude of different combinations of the clinical signs. For some of these combinations, the number of available sites was insufficient for interpretation. This was especially true for combinations with suppuration on probing. For other combinations, e.g. those with plaque scores, no improvement of predictability was observed.

Diagnostic predictability of residual probing depth was only slightly enhanced by combination with bleeding frequency ≥ 75 % or with suppuration ≥ 1 times. Combinations of residual probing depth and increase in probing depth elevated the predictability somewhat over that of increase in probing depth alone.

Addition of bleeding frequency or suppuration to the combinations of residual probing depth and increase in probing depth did not enhance the diagnostic predictability.

Discussion

Plaque and bleeding frequencies seem to have modest predictive power in both studies. There may be limited reasons to expect that frequent occurrence of supragingival plaque should result in attachment loss within 3½ to 5 years in the majority of sites in patients on maintenance. The results seem to support this notion. Frequent bleeding on probing, on the other hand, could conceivably have been expected to show higher predictability. However, it is possible that the modest predictive value of bleeding is related to the dicotomous type of score that was used (bleeding/no bleeding). Minimal bleeding may often have occurred after probing of many sites, thus giving high bleeding frequency to sites with limited subgingival inflammation. A scoring system selecting sites with marked bleeding only might have improved the predictive power of bleeding upon probing.

The predictive power of residual probing depth was found to be related to the baseline probing depth of the investigated sites. Residual probing depth ≥ 7.0 mm had limited predictive value if probing depth had been ≥ 8.0 at baseline.

Increase in probing depth compared to baseline (prior to therapy) seem to be the single criterion with best predictive value. The combination of residual probing depth and increase in probing depth gave only slightly higher predictability than increase in depth alone. No other combinations of clinical signs were observed in these studies yielding higher predictive values than increase in probing depth alone, or its combination with residual probing depth.

The high predictive power of increase in probing depth at a later interval like 36 months could be considered to be "a finding of the obvious": Probing attachment loss in periodontal disease would be expected to be associated with increased probing depth. For clinical purposes, however, these observations may have some affirmative value. Probing attachment level measurements are time consuming and may not be regularly used. In the absence of these measurements periodontal deterioration can be detected with a reasonably good accuracy by the observation of an increase in probing depth after a few years of observations.

Opinions may vary about what constitutes an acceptable diagnostic predictability of probing attachment loss. In a situation that deals with the provision of supplementary surgical therapy following reevaluation of the results of initial therapy, an acceptance of low predictability levels may result in overtreatment. Conversely, the requirement of high predictability values prior to institution of surgical therapy involves the risk of attachment loss due to the withholding of therapy (provided the surgical therapy would correct the problem). An attempt at summarizing the findings of the 2 studies for clinical application is presented in the following table:

Table VII. Time point for reevaluation and clinical criterion to be used to meet various diagnostic predictability levels

Diagnostic predictability level	Time point for reevaluation	Clinical criterion
≥ 33 %	24 months	Increase in probing depth
≥ 50 %	36 months	Increase in probing depth

Based upon the findings of the present studies, it appears that the use of increase in probing depth alone among available clinical signs seem practical and justified. A clinician who may prefer a predictability level of ≥ 33 % would be recommended to perform his reevaluation 24 months after initial therapy. If a predictability level of ≥ 50 % is preferred, reevaluation could be postponed until 36 months.

The results of these 2 studies highlight the slow nature of progressive periodontal disease in adults and the usefulness of probing depth measurement, particularly the evaluation of increase in probing depth. However, the results should not be interpreted as an indication of the lack of usefulness of inflammatory signs for monitoring purposes. As discussed above, the bleeding scores used may have limitations. Suppuration on probing did not occur often enough among these patients for conclusive evaluation.

Also, the goal of periodontal maintenance may also be the control of gingival inflammation, not only measures focused on attachment loss.

References

BADERSTEN, A.; NILVEUS, R., and EGELBERG, J.: Effect of nonsurgical periodontal therapy. V. Patterns of probing attachment loss in non-responding sites. J. Clin. Periodontol. 12: 270-282 (1985a).

BADERSTEN, A.; NILVEUS, R., and EGELBERG, J.: Effect of nonsurgical periodontal therapy. VII. Bleeding, suppuration and probing depth in sites with probing attachment loss. J. Clin. Periodontol. 12: 432-440 (1985b).

BADERSTEN, A.; NILVEUS, R., and EGELBERG, J.: Effect of nonsurgical periodontal therapy. VIII. Probing attachment changes related to clinical characteristics. J. Clin. Periodontol. 14: 425-432 (1987).

BADERSTEN, A.; NILVEUS, R., and EGELBERG, J.: Scores of plaque, bleeding, suppuration and probing depth to predict probing attachment loss. 5 years of observation following nonsurgical periodontal therapy. Submitted for publication in J. Clin. Periodontol. (1988)

CLAFFEY, N.; NYLUND, K.; KIGER, R.; GARRETT, S., and EGELBERG, J.: Diagnostic predictability of scores of plaque, bleeding, suppuration and probing depth for probing attachment loss. 3½ years of observation following initial periodontal therapy. Submitted for publication in J. Clin. Periodontol. (1988).

GOODSON, J.M.; TANNER, A.C.R.; HAFFAJEE, A.D.; SORNBERGER, G.C., and SOCRANSKY, S.S.: Patterns of progression and regression of advanced destructive periodontal disease. J. Clin. Periodontol. 9: 472-481 (1982).

HAFFAJEE, A.D.; SOCRANSKY, S.S., and GOODSON, J.M.: Clinical parameters as predictors of destructive periodontal activity. J. Clin. Periodontol. 10: 257-265 (1983).

LANG, N.P.; JOSS, A.; ORSANIC, T.; GUSBERTI, F.A., and SIEGRIST, B.E.: Bleeding on probing. A predictor for the progression of periodontal disease? J. Clin. Periodontol. 13: 590-603 (1986).

VANOOTEGHEM, R.; HUTCHENS, L.H.; GARRETT, S.; KIGER, R., and EGELBERG, J.: Bleeding on probing and probing depth as indicators of the response to plaque control and root debridement. J. Clin. Periodontol. 14: 226-230 (1987).

Author's address

Jan Egelberg, Postgraduate Dental Education Center, Örebro County Council, Box 1126, S-701 11 Örebro, Sweden.

Periodontology Today. Int. Congr., Zürich 1988, pp. 244–250 (Karger, Basel 1988)

Response to Treatment, Our Chief Diagnostic Method?

Ubele Van der Velden

Department of Periodontology, Academic center for Dentistry Amsterdam, Amsterdam, The Netherlands

1. Introduction

The rational for treatment of inflammatory periodontal diseases is based upon the concept that the primary cause of these diseases is from bacterial origin (VAN PALENSTEIN HELDERMAN,1981). If this concept holds true parallels can be drawn with other diseases in the field of medical microbiology.

Among the vast numbers of species of microorganisms with which our lives are bound, there are a relative few whose properties and interaction with the human body may lead to development of disease. These microorganisms are of concern in the diagnosis, treatment and cure of diseases. In relation to this it is important to point out that colonization of the host usually represents a balanced relationship between microorganisms whereas infection results from a more damaging interplay between microorganisms with injurious properties and the "infected body's" responses to them.

Succesful treatment of a microbial infection depends in the first place on an accurate diagnosis. When the cause of the disease is established then an adequate therapy can be installed. Succesful treatment or complete cure of the disease can be defined as having after treatment a long term absence of the causal agent and/or a long term absence of disease. In the field of periodontology we are far away from a proper diagnosis and complete cure of the disease.

2. Clinical diagnosis

Proper diagnosis from a clinical point of view is extremely difficult since all infections of the periodontium result in inflammation of the periodontal tissues. A proper diagnosis would include a clear difference between an inflammation of the gingiva which will convert to periodontitis and a stable gingivitis.

Clinical evaluation of the degree of inflammation includes

redness and swelling of the gingiva together with bleeding on probing. During the last decade a tendency can be seen in the literature from evaluation by means of indices which include all 3 items, e.g. GI (LOE and SILNESS,1963) and SBI (MUHLEMANN and SON,1971), towards evaluation by means of bleeding on probing alone (POLSON and CATON,1985). However the bleeding can be provoked in different ways and in addition the degree of bleeding can be assessed in the relation to the amount of bleeding. Therefore the question: bleeding on probing what does it mean and which bleeding means what, seems to be relevant.

In general it was found that bleeding on probing is indicative of an inflammatory lesion in the connective tissue (GREENSTEIN et al.,1981, DAVENPORT et al.,1982). ENGELBERGER et al.(1983) reported that as the severity of the bleeding respons increased there was a concomitant increase in the size and intensity of the inflammatory infiltrate. Further studies evaluated the prognostic value of bleeding on probing in identifying sites at risk for periodontal breakdown (LANG et al.,1986, HARLEY et al.,1987). Unfortunately, conflicting results were reported and therefore only a limited value can be attributed to bleeding on probing in this respect.

In most studies the way bleeding is provoked varies greatly from one to the other. In principal two different methods are employed. The bleeding can be provoked: 1)at the marginal gingival tissues by e.g. running a probe along the soft tissue wall at the orifice of the pocket and 2)by probing to the "bottom" of the pocket. In the latter case the probing force is an important variable since it has been shown that with increasing probing force the bleeding index increases concomitant with an increasing probing depth (VAN DER VELDEN,1980).

As the base of the pocket seems to be the most critical area in the development of periodontal breakdown, probing at orifice of the pocket may not adequately diagnose inflammatory lesions in deeper pockets. However in shallow pockets no major differences should be present whether the bleeding is assessed either by probing to the bottom of the pocket or by running the probe along the soft tissue wall of the pocket.

Since in the literature no data are available in relation to this problem we investigated the bleeding tendency in 11 untreated patients suffering from severe periodontal disease. The bleeding was provoked first by entering a Merrit-B probe (HU-FRIEDY) 2mm into the pocket and then running the probe along the soft tissue wall back and forwards over a 2mm distance. This type of bleeding, present or absent, is further referred to as the MPBI (marginal pocket bleeding index). After a time lapse the same area was probed by means of a Borodontic® pressure probe calibrated to a 240 N/cm^2 probing pressure. Pocket depth and the PPBI (periodontal pocket bleeding index, VAN DER VELDEN,1979) were assessed.

The results are presented in table 1. It can be seen that in deep pockets the mean bleeding index as assessed by the PPBI is 0.31 higher compared to the results by means of the MPBI.

Table 1. Pocket depth (PD) in mm, periodontal pocket bleeding index (PPBI) and marginal pocket bleeding index /MPBI) of 11 untreated subjects suffering from severe periodontal disease.

	Deep pockets >3mm			Shallow pockets ⩽3mm		
subject	PD	PPBI	MPBI	PD	PPBI	MPBI
1	4.72	0.81	0.62	2.90	0.18	0.19
2	4.77	0.90	0.70	2.68	0.57	0.38
3	4.96	0.76	0.60	2.42	0.53	0.30
4	5.00	1.00	0.52	3.00	0.62	0.06
5	5.01	0.87	0.61	2.60	0.55	0.29
6	5.04	0.83	0.44	2.51	0.59	0.26
7	5.11	0.78	0.36	2.76	0.35	0.11
8	5.48	0.90	0.37	2.35	0.10	0.08
9	5.61	0.91	0.38	2.62	0.40	0.21
10	5.73	0.65	0.56	3.00	0.40	0.00
11	5.97	0.89	0.43	2.97	0.50	0.15
Mean(SD)	5.22(0.41)	0.85(0.09)	0.51(0.12)	2.71(0.23)	0.44(0.17)	0.18(0.12)
t-test		t=7.42; df=20; p<0.0001			t=4.03 df=20; p<0.0001	

More over in shallow pockets the mean value of the PPBI was 0.26 higher then the mean MPBI value. This result may indicate that bleeding provoked by exerting a considerable force at the base of the pocket has a different background then the bleeding provoked by running a probe along the pocket wall. It is likely that the latter is related to ulceration of the epithelium (ABRAMS et al, 1984), whereas the first may be a combination of the presence of ulceration of the epithelium and tissue damage due to the probing procedure. It may be hypothezised that probing in the latter case can be regarded as a tensile strength measurement comparable to e.g. the tensile strength measurements as assessed for healing skin incision wounds.

In conclusion it is far from being clear what bleeding on probing means, where the bleeding comes from and what type of bleeding is possibly related to future periodontal destruction. This shows clearly an urgent need for further research on the significance of bleeding on probing. This conclusion also implies that at present no proper diagnosis can be made in relation to the type of periodontal infection on the basis of clinical measurements.

3. Microbiological diagnosis

As stated in the introduction succesful treatment of a microbial infection depends in the first place on an accurate diagnosis. This statement, adopted from the field of medical microbiology, includes obviously extensive knowledge on the causing agent of a given disease. In relation to this, major progress has been made in the field of periodontology during the last decade. It seems that today several microbes may be regarded as periodontopathic microorganisms e.g. Actinobacillus actinomycetemcomitans, Bacteroides gingivalis and Bacteroides intermedius (SLOTS et al.,1986). It is likely that in the future evidence will be presented which shows that several other species may be regarded as periodontopathic microorganisms as well.

Nevertheless no definite ideas have taken shape in relation to the question as to whether periodontitis should be regarded as a classical infection in which colonization of the host by an agent is followed by disease or an opportunistic infection in which colonization is not necessarely followed by disease. Hypothetically there are for each agent or combination of agents 3 possibilities:

I All human beings are colonized of which a part develops disease

II Part of the population is colonized and all colonized subjects develop disease

III Part of the population is colonized of which a certain amount develops disease.

In order to be able to judge these hypotheses extensive knowledge must be obtained on the normal habitat of periodontopathic microorganisms.

Recently it has been suggested that not only the periodontal pocket but also the oral mucosa membranes may be regarded as a habitat of periodontopathic microorganisms (VAN DER VELDEN et al.,1986, VAN WINKELHOFF et al.,1986). Therefore e.g. the finding of ASIKAINEN et al.(1986) that A. actinomycetemcomitans is rarely detected in teenagers with healthy periodontal conditions does not necessarely mean that these individuals are not colonized since the autor investigated only the subgingival area. Obviously, it is of great importance to know whether the subjects with a healthy periodontal condition are not colonized at all or whether they are colonized but as yet have not developed disease.

In relation to the 3 proposed hypotheses the study of LOE et al.(1986) on the natural history of periodontal disease is of interest. In this study they identified within their studied population 3 subpopulations: a group with rapid progression (10%), a group with moderate progression (80%) and a group with no progression (10%). It is tempting to speculate that for the group with rapid progression the hypothesis II is relevant: all individuals are colonized and all develop disease. It seems not unlikely that in this case the, at present, most obvious periodontopathic microorganisms are involved e.g. A. actinomycetemcomitans. For the group with no progression a combination of the hypotheses would fit. This group may be either not colonized or colonized but did not develop disease. The majority of the population (80%) developed moderate progression which may also be explained by a combination of hypotheses but does suggest that the major part of this population is indeed colonized with periodontopathic microorganisms.

In conclusion a proper diagnosis based on a microbiological test is still not available although promising results have been obtained during recent years.

4. Cure of the disease

Succesful treatment or complete cure of the disease is defined in the introduction as having after treatment a long term absence of the causal agent and/or a long term absence of disease. Applied to periodontal therapy this means that after cure there should be a long term absence of disease dispite the presence of plaque.

In relation to the results of periodontal treatment extensive research has been carried out during the period from 1970 to 1980. It can be concluded from the literature that if one is able to remove all subgingival plaque and prevents its reformation, progression of the periodontal lesion will not occur (LINDHE and NYMAN,1975, AXELSSON and LINDHE,1978, KNOWLES et al.,1979). In this respect elimination of supragingival plaque on a daily basis seems to be of crusial importance since periodontal treatment is unsuccesful in patients who are not able to maintain a plaque free dentition (KERR,1981, AXELSSON and LINDHE,1981). This finding implies that succesful treatment of periodontitis is today not possible. The reason for this may be that during periodontal treatment the periodontopathic microorganisms are not eliminated from the oral cavity. After treatment they may be still present on e.g. the dorsum of the tongue or on the tonsils causing reinfection of the periodontium when the plaque control is unsuffecient.

5. Conclusion

Since we are , at present, not able to make a proper diagnosis and are not able to cure periodontal disease, response to treatment is still our chief diagnostic method.

References

ABRAMS,K., CATON,J. and POLSON,A.: Histological comparisons of interproximal gingival tissues related to the presence or absence of bleeding. J.Periodontol.55:629-632 (1984).

ASIKAINEN,S., ALALUUSUA,S., KARI,K. and KLEEMOLA-KUJALA,E.: Subgingival microflora and periodontal conditions in healthy teenagers. J.Periodontol.57:505-509 (1986).

AXELSSON,P. and LINDHE,J.: Effect of controlled oral hygiene procedures on caries and periodontal disease in adults. J. Clin.Periodontol.5:133-151 (1978).

AXELSSON,P. and LINDHE,J.: The significance of maintenance care in the treatment of periodontal disease in adults. J.Clin. Periodontol.8:281-294 (1981).

DAVENPORT,R.H., SIMPSON,D.M. and HASSELL,T.M.: Histomatric comparison of active and inactive lesions of advanced periodontitis. J.Periodontol.53:285-295 (1982).

ENGELBERGER,T., HEFTI,A., KALLENBERGER,A. and RATEITSCHAK,K.H.: Correlations among Pappila Bleeding Index, other clinical indices and histologically determined inflammation of gingival papilla. J.Clin.Periodontol.10:579-589 (1983).

GREENSTEIN,G., CATON,J. and POLSON,A.M.: Histologic characteristics associated with bleeding after probing and visual signs of inflammation. J.Periodontol.52:420-425 (1981).

HARLEY,A., FLOYD,P. and WATTS,T.: Monitoring untreated periodontal disease. J.Clin.Periodontol.14:221-225 (1987).

KERR,N.W.: Treatment of chronic periodontitis. 45% failure rate after 5 years. Br.Dent.J.150:222-224 (1981).

KNOWLES,J.W., BURGETT,F.G., NISSLE,R.R., SHICK,R.A., MORRISON, E.C. ans RAMFJORD,S.P.: Results of periodontal treatment related to pocketdepth and attachment level. Eight years. J.Periodontol.50:225-233 (1979).

LANG,N.P., JOSS,A., ORSANIC,T., GUSBERTI,F.A. and SIEGRIST, B.E.: Bleeding on probing- A predictor for the progression of periodontal disease? J.Clin.Periodontol.13:590-596 (1986).

LINDHE,J. and NYMAN,S.: The effect of plaque control and surgical pocket elimination on the establishment and maintenance of periodontal health. A longitudinal study of periodontal therapy in cases of advanced disease. J.Clin.Periodontol.2:67-69 (1975).

Loe,H. and SILNESS,J.: Periodontal disease in pregnancy. I. Prevalence and severity. Acta Odont.Scand.21:533-551 (1963).

LOE,H., ANERUD,A., BOYSON,H. and MORRISON,E.: Natural history of periodontal disease in man. Rapid, moderate and no loss of attachment in Sri Lankan Laborers 14 to 46 years of age. J.Clin.Periodontol.13:431-440 (1986).

MUHLEMAN,H.R. and SON,S.: Gingival sulcus bleeding- a leeding symptom in initial gingivitis. Helv.Odont.Acta 15:105-113 (1971).

POLSON,A.M. and CATON,J.G.: Current status of bleeding in the diagnosis of periodontal diseases. J.Periodont.Special Issue:1-3 (1985).

SLOTS,J., BRAGD,L., WIKSTROM,M. and DAHLEN,G.: The occurence of Actinobacillus actinomycetemcomitans, Bacteroides gingivalis and Bacteroides intermedius in detructive periodontal disease in adults. J.Clin.Periodontol.13:570-577 (1986).

VAN DER VELDEN,U.: Probing force and the relationship of the probe tip to the periodontal tissues. J.Clin.Periodontol. 6:106-114 (1979).

VAN DER VELDEN,U.: The influence of periodontal health on probing depth and bleeding tendency. J.Clin.Periodontol.7: 129-139 (1980).

VAN DER VELDEN,U., VAN WINKELHOFF,A-J., ABBAS,F. and DE GRAAFF, J.: The habitat of periodontopathic microorganisms. J.Clin.Periodontol.13:243-248 (1986).
VAN PALENSTEIN HELDERMAN,W.H.: Microbial etiology of periodontal disease. J.Clin.Periodontol.8:261-280 (1980).
VAN WINKELHOFF,A-J., VAN DER VELDEN,U., WINKEL,E.G. and DE GRAAFF,J.: Black-pigmented *Bacteroides* and motile organisms on oral mucosal surfaces in individuals with and without periodontal breakdown. J.Periodont.Res.21:434-439 (1986).

Ubele Van der Velden, Depeartment of Periodontology, Academic Center for Dentistry Amsterdam, Louwesweg 1, 1066 EA Amsterda, The Netherlands.

Periodontology Today. Int. Congr., Zürich 1988, pp. 251–259 (Karger, Basel 1988)

Does Supragingival Plaque Removal Prevent Further Breakdown?

Rolf Attström

Department of Periodontology, School of Dentistry, Lund University, Malmö, Sweden

Introduction

Experimental and epidemiological studies indicate an association between the presence of bacteria above and below the gingival margin and the occurrence of gingival inflammation,"gingivitis",and the development of periodontal attachment loss,"periodontitis".The bacterial activity elicits inflammatory processes in the gingival tissue.The reactions are limited to the junctional and pocket epithelium and to a narrow zone of the adjacent connective tissue.The tissue alterations in this defense reaction are considered to be the cause of periodontal attachment loss.Gingivitis is the stereo typed response to irritation of the gingival margin(2,21).In animals and humans gingivitis can be provoked and cured, respectively,by abstaing from or performing supragingival cleaning.Clinically, the gingival lesion is a summary of all "histopathological" events that at a given time have taken place in the marginal gingiva.No evidence indicates that the clinical appearance of the gingival tissue predicts further attachment loss.It should be realized that so far periodontitis has not been demonstrated without a past or simultaneous inflammation - infection of the gingiva. Periodontitis could thus from a logical point of view always be seen as the consequence of an ongoing gingivitis.This means that gingivitis is the disease and periodontal attachment loss the result of the disease.The fact that some gingival infections do not proceed to periodontitis does not contradict the conclusion that gingivitis gives rise to periodontal attachment loss.

The complexity of the bacterial flora,the lack of criteria with diagnostic precision and the nature of the disease interfere with the researcher´s ambition to describe the cause and effects in periodontal disease(19).Bearing this in mind, it is the purpose of the present paper to review and evaluate the role of supragingival plaque removal for the prevention of periodontal attachment loss.

The healthy dentogingival region

The healthy gingival margin is firmly attached to the tooth, and the clinical appearance of the tissue may vary depending on anatomical factors.In humans, monkeys and dogs a supragingival plaque removal frequency of once every 24-48 hours is sufficient to preserve gingival health on a clinical level(2,29).Likewise, gingival healing following treatment requires supragingival plaque removal to proceed optimally(32).

Bacterial invasion of the dentogingival region

The anatomy and physiology of the gingival margin favour accumulation and growth of bacteria in the gingival sulcus region.Once the bacteria have been established subgingivally they will spread in the apical/lateral direction. The junctional epithelium may be detached from the tooth surface by the combined effect of bacterial proliferation and inflammatory exudation(25).The microbes also seem to colonize the surfaces of the superficial epithelial cells as well as to thrive in the exudate of the gingival pocket(28).Bacterial invasion of the gingival-periodontal tissues may occur subgingivally at advanced periodontal disease stages(6).

A close relation between the subgingival location of the advancing bacterial front and the level of connective tissue attachment has been noted(31).The bacteria elicit an inflammatory reaction apical/lateral to the junctional epithelium. The connective tissue is decomposed as a consequence of the local release of tissue damaging substances from components of the inflammatory reaction or from the advancing bacteria. Epithelial proliferation ensues along the root surface(2). Supragingival plaque removal may have a limited effect on periodontal pathology once the microorganisms have become established subgingivally.

Periodontal attachment loss

It has long been believed that periodontal disease is a slow, continuous process.Once initiated it was supposed to continue until treatment was undertaken or the tooth lost. During recent years this view on the progression pattern of periodontal disease been modified. Experiments in animals and longitudinal studies in humans suggest periodontal disease may progress by bursts of increased inflammatory activity(2, 8).Dental plaque,gingival redness, and bleeding on probing and initial pocket depth probing have been found not to relate to the occurrence of probing attachment loss. The frequency of periodontal sites with active disease in untreated patients seems to be low(8).These findings have been taken to indicate that progression of periodontal disease does not relate to the presence of supra- and subgingival bacterial colonization as such but to the activity of specific bacteria (26).Variations in host response have also been suggested as contributing causes(21). Progression of periodontal disease is clinically determined by measurements of changes in the probing of attachment level.Attachment loss on an individual tooth surface is considered to have occurred when an increase in probing attachment distance of 1.5-2 mm or more can be measured from base-line data.The measurement error of the probing method for the determination of attachment loss is significant and relates to biological and technical factors(22).The burst model for periodontal disease may be a consequence of the fact that it´s only the major changes in attachment level which can be identified and separated from the measurment errors.This does not mean that rapid burstlike progressions of periodontal disease do not occur.Likewise a slow continuous progression of periodontal disease cannot be ruled out.The methods used for the identification of sites losing attachment do not allow precise determination of the day to day tissue loss.The progression rate may be as low as fractions of a millimeter per year and it will thus take several years until a significant change has occurred with a detection limit of 2 mm(31).The inflammatory burst hypothesis may have arisen from the ease of observing attachment loss in connection with the development of periodontal abscesses.Supragingival plaque removal at sites with periodontal abscess formation may have a limited effect on the cause of the disease.

Supragingival plaque and periodontal attachment loss

The incidence of periodontal disease seems to be related to poor oral hygiene and calculus formation(16).A correlation between the oral hygiene level and the severity of periodontal disease has also been observed(24).It should be noted that in subjects practising some oral hygiene procedures, the disease distribution in the individual´s mouth and around a single tooth has a consistent pattern and reflects the efficacy of supragingival plaque removal.Periodontal pathology and attachment loss is most severe in the interproximal regions and least in the buccal one.

The natural history of periodontal disease in a population from Sri Lanka and in a population from Norway was studied over an extended period of time(14,15).All individuals in Sri Lanka had gingival inflammation and sub- and supragingival calculus.Few persons if any were free from periodontal disease.Measurements of the calculus index indicated that those with slowly progressing periodontitis had less calculus than those with a rapid progression of the disease. The subjects had not recieved dental care,nor had they practised systematic oral hygiene measures.In the Norwegian population dental care was given on a regular basis, and the subjects performed daily oral hygiene procedures.The plaque and gingival scores were low, and the loss of periodontal attachment was insignificant during the investigated time periods. Although there are a number of factors which may have influenced the disease rates in the two populations, the differences in oral hygiene level is a significant condition which may explain the large difference in the rate of periodontal attachment loss.

Recently reported studies of large populations from industrialized countries also indicate that the incidence of periodontitis increased with age.The increase seems to be more pronounced in individuals with poor oral hygiene than in those with good(1,18).Supragingival plaque removal by self-performed oral hygiene procedures seems to reduce the progression of periodontal disease.

Supragingival plaque removal and subgingival bacteria

The composition of the subgingival flora and the extent of periodontal disease progression varies from individual to individual,from tooth to tooth and from site to site around a tooth(19,21).The distance from the apical plaque border to the connective tissue attachment also varies(31).Elimination of the subgingival bacteria combined with efficient supragingival plaque removal will arrest the pathological process and readapt the tissue to the tooth by epithelial attachment(30). Supragingival plaque removal affects bacterial plaque a short distance apical to the gingival margin.Subgingival plaque is more or less unaffected by supragingival cleaning once the subgingival plaque has become established in the more apical regions of the dentogingival area(5,31).

Subgingival root debridment by instrumentation appears difficult in moderate and advanced periodontitis and chances of removing all subgingival bacteria seem small. The incomplete subgingival cleaning may be masked by the patient´s own supragingival plaque removal,which induces gingival health,but does not eliminate the subgingival bacteria(31).

If the subgingival bacterial elimination has been efficient, supragingival plaque removal prevents reinfection of the subgingival region(12,17,30).When supragingival plaque is present, the subgingival flora tends to return to its preoperative composition around 4-8 weeks after treatment.In deeper pockets, > 8mm at treatment,the supragingival plaquecontrol does not result in a sustained alteration of the subgingival flora(17).Those studies which show a rapid regrowth of subgingival plaque despite seemingly efficient supragingival plaque control may be suspected to have been ineffective in the elimination of the subgingival bacteria(4,10).

Supragingival plaque removal has been observed to reduce the subgingival presence of periodontitis associated bacteria and induce improvements in clinical parameters(27).In a recent study the presence of Bacteroides gingivalis was determined subgingivally around molar teeth with varying degrees of attachment loss(9).Paperpoint samples were taken at 8 sites around each molar. The presence of the organism in the samples was determined by immunocytochemistry using monoclonal antibodies.A total of 216 samples were obtained from 7 untreated patients, each contributing with 4 molars, 2 upper and 2 lower. B.gingivalis was found in 62 % of the samples.The organism was more frequent in samples from the proximal areas than in samples from buccal and lingual regions.(Figure 1).The presence of the supragingival plaque and bleeding in cumulated data related to the presence of B.gingivalis, and a weak association was found between the bacteria and probing pocket depth and level of attachment loss.The observations indicate that in untreated patients the composition of the subgingival flora is influenced by the presence of supragingival plaque.

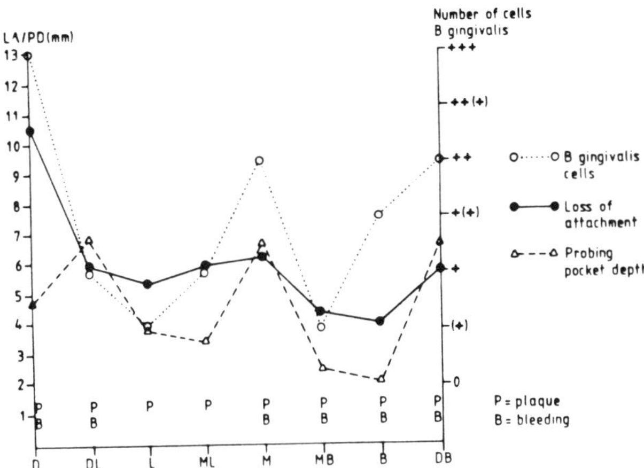

Figure 1.Variations in the presence of B.gingivalis cells, probing attachment loss,probing pocket depth, supragingival plaque(P) and bleeding(B) on probing at 8 sites around a molar in a patient with untreated periodontal disease. D:distal, DL:distolingual, L:lingual, ML:mesiolingual M:mesial, MB:mesiobuccal, B:buccal, DB:distobuccal

As I have mentioned above, regular supragingival plaque removal prevents infection of the subgingival region and maintains gingival health.However, in both animals and humans with compromised defense systems supragingival plaque removal does not counteract subgingival bacterial colonization to the same extent(25,34).In particular, defects of neutrophilic granulocytes seem to have a deleterious effect on the efficiency of the defense of the dentogingival region.The rapid subgingival bacterial growth in dogs rendered neutropenic illustrates the role of this cell in the defense of the periodontal tissues(25).However in humans the consequences of a defective defense may be counteracted by treatment and supragingival plaque removal.

Supragingival plaque removal and periodontal treatment

In dogs supragingival plaque removal prevents on a long-term basis the development as well as the progression of periodontal attachment loss(11).Futhermore, Beagle dogs subjected to regular supragingival plaque removal subsequent to treatment by scaling and root planing maintain periodontal attachment.Repeated scaling did not add significantly to the effect of the supragingival plaque control.In a no oral hygiene control group periodontal attachment loss continued in the animals despite repeated scaling sessions during a 36 months study period.A reduced progression rate, however, was observed in the scaled regions compared to the untreated areas(20).

In patients treated for periodontal disease the personal oral hygiene seems,to be of importance for pocket reduction and maintenance of attachment following treatment(23).In those with less than perfect postoperative plaquecontrol the attachment level can be maintained by supporting the patient´s plaque removal by regular subgingival debridments. Probably these treatments cause a shift in the subgingival flora to a less pathogenic composition.

Professional plaque control programs have been used in order to secure a plaque-free dentition and compliance with recommended oral hygiene procedures.This treatment includes careful mechanical cleaning of the teeth at regular intervals and reinstruction of the patient in adequate oral hygiene procedures.Using this technique the importance of self-performed oral hygiene for the maintenance of treatment results following periodontal therapy has been documented(13,32). Supragingival plaque removal seems to be a determining factor for the prevention of periodontal pathology and continued attachment loss following treatment(12,13,32).The mechanical plaque removal has even been found superior to chemical plaque control by chlorhexidine(32).Patients who participate in a professional plaque removal program have fewer sites with attachment loss postoperatively than those who are left on their own. Compliance with given recommendations seems to be better in patients who participate in the professional plaque control program.

Treatment of moderate and advanced periodontal disease by careful subgingival root debridment and oral hygiene instructions results in significant reductions of pocket depths and gain of probing attachment in deep pockets, while attachment loss was found in pockets less than 4 mm initially (3).Most patients reached a high standard of plaque control. Despite this several of them demonstrated continued attachment loss at one or several sites.This attachment loss had a limited relation to various clinical parameters. However, persistent soft tissue pathology seemed to have some relevance for the continued attachment loss.The clinical implication of these findings must await further studies including bacteriologic analysis of the subgingival flora in order to determine the efficacy of root debridment in relation to the treatment result.

General comments on compliance

In analysing the role of supragingival plaque removal for the prevention of periodontal disease and for the maintenance of periodontal attachment level following treatment phsycological factors -compliance- must be considered(33). Patients rapidly learn the techniques of proper plaque removal.This does not mean they practise the habit at home to a satisfactory degree. The interest they receive when they participate in a research project may stimulate the patients to increased compliance while the study is running.Studies indicate that many patients relapse to previous oral hygiene habits at varying times following the instruction in oral hygiene procedures(7).Frequent reinstructions are therefore recommended in order to achieve optimal oral cleanliness.The succesful treatment results from the Gothenburg group may be related to their intense postoperative professional plaque control programs(12).Another factor of importance is that most patients actually develop the skills to clean their teeth efficiently.In the time period up to a check-up visit they increase their efforts to clean their teeth, with the result that the researcher will be presented with a clinical condition of fairly clean teeth but persistent periodontal pathology.The risk of biased conclusions is obvious.

Summary and conclusions

Periodontal disease is caused by subgingival bacterial activity and progresses over time.The clinical methods for the determination of periodontal attachment loss do not allow longitudinal measurements of minor attachment changes. Occassionally the disease process may be accelerated by the formation of periodontal abscesses. Epidemiological studies show an association between oral cleanliness and the prevalence and severity of periodontal disease.The effect of age on peridontal disease seems less than the effect of oral cleanliness. Supragingival plaque removal by oral hygiene procedures in a population,therefore,may be one way to limit the incidence and progression of periodontal disease.
The efficient supragingival plaque removal prevents infection of the dentogingival region if the subgingival area is free from bacterial colonization.Individuals with compromised defense mechanisms may not be able to counteract subgingival bacterial colonization by supragingival plaque removal to the same extent.

References

1. ABDELLATIF, H.M. and BURT, B.A.: An epidemiological investigation into the relative importance of age and oral hygiene status as determinants of periodontitis. J. Den. Res. 66: 13-18 (1987).
2. ATTSTRÖM,R. and LINDHE,J.Pathogenesis of plaque associated periodontal disease;in LINDHE,Textbook of clinical periodontitis;1st ed.,pp.154-187(Munksgaard,Copenhagen 1983)
3. BADERSTEN,A.NILVEUS,R.and EGELBERG,J.:Effect of nonsurgical periodontal therapy(VIII).Probing attachment changes related to clinical charecteristics.J.Clin.Periodontol.14: 425-432(1987).

4.BELTRAMI, M.; BICKEL, M. and BAEHNI, P.C.: The effect of supragingival plaque control on the composition of the subgingival microflora in human periodontitis. J. Clin. Periodontol. 14: 161-164 (1987).
5.CERCEK, J.F.; KIGER, R.D.; GARRETT, S. and EGELBERG, J.: Relative effects of plaque control and instrumentation on the clinical parameters of human periodontal disease. J. Clin. Periodontol. 10: 46-56 (1983).
6.FRANK,R.M.;Bacterial penetration in the apical pocket wall of advanced human periodontitis.J.Periodontal Res.15: 563-432(1981).
7.GLAVIND, L.: The result of periodontal treatment in relationship to various background factors. J. Clin. Periodontol. 13: 789-794 (1986).
8.HAFFAJEE, A.D. and SOCRANSKY, S.S.: Frequency distributions of periodontal attachment loss. Clinical and microbiological features. J. Clin. Periodontol. 13: 625-637(1986)
9.HARARI, S.; SJÖGREN, S. and ATTSTRÖM, R.: Bacteroides gingivalis frequency in healthy and diseased periodontal pockets.To be published(1988).
10.LAVANCHY, D.L.; BICKEL, M. and BAEHNI, P.C.: The effect of plaque control after scaling and root planing on the subgingival microflora in human periodontitis. J.Clin. Periodontol. 14: 295-299 (1987).
11.LINDHE,J.;HAMP,S.E.and LÖE,H.Plaque induced periodontal disease in beagle dogs.A 4-years clinical roentgenografical and histometric study.J.Periodontal Res.10:243-255 (1975).
12.LINDHE,J.and NYMAN,S.;Long-term maintenance of patients treated for advanced periodontal disease.J.Clin.Periodontol.11:448-458 (1984).
13.LINDHE, J.; WESTFELT, E.; NYMAN, S.; SOCRANSKY, S.S. and HAFFAJEE, A.D.: Long-term effect of surgical/non-surgical treatment of periodontal disease. J. Clin. Periodontol. 11: 448-458 (1984).
14.LÖE, H.; ÅNERUD, Å.; BOYSEN, H. and MORRISON,E.: The natural history of periodontal disease in man.Rapid,moderate andno loss of attachment in Sri Lankan laborers 14-46 years of age.J.Clin.Periodontol.13:431-440.(1986)
15.LÖE,H.;ÅNERUD,A.;BOYSEN,H.and SMITH,M.R.:The natural history of peridontal disease in man.The rate of periodontal destruction before 40 yearsage.J.Periodontol.49: 607-620(1978).
16.LÖVDAHL, A.; ARNO, A. and WAERHAUG, J.: Incidence of clinical manifestations of periodontal disease in light of oral hygiene and calculus formation. JADA 56: 21-33 (1958).
17.MAGNUSSON, I.; LINDHE, J.; YONEYAMA, T. and LILJENBERG, B.:Recolonization of a subgingival microbiota following scaling in deep pockets.J.Clin.Periodontol.11:193-207 (1984).
18.MAIZELS, A. and SHEIHAM A.:A new measure of teeth-cleaning efficiency and periodontal disease. J. Clin.Periodontol

14: 105-109 (1987)
19.MOORE, W.E.C.: Microbiology of periodontal disease. J. Periodontal Res. 22: 335-341 (1987).
20.MORRISON, E.C.; LANG, N.P.; LÖE, H. and RAMFJORD, S.P.: Effects of repeated scaling and root planing and/or controlled oral hygiene on the periodontal attachment level and pocket depth in beagle dogs. J. Periodontal Res. 14: 428-437 (1979).
21.PAGE,R.and SCHRÖDER,H.E.:Periodontitis in man and other animals;(Karger,Basel 1982)
22.RALLS,A.S.and COHEN,M.E.:Problems in identifying bursts of periodontal attachment loss.J.Periodontol. 57:746-752(1986)
23.RAMFJORD, S.P.; MORRISON, E.C.; BURGETT, F.G.; NISSLE,R.R. ;SHICK, R.A.; ZANN, G.J. and KNOWLES, J.W.: Oral hygiene and maintenance of periodontal support.J. Periodontol. 53: 26-30 (1982).
24.SCHEI, O.; WAERHAUG, J.; LOVDAH, A. and ARNO, A.: Alveolar bone loss as related to oral hygiene and age.J.Periodontol.30:7-16(1959).
25.SCHROEDER, H.E. and ATTSTRÖM, R.: Pocket formation: An hypothesis.In Lehner and Cimasoni.The borderland between caries and periodontal disease.Vol II.pp. 99-123(1980).
26.SLOTS, J.: Bacterial specificity in adult periodontitis a summary of recent work. J. Clin. Periodontol. 13: 912-917 (1986).
27.SMULOW, J.B.; TURESKY, S.S. and HILL, R.G.: The effect of supragingival plaque removal on anaerobic bacteria in deep periodontal pockets. JADA 107: 737-742 (1983).
28.THEILADE, J. and ATTSTRÖM, R.: Distribution and ultrastructure of subgingival plaque in beagle dogs with gingival inflammation. J. Periodontal Res. 20: 131-145 (1985).
29.TROMP, J.A.H.; JANSEN, J. and PILOT, T.: Gingival health and frequency of tooth brushing in the beagle dog model. Clinical findings. J. Clin. Periodontol. 13: 164-168 (1986).
30.WAERHAUG, J.: Healing of the dento-epithelial junction following subgingival plaque control. I. As observed in human biopsy material. J. Periodontol. 49: 1-8 (1978).
31.WAERHAUG, J.: Healing of the dento-epithelial junction following subgingival plaque control. II: As observed on extracted teeth. J. Periodontol. 49: 119-134 (1978).
32.WESTFELT,E.;NYMAN,S.;LINDHE,J.and SOCRANSKY,S:Use of chlorhexidine as plaque control measure following surgical treatment of periodontal disease.Clin.Periodontol. 10:22-36(1983).
33.WILSON, T.G., jr.: Compliance. A review of the literature with possible applications to periodontics. J. Periodontol. 58: 706-714 (1987).
34.WRIGHT, W.E.: Periodontium destruction associated with oncology therapy. J. Periodontol. 58: 559-563 (1987).
School of Dentistry,Karl Gustavs väg 34,214 21 Malmö,Sweden.

Dr. R. Attström, Department of Periodontology, School of Dentistry, University of Lund, Carl Gustav Väg 34, 214 21 Malmö, Sweden

Periodontology Today. Int. Congr., Zürich 1988, pp. 260–270 (Karger, Basel 1988)

Can Crevicular Fluid Component Analysis Assist in Diagnosis and Monitoring Periodontal Breakdown?

Giorgio Cimasoni and Catherine Giannopoulou

Dental School, Division of Physiopathology and Periodontology, Medical Faculty, University of Geneva, Geneva, Switzerland

Many efforts have been aimed in finding biochemical parameters in gingival crevicular fluid which could supplement or replace the inadequate traditional clinical indices of diagnosis and prognosis. Most of our investigations however have tested the validity of biochemical measurements by using, in cross-sectional studies, these very same inadequate indices.

The present review will cover some of the problems related to procedures of collection, analysis and data reporting on gingival crevicular fluid (GCF). Findings of clinical significance will be discussed and results from our laboratory on GCF collection and analysis will be presented.

1. Collection and analysis of GCF: a critical appraisal

1.1. Procedure of GCF collection

The nature and significance of GCF might be different depending on the collection procedure. When inserting the tip of a filter paper in an undisturbed sulcus, one probably collects the pool of fluid present in that sulcus (BINDER, GOODSON and SOCRANSKY, 1987; LAMSTER, HARTLEY and VOGEL, 1985). In order to sample fluid produced at a constant flow one should standardize the sampling technique in regards to two points: depth of insertion below the gingival margin and time of collection. The possibility of dilution or "contamination" of GCF by serum should also be mentioned: whenever collecting fluid for long periods of time by an intracrevicular technique, the flow is known to increase due to an increased passage of serum caused by irritation (EGELBERG, 1966; CIMASONI, 1983). Such a dilution probably also takes place when using capillaries for the collection of several µl of fluid (LAMSTER et al., 1985).

1.2. Evaluation of the amount of fluid collected

With the exception of at least one report (SCHIFTER and CHILTON, 1985) most of the investigators agree that the electronic machine Periotron 6000 appears to be a reliable device for measuring the fluid absorbed by a filter paper strip (BICKEL and CIMASONI, 1984; HINRICHS et al., 1984). The amount of GCF collected on such a strip might however be too high to be measured correctly with this machine: satisfactory correlations between Periotron readings and volumes of GCF are found between 0 and 400 nl of fluid, (BICKEL and CIMASONI, 1984) but greater volumes can easily be reached. It is felt that alternative methods, such as weighing, should be available (VALAZZA et al., 1972).

1.3. Reporting of biochemical data

Traditionally, biochemical data on GCF have been expressed as concentrations (activity or amount per unit volume), as when reporting data for biological fluids (for review see CIMASONI, 1983). However, this has been recently challenged and several reports have suggested that the total activity or amount in a given sample would be a more appropriate way of expressing biochemical data on GCF (OSHRAIN et al., 1984; LAMSTER, OSHRAIN and GORDON, 1986; LAMSTER et al., 1987; SMITH, HINRICHS and MELNYK, 1986; BINDER et al., 1987). Before such a way of presenting data becomes widely accepted, at least two points should be further clarified: the influence of the volume of fluid and, for enzymes, the influence of the number of polymorphonuclear leucocytes (PMNs). A recent investigation on mammalian collagenase has shown that there is no correlation between collagenase activity and collected volume (VILLELA et al., 1987). Furthermore BINDER et al. (1987) have shown that alkaline phosphatase levels varied inversely to GCF volume. This problem has been further investigated in the present research, by comparing concentrations of 2 proteases in increasing volumes of fluid from the same sites.

Although the volume of fluid and the number of PMNs that can be recovered at the gingival margin are largely independent (KOWASHI, JACCARD and CIMASONI, 1980) it remains true that more PMNs, and thus more lysosomal enzyme, will be present on a strip collecting fluid from a more inflamed gingiva. Unfortunately, except for the semiquantitative techniques of washings (SKAPSKI and LEHNER, 1976; KOWASHI et al., 1980) and the one of ATTSTRÖM (1970) using styroflex films, no precise procedure is available for counting PMNs in a given site.

2. Biochemical data of clinical significance

Ideally, diagnosis of periodontal disease activity should be studied in man by a longitudinal approach, including repeated measurements of attachment level changes and monitoring of pathogenic bacteria. Standardized techniques of GCF collection should be used, allowing the evaluation of the amount of fluid and the counting of PMNs. The present review will thus be limited to investigations which have taken into account most if not all of these prerequisites. Enzymes in GCF will be considered first, followed by metabolic and bacterial products and, finally, by host response factors.

The enzymes β-glucuronidase and arylsulfatase, markers for ground substance degradation, have been monitoried, together with loss of attachment, in a longitudinal study of patients with periodontitis by LAMSTER et al. (1987): preliminary results indicate that total activity of β-glucuronidase in samples of GCF, however not related to the number of PMNs, is significantly higher in sites showing rapid attachment loss. Interesting findings have been reported by BINDER et al. (1987) on GCF levels of phosphatases in subjects monitored longitudinally: alkaline phosphatase concentration was shown to be positively associated with periodontal disease activity. Among the proteases of GCF, collagenase and elastase have received much attention (for review see CIMASONI, 1983 and FINE and MANDEL, 1987) but, so far, not in longitudinal studies. Collagenase has been shown to be highly correlated with pocket depth (GOLUB et al., 1976, VILLELA et al., 1987). Further longitudinal investigations on this enzyme should be encouraged. Kits for neutral proteases have been recently tested (ZAHRADNIK and DANKERS, 1987) and, ELISA techniques are now available for PMN elastase and for elastase-inhibitors complexes (NEUMANN, 1984).

GCF contains metabolic products from periodontal tissues. Degradation of collagen, for instance, can be monitored by the release of hydroxyproline (SVANBERG, 1987). In a recent study, COIL, TONZETICH and BEAGRIE (1987) found that the hydroxyproline content of GCF from periodontitis patients decreased during a 24 weeks period of periodontal therapy. Metabolic products from connective tissue ground substance were also identified in human GCF and one of these components, chondroitin-4-sulfate, was found to disappear in GCF after completion of periodontal therapy (LAST, STANBURY and EMBERY, 1985). ELISA assay techniques for the determination of such products could hopefully provide a convenient means of monitoring periodontal conditions (ROBINSON, AYTON and BATE, 1987).

Several bacterial products, such as endotoxin, hydrogen sulfide, butyrate, proprionate and polyamines have been studied in human GCF (for review see FINE and MANDEL, 1986). Recently, the availability of new synthetic substrates specific for bacterial proteases has made it possible to diagnose the presence of pathogenic bacteria in subgingival plaque by detecting their proteolytic activity (LOESCHE, SYED and STOLL, 1987). Such a detection appears to be possible through a simple colorimetric procedure which could give a potential test for active periodontitis.

Among host response factors one should mention complement, prostaglandins and antibodies. It is known that a functional complement system is present in GCF and recent studies have shown a correlation between the percentage of C3 conversion and the degree of gingival inflammation or the depth of pockets (PATTERS, NIEKRASH and LANG, 1985; NIEKRASH, 1985). A recent study on prostaglandin was longitudinal in nature and lasted for 3 years: interestingly, PGE2 levels were found to be much higher in GCF from sites with loss of attachment as compared to control, stable sites (OFFENBACHER, ODLE and VAN DYKE, 1985). As reviewed by CHALLACOMBE and WILTON (1984), antibodies against pathogenic bacteria are found in GCF. They might be more closely related to disease experience than serum antibodies.

3. Material and methods

3.1. Evaluation of the amount of fluid on a strip

Known volumes of serum, increasing from 250 to 1000 nl were blown out from Minicaps capillaries on strips of periopaper (Harco Electronics Ltd., Winnipeg, Manitoba, Canada) or strips of filter paper (Schleicher & Schell No 595), having a dimension of 2 x 5 mm. The amount of serum on the periopapers was measured with the Periotron 6000, while the amount of serum on the filter paper strips was measured by weighing. Each filter paper strip was weighed before the collection within a sealed microcentrifugation plastic tube and the weighing repeated immediately after the collection, the strip having been reintroduced and sealed in the same tube (VALAZZA et al., 1972). Measurements were also performed by weighing the dry strip together with a sealed microtube containing 150 µl of buffer and repeating the weighing immediately after collection, the strip having been introduced and sealed with the buffer in the same microtube. Rubber gloves were used throughout the procedure to avoid contamination. Evaporation of the buffer and of GCF was kept to a minimum by limiting to a few seconds the time during which the tube remained open.

3.2. Procedure of GCF collection

Strips of filter paper 2 mm wide and 5 mm long were used in 2 trials. In the first trial, GCF was collected from 6 sites along the upper arch in 3 volunteers, by inserting the tip of a filter paper 1 mm below the gingival margin. The sites showed mild inflammation (GI = 1 or 2) and a sulcus depth from 2 to 4 mm. In one experiment, performed in the afternoon (4 pm), each strip was left _in situ_ for 30 s and immediately replaced by the following; the procedure was repeated 5 times (continuous sampling). In a second experiment, performed in the morning (10 am), the strip was also left _in situ_ for 30 s but was replaced only after a 30 s interval, also for a total of 5 collections (discontinuous sampling). Each series was repeated for 4 consecutive days. The following week, the same sites and the same procedure were used, except that the strips were inserted deeper into the sulci, until mild resistance was felt.

For the second trial, a short-term experimental gingivitis was performed: GCF was collected from 8 sites showing a very mild inflammation (GI = 0 or 1) on one side of the upper arch in 4 volunteers. The strips were inserted deeply into the sulci, left in place for 30 s and the collected fluid measured by weighing. To obtain baseline values two collections were performed, with a 24 h interval. Then the volunteers refrained from brushing for 4 days and a third collection was performed immediately after removal of plaque.

3.3. Counting of polymorphonuclear leucocytes

Counting of PMNs was performed only for the trial of experimental gingivitis. After the introduction of the strip into the tube containing 100 µl of phosphate-buffer-saline, sealing and weighing, the tube was shaken on a vortex for 30 s. A fifteen µl sample of buffer was then transferred to a Neubauer chamber for counting the PMNs. This allowed the approximative determination of the number of cells contained in the original sample of GCF.

3.4. Biochemical analysis

An ELISA assay has been developed for quantitation of PMN elastase and cathepsin G in microamounts of GCF. The wells of the immunoplates were coated with 200 µl of rabbit antisera (0,65 µg/ml) and stored at 4°C for at least 15 h before use. For the standard curves, 100 µl of elastase and cathepsin G, obtained from human PMNs (BAUGH and TRAVIS, 1976) were both applied at the concentration of 0,132 mg/ml (dilution range: 1:2000 - 1:512,000). The GCF was applied in the dilution range from 1:2800 to 1:16,800. After 2 h incubation the plates were coated with 200 µl of antiserum conjugated with alkaline-phosphatase (dilutions: anti-cathepsin G = 1:16,000; anti-elastase = 1:4000). Finally, 200 µl of the substrate p-nitrophenylphosphate (1mg/ml) was added to each well and the reaction stopped with 50 µl of a 3M solution of NaOH.

4. Results

4.1. Weighing and Periotron

A linear relationship was obtained between volume and weight (t = 13,52) when weighing increasing amounts of serum eluted from filter paper strips, in the range of the relatively high volumes of serum tested.

As for the Periotron, the measurements reached a plateau for volumes above 700 nl.

4.2. Continuous or discontinuous sampling

When collecting GCF for 5 successive 30 s period without intervals, a decrease of the amount of fluid was observed. The difference between the first and the last sample collected was statistically significant with both the 1 mm ($p < 0.01$) and the deep intracrevicular technique ($p < 0.001$).

On the contrary, when a discontinuous sampling was performed on the same sites, with 30 s intervals between each collection, the volume of GCF increased but a constant flow rate was not achieved. The difference between the first and the last amount collected was significant for both the 1 mm and the deep intracrevicular technique ($p < 0.05$).

4.3. Experimental gingivitis

The volume of GCF and the number of PMNs were measured in 8 sites from 4 patients before and after a 4 day period of plaque accumulation. The average GCF flow at baseline, calculated from all the measurements at days -1 and 0, increased about two fold after 4 days of no-brushing. In some of the sites however there was no increase of GCF flow and, in general, the values at baseline were quite variable. The number of PMNs increased in all sites by a factor of about 3. The average total amount of elastase found initially increased about two fold after 4 days of plaque accumulation. The average concentration however (µg/nl of GCF) showed only a slight variation. As for the specific activity (µg/No of PMNs), this parameter decreased by an average of about 50% at the end of of the observation period. The same tendency was found for cathepsin G.

The changes of these parameters in 2 sites from 2 different patients are shown in figures 1 and 2 as percentages of their values at day 0.

8 sites from 4 patients before and after a 4 day period of plaque accumulation. The average GCF flow at baseline, calculated from all the measurements at days -1 and 0, increased

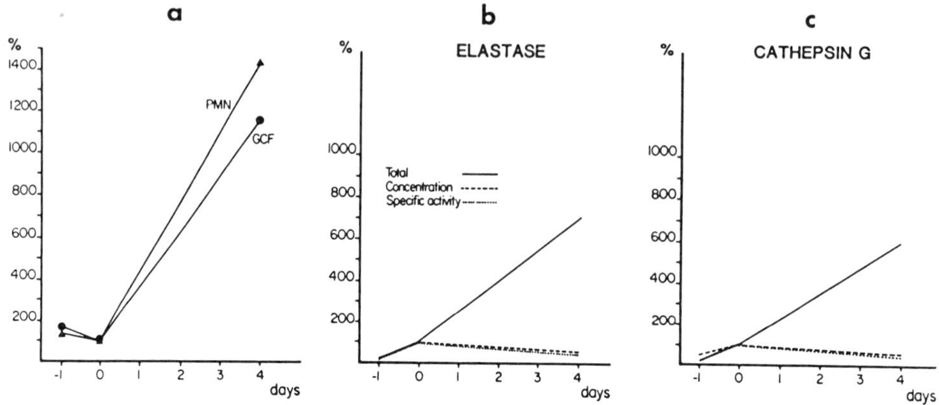

Fig. 1. Variations of parameters in one given site, as percentages of their values at time 0, during a short-term experimental gingivitis. a) PMN number and GCF volume; b) total amount, concentration and specific activity of elastase; c) total amount, concentration and specific activity of cathepsin G.

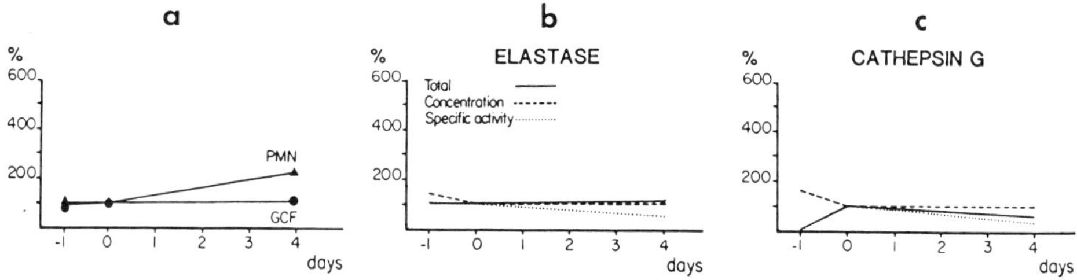

Fig. 2. Variations of PMN number, GCF volume (a) and of the two proteases (b and c) in a given site.

The first site (figure 1a) showed a strong increase both in the GCF flow and PMN number while the second site (figure 2a) was characterized by a stable GCF flow and an increase in PMN number. As can be seen in figures 1b, 1c and 2b and 2c, the total amounts of elastase and cathepsin G varied at both sites in a fashion which was parallel to the flow of GCF. On the contrary, the concentrations and the specific activities of the two enzymes decreased (figures 1b and 1c) or remained fairly stable (figures 2b and 2c).

5. Conclusions

The present investigation has tried to further clarify some of the drawbacks in the sampling procedures and analysis of GCF, in an effort of standardization. We have shown that, at least for very shallow pockets, the depth of insertion of the paper strip does not seem to play a role in the dynamics of fluid production (continuous or discontinuous sampling). Concerning the flow of GCF we have shown that intervals of 30 s in a discontinuous sampling procedure are still too long to obtain a constant flow rate. Unfortunately, our results with the discontinuous sampling do not support the concept of a pool of fluid being present in a given sulcus. The techniques of weighing should help investigators in dealing with amounts of GCF higher than those measurable with the Periotron. We have also shown that the number of PMNs in a given sample of GCF can be counted, although the procedure requires further refinement.

In a short term experimental gingivitis the total amounts of two lysosomal proteases increased in GCF during inflammation, parallel to the increase in GCF volume. Their concentrations on the contrary, as well as their specific activities remained constant or tended to decrease: we feel that biochemical data on GCF should take into account the volume of fluid collected and, for lysosomal enzymes, the number of PMNs.

A partial answer to the question raised by the present title has been given under section 2: some of the studies on biochemical parameters in GCF have given promising results but much remains to be done before a chairside procedure can be offered to the practitioner.

Acknowledgements: We thank Mrs. I. Condacci and E. Andersen for their skillfull technical assistance and Prof. P. Baehni for reading the manuscript.

References

ATTSTRÖM, R.: Presence of leukocytes in crevices of healthy and chronically inflamed gingivae. J. periodont. Res. 5: 42-47 (1970).

BAUGH, R.J. and TRAVIS, J.: Human leucocyte granule elastase: rapid isolation and characterization. Biochemistry 15: 836-841 (1976).

BICKEL, M. and CIMASONI, G.: Reliability of volume measurements with the new Periotron 6000. J. periodont. Res. 20: 35-40 (1985).

BINDER, T.A.; GOODSON, J.M. and SOCRANSKY, S.S.: Gingival fluid levels of acid and alkaline phosphatase. J. periodont. Res. 22: 14-19 (1987).

CHALLACOMBE, S.J. and WILTON, J.M.A.: A study of antibodies and opsonic activity in human crevicular fluid in relation to periodontal disease. J. periodont. Res. 19: 604-608 (1984).

CIMASONI, G.: Crevicular fluid updated. Monographs in Oral Science, Vol. 12 (Karger Press, Basel 1983).

COIL, J.; TONZETICH, J. and BEAGRIE, G.S.: Hydroxyproline content of crevicular fluid collected from periodontally involved sites. J. dent. Res. 66: 233 (abstract No 1011) (1987).

EGELBERG, J.: Permeability of the dento-gingival blood vessels. II. Clinically healthy gingivae. J. periodont. Res. 1: 276-286 (1966).

FINE, D.H. and MANDEL, I.D.: Indicators of periodontal disease activity: an evaluation. J. clin. Periodontol. 13: 533-546 (1986).

GOLUB, L.M.: SIEGEL, K.; RAMAMURTHY, N.S. and MANDEL, I.D.: Some characteristics of collagenase activity in gingival crevicular fluid and its relationship to gingival diseases in humans. J. dent. Res. 55: 1049-1057 (1976).

HINRICHS, J.E.; BRANDT, C.L.; SMITH, J.A. and GOLUB, L.M.: A comparison of 3 systems for quantifying gingival crevicular fluid with respect to linearity and the effects of qualitative differences in fluids. J. clin. Periodontol. 11: 652-661 (1984).

KOWASHI, Y.; JACCARD, F. and CIMASONI, G.: Sulcular polymorphonuclear leucocytes and gingival exudate during experimental gingivitis in man. J. periodont. Res. 15: 152-158 (1980).

LAMSTER, I.B.; HARPER, D.S.; FIORELLO, L.A.; OSHRAIN, R.L.; CELENTI, R.S. and GORDON, J.M.: Lysosomal and cytoplasmic enzyme activity, crevicular fluid volume and clinical parameters characterizing gingival sites with shallow to intermediate probing depths. J. periodont. Res. 58: 614-621 (1987).

LAMSTER, I.B.; HARTLEY, L.J. and VOGEL, R.I.: Development of a biochemical profile for gingival crevicular fluid. J. Periodontol. 56: 13-21 (1985).

LAMSTER, I.B.; OSHRAIN, R.L. and GORDON, J.M.: Enyzme activity in human gingival crevicular fluid: considerations in data reporting based on analysis of individual crevicular sites. J. clin. Periodontol. 13: 799-804 (1986).

LAST, K.S.; STANBURY, J.B. and EMBERY, G.: Glycosaminoglycans in human gingival crevicular fluid as indicators of active periodontal disease. Archs oral Biol. 30: 275-281 (1985).

LOESCHE, W.J.; SYED, S.A. and STOLL, J.: Trypsin-like activity in subgingival plaque. A diagnosis marker for spirochetes and periodontal disease? J. Periodontol. 58: 266-273 (1987).

NEUMANN, S.: Granulocyten-elastase als marker für entzündliche Prozesse; in Pathobiochemie der Entzündung. Ed. by H. Lang and H. Greiling, pp. 94-101 (Springer, Berlin 1984).

NIEKRASH; C.E.: Assessement of complement cleavage in gingival fluid with and without periodontal disease. J. dent. Res. 64: 164 (abstract No H 15) (1985).

OFFENBACHER, S.; ODLE, B. and VAN DYKE, T.E.: Crevicular fluid prostaglandin E2 levels predict periodontal attachment loss. J. dent. Res. 64: 374 (abstract No 1797) (1985).

OSHRAIN, R.L.; LAMSTER, I.B.; HARTLEY, L.J. and GORDON, J.M.: Arylsulphatase activity in human gingival crevicular fluid. Archs oral Biol. 29: 399-402 (1984).

PATTERS, M.; NIEKRASH, C.E. and LANG, N.P.: Assessement of complement cleavage in gingival fluid during experimental gingivitis in humans. J. dent. Res. 64: 360 (abstract No 1674) (1985).

ROBINSON, C.; AYTON, F.D. and BATE, A.S.: Immunological analysis of crevicular fluid as a basis for assessment of periodontal condition. J. dent. Res. 66: 855 (abstract No 184) (1987).

SCHIFTER, C.S. and CHILTON, N.W.: Reproducibility of gingival crevicular fluid volume measurements. J. dent. Res. 20: 375 (abstract No 1803) (1985).

SKAPSKI, H. and LEHNER, T.: A crevicular washing method for investigating immune components of crevicular fluid in man. J. periodont. Res. 11: 19-24 (1976).

SMITH, Q.T.; HINRICHS, J.E. and MELNYK, R.S.: Gingival crevicular fluid myeloperoxidase at periodontitis sites. J. periodont. Res. 21: 45-55 (1986).

SVANBERG, G.K.: Hydroxyproline titers in gingival crevicular fluid. J. periodont. Res. 22: 212-214 (1987).

VALAZZA, A.; MATTER, J.; OGILVIE, A. and CIMASONI, G.: Fluide gingival, inflammation gingivale, profondeur des poches et perte osseuse. Revue mens. suisse Odonto-stomat. 82: 824-832 (1972).

VILLELA, B.; COGEN, R.B.; BARTOLUCCI, A.A. and BIRKEDAL-HANSEN, H.: Crevicular fluid collagenase activity in healthy, gingivitis, chronic adult periodontitis and localized juvenile periodontitis patients. J. periodont. Res. 22: 209-211 (1987).

ZAHRADNIK, R.T. and DANKERS, I.: Reproducibility of neutral protease measurements in healthy and periodontal patients. J. dent. Res. 66: 233 (abstract No 1012) (1987).

Prof. Giorgio Cimasoni, Dental School, University of Geneva, 19, rue Barthélemy Menn, 1211 Geneva 4, Switzerland

Periodontology Today. Int. Congr., Zürich 1988, pp. 271–280 (Karger, Basel 1988)

Repair or Regeneration, Does it Matter?

Thorkild Karring

Department of Periodontology, Royal Dental College, Aarhus, Denmark

Introduction

Several longitudinal studies have documented that irrespective of surgical or nonsurgical periodontal treatment, pocket probing depth reductions and clinical attachment levels can be maintained over several years provided that scaling is applied at regular intervals and provided a high standard of oral hygiene is maintained (PHILSTRÖM et al. 1983, ISIDOR and KARRING 1986, RAMFJORD et al. 1987). It should be noticed that the magnitude of pocket reduction and gingival recession in these studies is similar following surgical and nonsurgical treatment and that the findings are mainly obtained on single-rooted teeth. Specific data on the effect of surgical and non-surgical treatment on multirooted teeth with deep pockets extending into the furcation area are limited.

Regardless of the type of periodontal treatment healing results in recession of the gingival margin which in advanced cases of periodontitis may present a serious cosmetic problem. During maintenance care following treatment it is also important to be able to get access for retreatment of pockets with signs of disease, i.e. inflammation, exudation and bleeding on probing. In the presence of deep pockets in association with angular bony defects it may be difficult or even impossible to remove accretions from the root surface. For such reasons it is an optimal goal of periodontal therapy to restore those parts of the periodontium which have been destructed because of periodontitis.

Reconstructive periodontal surgery

Reconstructive periodontal surgery has been used for more than two decades in attempts to restore lost tooth support. The results have been varying and for those cases which clinically have been evaluated as successful the result of healing has been a subject of speculation. Did healing result in regeneration or repair? According to MELCHER (1969) does <u>regenera-</u>

tion imply that the architecture and function of the lost tissue is completely restored. Repair, on the other hand, involves that the disrupted tissue is restored by a tissue which does not replicate the structure and function of the lost tissue. As far as regeneration of the periodontium is concerned, this must require that new cementum with inserting collagen fibers are formed on the previously periodontitis involved root surfaces and that this formation of a new connective tissue attachment is accompanied by regrowth of the alveolar bone.

In attempts to restore lost tooth support particular attention has been directed towards the regeneration of the alveolar bone. The effect of osseous grafting has been evaluated in many studies and there are several reports indicating that healing of periodontal angular bony defects is promoted following flap procedures which include the placement of bone grafts or bone substitutes in the defects (for review see GARA and ADAMS 1981). In a discussion of the significance of regeneration or repair it may be of interest to look upon the results of some studies in which the fate and effect of bone grafts were evaluated in periodontal lesions in monkeys. Following placement of iliac bone marrow grafts in experimentally created angular bony defects in monkeys ELLEGAARD et al.(1974) observed that bone fill had occurred almost consistently. However, this regeneration of bone was not accompanied by the formation of cementum on the root surface and healing did always result in ankylosis and root resorption. In a previous study (ELLEGAARD et al. 1973), where iliac bone marrow grafts and bone grafts taken from edentulous areas of the jaw were placed in interradicular periodontal lesions, it was revealed that only the iliac bone marrow grafts survive transplantation. On the basis of this observation it was suggested that it is the surviving iliac bone marrow cells which are responsible for the induction of root resorption.

Jaw bone grafts placed in periodontal lesions fail to survive transplantation and show the same behaviour during healing as nonvital bone grafts (ELLEGAARD, KARRING and LÖE 1975, NIELSEN, KARRING and LÖE 1980). They do not actively contribute to bone formation but may serve as a scaffold for bone regeneration when reached by bone growing out from the host. Most grafts in these studies, however, were never reached by bone (fig. 1), but occurred as isolated particles surrounded by a cementum-like substance (fig. 2). Judged from the course of the blood vessels during healing of the treated defects it appeared like a major portion of the granulation tissue in the bifurcation area developed from the periodontal ligament (fig. 3). On the basis of this observation and because the periodontal ligament tissue is known to inhibit osteogenesis (MELCHER 1976) it was suggested that the negligible amount of bone regeneration in the bifurcation defects following healing could be due to the fact that the area had become occupied by tissue derived from the periodontal ligament (NIELSEN, KARRING and LÖE 1980). Since the periodontal ligament is also known to contain cells with cementum forming potentials, it was suggested that it was these cells which were responsible for the formation of the new cementum in the bifurcation defect including the cementum-like substance observed around the transplanted bone particles (fig. 1,2).

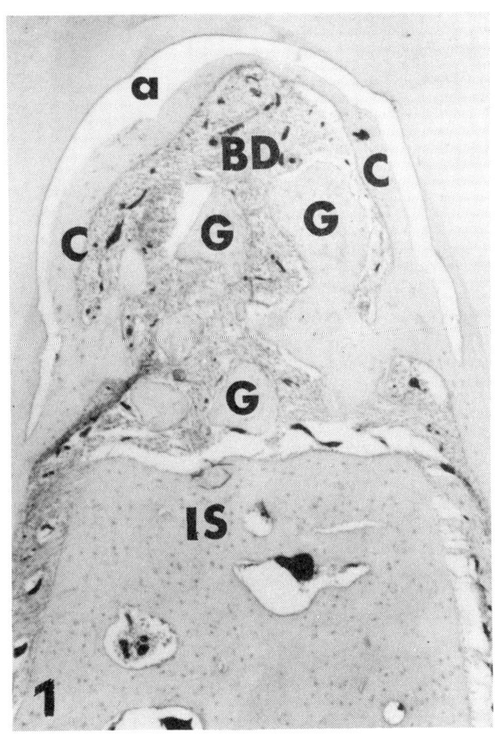

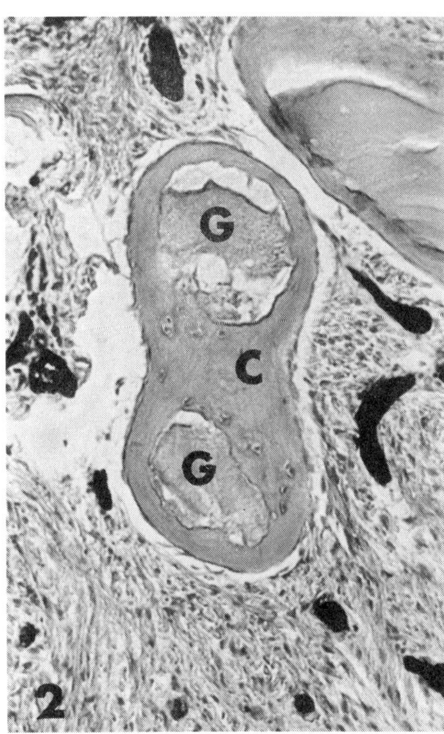

Fig. 1. Photomicrograph of a healed bifurcation defect (BD) following transplantation of autogenous bone grafts. The bone grafts (G) have not been reached by bone formation from the interradicular septum (IS) but occur as isolated particles surrounded by a cementum-like substance. Cementum (C) formation and new connective tissue attachment have taken place along the entire circumference of the bifurcation. A split (a) has occurred between the root surface and the new cementum during preparation of the specimen.

Fig. 2. Photomicrograph showing isolated bone grafts (G) surrounded by a cementum-like substance (C).

Practically all bifurcation defects treated in the studies mentioned above healed with repair rather than regeneration. The majority of the defects failed to heal with a fibrous attachment but demonstrated an epithelial lining along the circumference of the furcation coronal to the apical termination of root instrumentation.

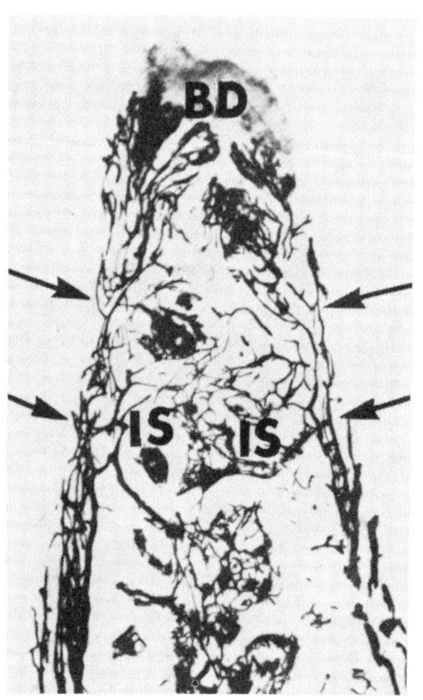

Fig. 3. Cleared specimen from a one week old bifurcation defect (BF) treated with bone grafts. Judged from the course of the blood vessels the granulation tissue in the defect is developing mainly from the periodontal ligament (arrows) and only to a minor extent from the interradicular septum (IS).

In an experiment in monkeys CATON, NYMAN and ZANDER (1980) studied healing after treatment of periodontal lesions with 4 different modalities of periodontal therapy. These were root planing and soft tissue curettage, Widman flap surgery without bone grafting and Widman flap surgery with the placement of frozen autogenous red marrow and cancellous bone or a bone substitute, beta tricalcium phosphate in the angular bony defects. The histological analysis demonstrated that healing following all treatment modalities had resulted in the formation of a long junctional epithelium extending to or close to the attachment level prior to the treatment. The results of this study and other studies indicate that healing following commonly used reconstructive surgical procedures results in repair by means of a long junctional epithelium facing the instrumented root surfaces.

Regenerative capacity of periodontal tissues

From the studies described above it appears like the type of repair or regeneration which occur after surgical treatment of periodontal lesions is depending on the type of tissue which invade the wound area during healing. A number of experiments in recent years have revealed that the various periodontal tissues involved in periodontal wound healing differs in their regenerative capacity.

Bone tissue does not produce new attachment

Periodontitis was induced in dogs by placing ligatures around their teeth (KARRING et al. 1980). When the destruction had reached to almost half of the root length, the ligatures were removed and the teeth were cleaned. After a tissue flap was raised on the buccal and lingual aspect of each experimental tooth, the root surface was scaled. The bone level was indicated by producing a notch in the root surface with a bur. Then, the roots were extracted and placed in sockets created surgically in edentulous areas after raising a tissue flap. The roots, completely surrounded by bone, were then covered by the tissue flap. This closure of the wound prevents infection and epithelial downgrowth along the root surface during healing. After 3 months of healing it was observed that a periodontal ligament had become reestablished in the apical portion of the reimplanted roots. However, in the coronal portion which had been previously exposed to periodontitis, healing consistently had resulted in ankylosis and root resorption (fig. 4). Only a very small amount of new connective tissue attachment was observed at the border between the exposed root portion and the apical portion (fig. 5) on which remnants of periodontal ligament tissue was retained at the time of reimplantation.

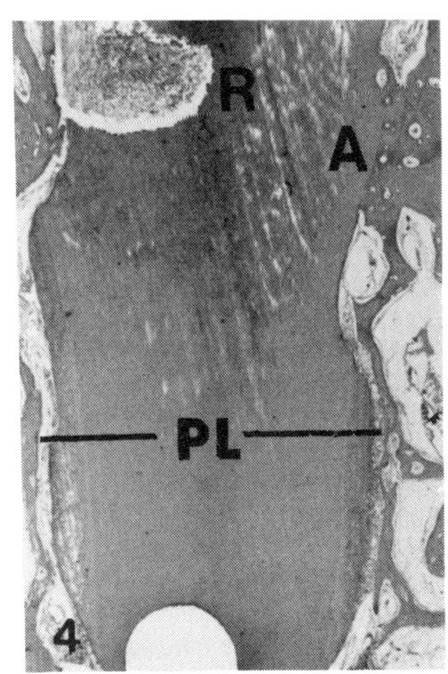

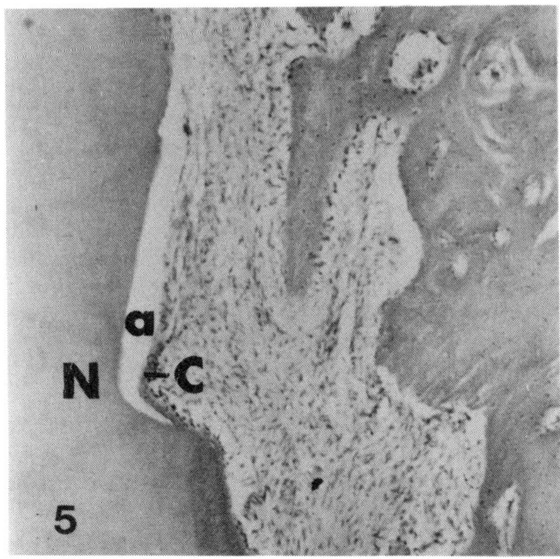

Fig. 4. Reimplanted root after healing. A periodontal ligament (PL) has become reestablished in the apical portion of the root whereas ankylosis (A) and root resorption (R) is the predominant feature in the coronal portion.

Fig. 5. New cementum (C) with inserting connective tissue fibers has formed within the notch (N) prepared in the root surface to indicate the bone level prior to extraction of the reimplanted root. a: split artifact.

Apparently, this remaining periodontal ligament tissue was the origin of the granulation tissue which had grown coronally along the exposed root surface and formed a small amount of new connective tissue attachment. The consistent finding of root resorption and ankylosis in the coronal portion of the reimplanted roots where bone tissue had reached contact with the surface indicates that granulation tissue originating from bone is incapable to produce a new connective tissue attachment.

Gingival connective tissue does not produce new attachment

Another tissue involved in periodontal wound healing is the gingival connective tissue. Therefore, another experiment was carried out in which the model was slightly modified (NYMAN et al. 1980). Instead of placing the roots completely in bone they were placed in such a way that only half of their circumference was in the bone. The remaining part was facing gingival connective tissue on the subsurface of the covering tissue flap. In histologic sections of these roots after 3 months of healing it was found that resorption was the characteristic feature on the surfaces facing the gingival connective tissue, like it was on the surfaces facing the bone tissue. Based on this observation it was concluded that also the gingival connective tissue lacks the ability to form a new connective tissue attachment to a root surface previously attacked by periodontitis.

Periodontal ligament tissue produces new attachment

In the studies mentioned above ankylosis and root resorption was sometimes observed also in the apical portion of the roots. This suggests that the periodontal ligament tissue retained in this area had become damaged due to the extraction procedure, thereby allowing bone tissue to reach contact with the root surface and cause resorption. This in turn means that this damage may also have limited the possibilities for coronal growth of periodontal ligament tissue.

In a later study (KARRING et al. 1985), where periodontitis involved roots were retained in their own sockets and covered by tissue flaps, significant amounts of new attachment had formed on the coronal portion of the roots (fig. 6). The finding of significant amounts of new attachment on these roots with a non-impaired periodontal ligament, while practically no new attachment had been formed on the extracted and reimplanted roots with an injuried periodontal ligament indicates that the periodontal ligament can produce a new connective tissue attachment on a root surface, which has been exposed due to periodontitis.

The role of epithelium

Some of the roots in the previous experiment (KARRING et al. 1985) had penetrated the mucosa during the first week of healing in such a way that the epithelium was allowed to migrate apically along the root surface. The length of newly formed attachment on the root surfaces attacked previously by periodontitis was much smaller on these where epithelium was allowed to grow down along the root, than on those which were covered throughout the study. Thus, the finding that the reexposed roots exhibited less new attachment than the covered roots indicates that the downgrowth of epithelium jeopardize the formation of a new connective tissue attachment.

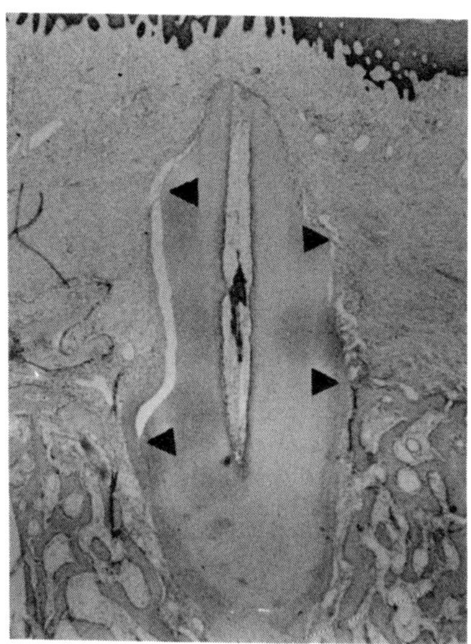

Fig. 6. Photomicrograph showing new attachment formation (between the arrows) on a submerged root with a non-impaired periodontal ligament.

Regeneration or repair - Sometimes it does matter!

The studies described above have indicated that granulation tissue derived from bone or gingival connective tissue induces root resorption when reaching contact with the curetted root surface during healing. Repair which includes such a contact is unacceptable since it may lead to loss of the involved tooth. It is apparent from the studies mentioned above that reestablishment of lost connective tissue attachment requires coronal growth of granulation tissue derived from the periodontal ligament at the same time as other tissues are prevented from reaching contact with the root surface during healing. Results of studies in experimental animals and humans have confirmed that new connective tissue attachment can indeed be achieved if this requirement is fulfilled (NYMAN et al. 1982, GOTTLOW et al. 1984, 1986).

The results of a study in dogs have indicated that the reestablishment of fibrous attachment to a root surface is not necessarily accompanied by regrowth of the alveolar bone (NYMAN and KARRING 1979). This rises the question whether repair by means of a long supra-alveolar connective tissue attachment is comparable to a situation where regrowth of the alveolar bone has resulted in a short distance between the apical extension of the junctional epithelium and the bone crest (regeneration). In an experimental study in the dog it was examined if a gingival unit with a long supraalveolar connective tissue attachment provides less resistance against progression of periodontal disease than a unit with a supraalveolar connective tissue attachment of normal length (NYMAN et al. 1984). It was found that the attachment loss was similar in sites with a long supraalveolar connective attachment and in sites with a supraalveolar connective tissue attachment of normal length. This finding suggests that the loss of attachment in periodontal disease is unrelated to the presence or absence of the bony component of the periodontium. Thus, regarding resistance to attachment loss, repair which involve reestablishment of a new connective tissue attachment without a concommitant regrowth of bone does not seem to be inferior to complete regeneration. However, under certain conditions a lack of bone formation may obviously influence tooth mobility. Also, it remains to be shown that a new formed connective tissue attachment exerts the same resistance to attachment loss in periodontal disease as the original attachment.

Following commonly used reconstructive surgical procedures healing does almost invariably result in repair with the presence of a long junctional epithelium (LISTGARTEN and ROSENBERG 1979). According to these authors "a long junctional epithelium" may well facilitate the passage of microbial products into the underlying connective tissue. The inflammatory infiltrate which may result from such a process, particular if the oral hygiene is inadequate, may lead to the sudden occurrence of probable defects at sites which initially appear to have responded well to therapy aimed at creating new attachment. Also, BARRINGTON (1981) has expressed that "repair by means of a long junctional epithelium and not by new attachment of connective tissue, may be a disadvantage in that the area may be prone to new pocket formation and reinstitution of disease activity". On the other hand, it has been examined in monkeys whether a gingival unit with a long junctional epithelium provides a less efficient seal against plaque infection than a unit with a junctional epithelium of normal length (MAGNUSSON et al. 1983). It was found that the inflammatory lesion in the gingival connective tissue resulting from plaque infection did not extend deeper into the periodontal tissues in sites with a long junctional epithelium than in gingival units with an epithelium of normal length. This result was interpreted to mean that a long junctional epithelium does not provide a less efficient seal against plaque infection than a unit with a junctional epithelium of normal length.

Although the quality of repair by a long junctional epithelium is not completely clarified it seems reasonable to assume that from a functional point of view a long junctional epithelium is inferior to a connective tissue attachment. This assumption is based on the fact that when a force is applied on a tooth it is the fibers inserting at the tooth surface opposite the direction of the force which become streched and prevents the tooth from further movement. The attachment of the junctional epithelium to the tooth surface may not nearly exert the same resistance to tooth movement as a fibrous attachment. Regarding the issue repair or regeneration there are still many aspects which need further investigation.

References

BARRINGTON, E.: An overview of periodontal surgical procedures. J. Periodontol. 52: 518-528 (1981).

CATON, J.; NYMAN, S. and ZANDER, H.: Histometric evaluation of periodontal surgery. II Connective tissue attachment levels after four regenerative procedures. J. Clin. Periodont. 7: 224-231 (1980).

ELLEGAARD, B.; KARRING, T.; LISTGARTEN, M. and LÖE, H.: New attachment after treatment of interradicular lesions. J. Periodontol. 44: 209-217 (1973).

ELLEGAARD, B.; KARRING, T.; DAVIES, R. and LÖE, H.: New attachment after treatment of intrabony defects in monkeys. J. Periodontol. 45: 368-377 (1974).

ELLEGAARD, B.; KARRING, T. and LÖE, H.: The fate of vital and devitalized bone grafts in the healing of interradicular lesions. J. Periodontol. Res. 10: 88-97 (1975).

GARA, G.G. and ADAMS, D.F.: Implant therapy in human intrabony pockets. A review of the literature. J. West. Soc. Periodont. 29: 32-47 (1981).

GOTTLOW, J.; NYMAN, S.; KARRING; T. and LINDHE, J.: New attachment formation as the result of controlled tissue regeneration. J. Clin. Periodontol 11: 494-503 (1984).

GOTTLOW, J.; NYMAN, S.; LINDHE, J.; KARRING, T. and WENNSTRÖM, J.: New attachment formation in the human periodontium by guided tissue regeneration. J. Clin. Periodont. 13: 604-616 (1986).

ISIDOR, F. and KARRING, T.: Long term effect of surgical and non-surgical periodontal treatment. A 5-year clinical study. J. Periodont. Res. 21: 462-472 (1986).

KARRING, T.; NYMAN, S. and LINDHE, J.: Healing following implantation of periodontitis affected roots into bone tissue. J. Clin. Periodont. 7: 96-105 (1980).

KARRING, T.; ISIDOR, F.; NYMAN, S. & LINDHE, J.: New attachment formation on teeth with a reduced but healthy periodontal ligament. J. Clin. Periodont. 12: 51-60 (1985).

LISTGARTEN, M.A. and ROSENBERG, M.M.: Histological study of repair following new attachment procedures in human periodontal lesions. J. Periodontol. 50: 333-344 (1979).

MAGNUSSON, I.; RUNSTAD, L.; NYMAN, S. and LINDHE, J.: A long junctional epithelium - A locus minoris resistentiae in plaque infection. J. Clin. Periodont. 10: 333-340 (1983).

MELCHER, A.H.: Healing of wounds in the periodontium; in MELCHER and BOWEN, The Biology of the periodontium., pp. 497-529 (Academic press, London 1969).

MELCHER, A.H.: On the repair potential of periodontal tissues. J. Periodontol. 47: 256-260 (1976).

NIELSEN, I.M.; ELLEGAARD, B. and KARRING, T.: Kielbone[R] in healing interradicular lesions in monkeys. J. Periodont. Res. 15: 328-337 (1980).

NYMAN, S. and KARRING, T.: Regeneration of surgically removed buccal alveolar bone in dogs. J. Periodont. Res. 14: 86-92 (1979).

NYMAN, S.; KARRING, T.; LINDHE, J. and PLANTEN, S.: Healing following implantation of periodontitis affected roots into gingival connective tissue. J. Clin. Periodontol. 7: 394-401 (1980).
NYMAN, S.; LINDHE, J.; KARRING, T. and RYLANDER, H.: New attachment following surgical treatment of human periodontal disease. J. Clin. Periodont. 9: 290-296 (1982).
NYMAN, S.; ERICSSON, I.; RUNSTAD, L. and KARRING, T.: The significance of alveolar bone in periodontal disease. An experimental study in the dog. J. Periodont. Res. 19: 520-525 (1984).
PHILSTRÖM, B.L.; McHUGH, R.B.; OLIPHANT, T.H. and ORTIZ-CAMPOS, C.: Comparison of surgical and non-surgical treatment of periodontal disease. J. Clin. Periodont. 10: 524-541 (1983).
RAMFJORD, S.P.; CAFFESSE, R.G.; MORRISON, E.C.; HILL, R.W.; KERRY, G.J.; APPLEBURRY, E.A.; NISSLE, R.R. and STULTS, D.L.: 4 modalities of periodontal treatment compared over 5 years. J. Clin. Periodont. 14: 445-452 (1987).

AUTHOR's ADDRESS:
Thorkild Karring
Department of Periodontology
Royal Dental College
Vennelyst Boulevard
DK-8000 Aarhus C
Denmark

Periodontology Today. Int. Congr., Zürich 1988, pp. 281–289 (Karger, Basel 1988)

Rational for Chemotherapy in the Treatment of Periodontal Disease

Martin Addy

Department of Periodontology, Dental School, University of Wales College of Medicine, Cardiff, South Wales, UK

In simple terms the initiation and progression of periodontal diseases are dependant upon the balance between the virulence of the associated microflora and the resistance of the host. Numerous variables influence these two main factors and in recent years much has been learnt concerning the aetiology and pathogenesis of peridontal diseases. In particular bacterial isolation, cultural and identification techniques have provided considerable information as to the bacteriology of progressing periodontal lesions (36,39). Unfortunately the specificity, or for that matter the non-specificity, of bacteria associated with periodontal disease has not been established and is still much debated (35,40).

The recognition of the importance of bacteria to advancing periodontal lesions has tended to consolidate periodontal treatment methods. However, reviews on the subject indicate that such methods were recommended many years ago and based on the same premise (12). Periodontal treatments are directed towards thorough debridement of the root surface using surgical or non-surgical techniques. But it is recognised that long term success is dependant upon maintained supragingival plaque control by the patient (27,31). Unfortunately, the clinical lesion of chronic periodontal disease, the pocket, is a considerable obstacle to the success of periodontal treatments. In the first place a pocket provides an apparently ideal environment for the proliferation of micro-organisms and protects the bacterial mass from routine oral hygiene methods including the use of antiplaque mouthrinses (9). Secondly, pocketing makes difficult mechanical debridement techniques and frequently surgical exposure is considered necessary to facilitate access. Failure to eliminate pocketing by treatment also makes difficult long term maintenance as recolonistion may be impossible to prevent.

In an attempt to ensure the success of periodontal treatments chemotherapy has been for a long time considered as an adjunct to mechanical methods and as a bolster to the maintenance of oral hygiene. Chemicals used to prevent plaque accumulation and the onset or re-establishment of periodontal diseases have so far been championed by chlorhexidine, and short to medium term regimens are established (1). Thus, whatever contrary opinions are held concerning the use of chemicals to prevent disease, researchers and commercial organisations will continue to strive to find compounds with minimal or no side effects which effectively prevent disease, and their use is almost certainly established for the forseeable future. However, the ideology for the routine use of chemotherapeutic agents in the treatment of periodontal disease is far from established and the benefits to be obtained not proven. Thus, it is important to state that in our present state of knowledge and expertise details of the microbial aetiologies of periodontal diseases are not precise enough, nor are antimicorbial drugs specific enough (10) to place chemotherapy on a firm scientific basis.

The rational for the use of chemotherapy in the treatment of inflammatory periodontal diseases is simply that most are bacterial associated. However, at best chemotherapy should be considered supportive to routine mechanical treatment methods. Because of this a decision to use chemotherapy must be made after weighing up the possible benefits against the potential disadvantages of use. Chemotherapeutic agents may produce harmful side effects and include the emergence of resistant bacterial strains, superinfection by resistant micro-organisms notably fungi, patient hypersensitivity reactions, specific toxicological effects and interactions with other drugs (6,8,22,38). Moreover clear benefits for adjunctive use of antimicrobial drugs have not always been established (20,23) and in the light of the chronic nature of most periodontal diseases it is unclear what influence chemotherapy has on recurrence of the disease process.

Chemotherapy is usually considered under two headings namely systemic and local, and both have the aim of drug delivery to the active periodontal lesion. Most of the bacterial mass lies within the pocket lumen and on the root surface and, therefore, should be accessible to chemotherapeutic agents introduced into the area via either the systemic or local route. This accessibility however may be compromised by several factors. Plaque has a finite thickness and, dependant upon the physico-chemical properties of the antimicrobial, diffusion into the plaque may not occur. Furthermore some bacteria may lie in the soft tissues (33) and certainly may be found in both subgingival calculus, cementum and even root dentine (5). An additional consideration in chemotherapy must also be the maintenance of activity of some antimicrobial drugs in the protein rich environment of the pocket. The action of some compounds, notably antiseptics may be reduced even vitiated by the presence of protein (4,30) and in vitro activity may not be a predictor of effects in vivo.

Systemic Chemotherapy

A number of chemotherapeutic agents, after systemic absorption, are excreted into the gingival crevicular fluid including tetracycline, metronidazole, erythromycin and spiromycin. Some, notably tetracycline, are concentrated in the crevicular fluid (17) and have properties other than antibacterial activity including the inhibition of host collagenase (14). Perhaps the most common use of chemotherapeutic agents in periodontology has been for acute diseases including acute ulcerative gingivitis, acute pericoronitis and acute periodontal abscesses (26). Many consider that use in such conditions should be reserved for patients with signs of systemic upset and/or evidence of local spread of infection. Moreover it must be remembered that chemotherapy will only resolve the acute phase and conventional methods are essential to prevent recurrence or progression to a chronic state.

In chronic periodontal disease there can be no doubt that systemic chemotherapy can be effective in treatment (11). However, alone the benefits were found of limited duration and adjunctive action to surgical or non-surgical techniques was minimal (20,23). One difficulty must be the choice of antimicrobial for use. With the present knowledge of bacterial specificity and limited availability of diagnostic bacteriological facilities drug prescribing is a matter of informed guesswork.

More specific uses of chemotherapy have been reported including tetracycline in the treatment of chronic juvenile periodontitis (37) and tetracyline and metronidazole in the treatment of refractory or rapidly advancing adult periodontitis (24,25). The encouraging findings may reflect the expected susceptibility of certain bacteria to the antimicrobial, notably in the case of chronic juvenile periodontitis the sensitivity of Actinobacillus actinomycetemcomitans to tetracycline (43). Even for these more specific conditions however there is evidence that mechanical treatments alone are just as effective (34). Nevertheless, factors other than the effectiveness of one treatment regimen over another may have to be taken into account. In particular chemotherapy alone or with non-surgical techniques may be required to avoid surgery for patients where this is contra-indicated for a variety of reasons. This could include in the young where surgery may interfere with the development of the alveolar process.

Least debated and researched must be the use of chemotherapy for periodontal patients with underlying systemic disease. Prophylactic chemotherapy has to be provided for patients at risk from systemic disease arising from periodontal treatments, notably those with congenital or acquired valvular heart defects. More unclear must be the need of adjunctive chemotherapy for patients predisposed to periodontal breakdown as a result of an underlying systemic disease. Each case has to be considered individually, a major factor being the nature and seriousness of the underlying disease. However, it is probable that if the underlying disease cannot be adequately treated the principle of using chemotherapy in the management of the periodontal treatment would be highly questionable since this would provide little if any long term benefit.

In summary and consistent with previous reviews (11,19) the use of systemic chemotherapy in the management of chronic periodontal diseases is open to doubt and should be reserved for those cases where the disease is rapid or refractory to conventional methods or where mechanical techniques are difficult or contraindicated. In those cases where systemic disease predisposes to periodontal breakdown careful consideration should be given to the actual benefits that might be obtained from the use of chemotherapy.

Local Chemotherapy

Due to the relative inaccessibility of the periodontal pocket to drugs delivered by conventional means, including mouthwashes (28), several vehicles have been developed to carry agents directly to the periodontal lesion. Such an approach is not new (12) but possesses some advantages over systemic chemotherapy. Drug dose is greatly reduced and, therefore, systemic side effects and drug interactions are minimised. Superinfection is unlikely and the emergence of resistant strains limited to a few sites. Additionally high concentration of drugs can be delivered directly to the lesions and most importantly drugs unsuitable for systemic use may be employed. Delivery methods to date have been i) direct irrigation (29) ii) drug impregnated vehicles including a) hollow fibres (15) b) monolithic fibres (16) c) acrylic strips (3) d) cellulose acetate strips (13). The drugs of choice have usually been chlorhexidine, metronidazole or tetracycline and perhaps surprisingly most reports of the various combinations of drugs and vehicles have indicated considerable success (2,18,21,42). Nevertheless the demonstration of a clear adjunctive effect to routine debridement techniques has only rarely been studied and demonstrated (32). The studies have themselves however raised some interesting points. Firstly some systems alone have produced clinical and microbiological effects comparable to root planing (18). Since the antimicrobials do not remove the subgingival acretions the importance of bacterial endotoxin in the hard subgingival tissues to maintenance of disease and healing is open to question. Secondly the data indicates that certain antimicrobials appear more effective than others. Thus in the acrylic delivery system metronidazole was more effective than tetracycline and chlorhexidine (2,18). Certain fundamental questions relating to local chemotherapy remain to be addressed. Notably for irrigation it is unclear whether a sufficient dose can be maintained in the pocket and whether results observed reflect merely a washing out rather than true antimicrobial action. The suitability of the subgingival environment for certain compounds has not been evaluated. Thus, chlorhexidine may be, inactivated by the protein rich environment (4,30), unable to penetrate plaque layers because of its cationic nature or relatively ineffective against some subgingival organisms (7). Finally a determination of the ideal vehicle for each drug and the optimum regimens of use has never been attempted. As with systemic drugs the choice of agent for a particular lesion can only be based on clinical experience. Thus, at present it would seem sensible to consider local antimicrobial therapy as an adjunct rather than replacement for mechanical debridement techniques. The approach does have the advantage that specific sites for treatment can be selected particularly those that remain refractory to conventional treatment and perhaps this should be the rational for their use.

In conclusion, chemotherapy would appear to have a small role in the treatment of periodontal disease and there is a need to improve diagnostic procedures before their use is expanded, and ideally, consideration should be given towards identifying effective and safe antimicrobials which have minimal or no use in the treatment of other human diseases (41).

References

1. ADDY, M.: Chlorhexidine compared with other locally delivered antimicrobials. A short review. J. clin. Periodontol. 13: 954-964 (1986).
2. ADDY, M. and LANGEROUDI, M.: Comparison of the immediate effects on the subgingival microflora of acrylic strips containing 40% chlorhexidine, metronidazole or tetracycline. J. clin. Periodontol. 11: 379-386 (1984).
3. ADDY, M.; RAWLE, L.; HANDLEY, R.; NEWMAN, H.N. and COVENTRY, R.: The development and in vitro evaluation of acrylic strips and dialysis tubing for

local drug delivery. J. Periodontol. 53: 693-698 (1982).

4. ADDY, M. and WRIGHT, R.: A comparison of the in vivo and in vitro antibacterial properties of povidone iodine and chlorhexidine gluconate mouthrinses. J. clin. Periodontol. 5: 198-205 (1978).

5. ADRIAENS, P.A.; LOESCHE, W.J. and DE BOEVER, J.A.: Bacterioloical study of the microbial flora invading the radicular dentine of periodontal diseased caries free human teeth; LEHNER and CIMANSONI, The borderland between caries and periodontal disease III; pp. 383-390 (Editions Medecine et Hygiene, Geneve 1986).

6. ALTMAN, E.G.: Rational use of metronidazole. Australian dent. J. 25: 135-138 (1980).

7. BAKER, P.J.; COBURN, R.A.; GENCO, R.J. and EVAN, R.T.: Structural determinants of activity of chlorhexidine and alkyl bisbiguanides against human oral flora. J. dent Res. 66: 1099-1106 (1987).

8. BURKE, A.C.; COMER, J.B. and JUMAS, M.: The tetracylines. Med. clin. North America. 66: 293-302 (1982).

9. FLOTRA, L.; GJERMO, P.; ROLLA, G. and WAERHAUG, J.: A 4-month study on the effects of chlorhexidine mouthwashes on 50 soldiers. Scand. J. dent Res. 80: 10-17 (1972).

10. GARROD, L.P.; LAMBERT, H.P.; O'GRADY, F. and WATERWORTH, P.M.: Antibiotics and chemotherapy; 5th ed., pp. 150-157 (Churchill Livingstone, Edinburgh 1981).

11. GENCO, R.J.: Antibiotics in the treatment of human periodontal disease. J. Periodontol. 52: 545-558 (1981).

12. GOLD, S.J.: Periodontics. The past - part III Microbiology. J. clin. Periodontol. 12: 257-269 (1985).

13. GOLOMB, G.; FRIEDMAN, M.; SOSKOLME, A.; STABHOLTZ, A. and SELA, M.N.: Sustained release device containing metronidazole for periodontal use. J. dent. Res. 63: 1149-1153. (1984).

14. GOLUB, L.M.; WOLFF, M.; LEE, H.M.; McNAMARRA, T.F.; RAMAMURTHYN, S.; ZAMBON, J. and CIANCIO, S.: Further evidence that tetracyline inhibits collagenase activity in human crevicular fluid and from other mammalian sources. J. Periodontol. Res. 20: 12-23 (1985).

15. GOODSON, J.M.; HAFFAJEE, A. and SOCRANSKY, S.S. Periodontal therapy by local delivery tetracylines. J. clin. Periodontol. 6: 83-92 (1974).

16. GOODSON, J.M.; HOLBOROW, D.; DUNN, R.; HOGAN, P and DUNHAM, S.: Monolithic tetracyline containing fibres for control delivery to periodontal pockets. J. Periodontol. 54: 575-579 (1983).

17. GORDON, J.M.; WALKER, C.B.; MURPHY, C.J.; GOODSON, J.M. and SOCRANSKY, S.S.: Tetracyline: Levels achievable in gingival crevice fluid and _in vitro_ effect on subgingival organisms. J. Periodontol. _10:_ 609-612 (1981).
18. HASSAN, H.; ADDY, M.; MORAN, J. and WADE, W.: A comparison of the effects of metronidazole, tetracyline and chlorhexidine containing acrylic strips and root planing on chronic periodontal pockets. J. dent. Res. _64:_ Ast. 682 (1985).
19. HELDERMAN van PALESTEIN, W.H.: Is antibiotic therapy justified in the treatment of human chronic inflammatory periodontal disease? J. clin. Periodontol. _13:_ 932-938 (1986).
20. HELLDEN, L.B.; LISTGARTEN, M.A. and LINDHE, J.: The effect of tetracycline and/or scaling on human periodontal disease. J. clin. Periodontol. _6:_ 222-230 (1979).
21. KHOO, J.G.L. and NEWMAN, H.N.: Subgingival plaque control by a simplified oral hygiene regime plus local chlorhexidine or metronidazole. J. Periodontol. Res. _18:_ 607-619. (1983).
22. KORNMAN, K.S. and KARL, E.H.: The effect of long term low dose tetracyline therapy on subgingival microflora in refractory adult periodontitis. J. Periodontol. _53:_ 504-509. (1982).
23. LISTGARTEN, M.A.; LINDHE, J. and HELLDEN, L.: Effect of tetracyline and/or scaling on human periodontal disease. Clinical, microbiological and histological observations. J. clin. Periodontol. _5:_ 246-271 (1978).
24. LOESCHE, W.; SYED, S.A.; MORRISON, E.C.; KERRY, G.A.; HIGGINS, I. and STOLL, J.: Metronidazole in periodontitis results after 15 to 30 weeks. J. Periodontol. _55:_ 325-335 (1984).
25. LUNDSTROM, A.; JOHANSSON, L.A. and HAMP, S.V.: Effect of combined systemic antimicrobial therapy and mechanical plaque control in patients with recurrent periodontal disease. J. clin. Periodontol. _11:_ 321-330 (1984).
26. MANSON, J.D.: Periodontics; 5th ed., pp. 196-206 (Kimpton Medical, Edinburgh and London 1986).
27. NYMAN, S.; LINDHE, J. and ROSLING, B.: Periodontal surgery in plaque infected dentitions. J. clin. Periodontol. _4:_ 240-249. (1977).
28. PITCHER, G.R.; NEWMAN, H.N. and STRAHAN J.D.: Access to subgingival plaque by disclosing agents using mouthrinsing and direct irrigation. J. clin. Periodontol. _7:_ 300-308 (1980).
29. RATHBUN, W.E.; CRIGGER, M. and OLIVER, R.: The effect of chlorhexidine and oxytetracycline irrigation on the subgingival microbiota. J. dent. Res. _53:_ 271 (1974).
30. ROBERTS, W.R. and ADDY, M.: Comparison of the _in vivo_ and _in vitro_ antibacterial properties of antiseptic

mouthrinses containing chlorhexidine, alexidine, cetylpyridinium chloride and hexetidine. Relevance to mode of action. J. clin. Periodontol. 8: 295-310 (1981).

31. ROSLING, B.; NYMAN, S.; LINDHE, J. and JERN, B.: The healing potential of periodontal soft tissues following different techniques of periodontal surgery in plaque free dentitions. J. clin. Periodontol. 3: 233-250 (1976).

32. ROSLING, B.G.; SLOTS, J.; CHRISTERSSON, L.A.; GRONDAHL, H.G. and GENCO, R.J.: Topical antimicrobial therapy and diagnosis of subgingival bacteria in the management of inflammatory periodontal disease. J. clin. Periodontol. 13: 975-981 (1986).

33. SAGLIE, R.; NEWMAN, M.G.; CARRANZA, F.A. and PATTISON, G.L.: Bacterial invasion of gingiva in advanced periodontitits in humans. J. Periodontol. 53: 217-222 (1982).

34. SAXEN, L.; ASIKAINEN, S.; SANDHOLM, L. and KARL, K.: Treatment of juvenile periodontitis without antibiotics. A follow up study. J. clin. Periodontol. 13: 714-719. (1986).

35. SLOTS, J.: Bacterial specificity in adult periodontitis. A summary of recent work. J. clin. Periodontol. 13: 912-917 (1986).

36. SLOTS, J. and GENCO, R.J.: Black-pigmented Bacteroides species, Capnocytophaga species and Actinobacillus actinomycetemcomitans in human periodontal disease: Virulence factors in colonisation survival and tissue destruction. J. dent. Res. 63: 412-421.

37. SLOTS, J. AND ROSLING, B.G.: Suppression of the periodontopathic microflora in localised juvenile periodontitis by systemic tetracycline. J. clin. Periodontol. 10: 465-486 (1983).

38. STOCKLEY, I.H.: Drug interaction alert; 4th ed., (Boehringer Ingelheim, Bracknell, Berkshire, U.K. 1980).

39. TANNER, A.C.R.; SOCRANSKY, S.S. and GOODSON, J.M.: Microbiota of periodontal pockets losing crestal alveolar bone. J. Periodont. Res. 19: 279 (1984).

40. THEILADE, E.: The non-specific theory in microbial aetiology of inflammatory periodontal disease. J. clin. Periodontol. 13: 905-911.

41. WADE, W. and ADDY, M.: A comparison in vitro of niridazole, metronidazole and tetracycline on subgingival bacteria associated with chronic periodontal disease. J. appl. Bacteriol. (in press).

42. YEUNG, F.I.S.; NEWMAN, H.N. and ADDY, M.: Subgingival metronidazole in acrylic resin versus chlorhexidine irrigation in the control of chronic periodontitis, J. Periodontol. 54: 651-657 (1983).

43. ZAMBON, J.J.: Actinobacillus actinomycetemcomitans in human periodontal disease. J. clin. Periodontol. 12; 1-20 (1985).

Martin Addy, PhD, Department of Periodontology, Dental School, University of Wales College of Medicine, Heath Park, Cardiff, South Wales, CF4 4XY, (U.K.)

Summaries of Panel Discussions

Periodontology Today. Int. Congr., Zürich 1988, pp. 291 (Karger, Basel 1989)

Note by the Editor

The last chapter of this volume contains the summaries of the discussions held during the 'Periodontology today' conference and were written by the respective moderators of each session. The moderators were permitted unlimited freedom to accomplish this difficult task. The only conditions requested were a limitation in the space and the request not to produce a mere transcript of the discussion. Due to this degree of liberty, the differences between the approaches made were rather pronounced. The reader will notice that the lack of a uniform format adds to the flavour of this chapter. Those who are personally acquainted with the various authors will remark with amusement, how well the form and style of their contributions reflect the different characters of their personalities.

B. Guggenheim

Periodontology Today. Int. Congr., Zürich 1988, pp. 292–303 (Karger, Basel 1989)

Anatomy and Physiology of the Periodontium troughout Life:

Philias R. Garant

Dean School of Dental Medicine, State University of New York at Stony Brook, New York, N.Y., USA

Anatomy and Physiology of the Periodontium Throughout Life, the title given to the first session of this conference, encompasses a wide body of knowledge. One would need several conferences dedicated solely to these subjects to summarize our state of understanding of the normal structure and function of the periodontium at the molecular, cellular, and gross anatomical level.

During this conference it was only possible to take six quick snapshots of recent activities in the general area of anatomy and physiology. From the discussion, it was evident that some of these snapshots were more controversial than others.

Certainly, our knowledge of periodontal anatomy and physiology has been advanced over the past several decades, primarily as we applied new technologies to old unanswered questions. For example, electron microscopy has increased our understanding of the complexity of cementum (Schroeder, this conference) and organ and cell culture techniques have permitted us to approach questions of cell differentiation and control at a more sophisticated level than was heretofore possible (see Melcher and Mackenzie, this conference). This process is likely to continue as the molecular biology of connective tissues, mineralization, and epithelial cell function continue to expand.

A rapidly growing subdivision of cell biology which is likely to have implications for our understanding of the structure and function of the periodontium has to do with cell matrix interactions. As a greater number of cell membrane receptors for matrix molecules, cytokines, and hormones are identified on cells of the periodontium, greater insight to the control of cellular differentiation will result. The identification of new molecules derived from oral tissues which act on cells via cell surface receptors is a related area of great promise. The periodontium is composed of a varied population of cells which are in communication with each other via chemical messengers. Discovery of this language of communication is the key to understanding the normal growth and development of the periodontal tissues as well as the basis for predictable tissue regeneration. It would be a mistake to think that there is nothing more to do in relation to the anatomy and physiology of the periodontium. In contrast, we have a long distance yet to travel; however, it will be a fascinating journey full of surprises.

The Clinically Healthy Periodontium

Dr. Wennstrom began the session by defining the clinical characteristics of a healthy periodontium. In reviewing the biologic factors affecting the color and texture of the gingiva, he stressed that sometimes color and texture do not reflect an underlying inflammation and that bleeding on probing is an earlier and more sensitive indicator of inflammation. Probing depths exceeding 4 to 5 mm were stated to be incompatible with health.

Referring to recent studies of the low prevalence of periodontitis in the population and to longitudinal studies of patients with untreated periodontitis, he noted that the gingiva is an effective defense barrier against most bacterial plaques. He posed the following key question: "...recognizing the low figures for development of destructive periodontal disease in the studies referred to, the question is whether the mere presence of clinical signs of gingival inflammation should be regarded as incompatible with periodontal health." Despite the suggestion that the term disease be restricted to cases with evidence of connective tissue destruction, Dr. Wennstrom stated that when it came to treatment, his goal was to eliminate all clinical signs of inflammation. "We have evidence from a number of studies showing that if we eliminate the clinical signs of inflammation then we reduce the risk for further development of destruction." During the discussion, Dr. Lang presented results indicating that even after six months of rigorous oral hygiene measures leading to the elimination of all visible signs of inflammation, it was still possible to demonstrate an inflammatory cell infiltrate adjacent to the junctional epithelium. He noted that leukocytes amounted to twenty percent of the cells in the test area of this super-clean gingiva. Dr. Lang posed the question of whether we should call this condition gingivitis, for in his view it was consistent with health. Dr. Schroeder responded by suggesting that what Dr. Lang had demonstrated was what, in the older literature, was described as physiological inflammation. He noted the importance of distinguishing between resident inflammatory cells and cells going through the tissue such as neutrophils. The presence of some level of activity within the peripheral defense system of the gingiva does not necessarily mean that we have a diseased gingiva. Dr. Schroeder noted that Dr. Wennstrom's criteria of health were "very useful for considering health in rather young people." "But what do you make of clinical health of the periodontium in elderly people with a case history of periodontitis, with a case history of treatment...recession, of atrophy?" Dr. Wennstrom replied that in a patient with a past experience of periodontal disease, there should be "definitely an absence of bleeding, no clinical signs of inflammation at all." He alluded to recent studies which indicated that patients previously treated for periodontitis which did not show bleeding on probing in subsequent examinations had a much better chance of avoiding further breakdown.

Dr. Soeder raised the issue that the patient's habits could have an effect on the clinical signs of gingival disease, for example smoking could mask the visible signs of inflammation. Dr. Wennstrom agreed that smoking could increase the thickness of the keratin layer leading to decreased appearance of vascularity; however, he noted that there was doubt that smoking had a direct effect of lowering gingival blood flow.

Developmental Origins

Dr. Melcher provided a thorough and insightful review of the status of our knowledge of the development of the periodontium and the control of phenotypic expression of cell types in the adult periodontal tissues. Although we have made good progress (much of it carried out by Melcher and his colleagues in Toronto), there is a great deal of basic information waiting to be discovered. It is not just biologic trivia devoid of clinical significance that we are after, but new information which is essential to identifying techniques of predictable and controlled periodontal tissue regeneration. The answers will come from the application of cell biological, biochemical, and genetic approaches to deciphering how various cell types of the periodontium regulate their environment, including exerting control of the differentiation of other cell lines. Specific areas of deficiency noted by Dr. Melcher included a "lack of direct evidence...that cells of periodontal ligament from fully erupted teeth have the capacity for osteogenesis or cementogenesis..." He concluded that we had insufficient knowledge of the fate of paravascular precursor cells and how the domain separating bone and cementum is maintained. Results of recent autoradiographic cell kinetic studies and *in vitro* experiments conducted by Melcher suggest that *alveolar bone* marrow may be a significant contributor of cells to the periodontal ligament.

In observing that most marrow spaces were located in the deeper (apical) regions of the alveolus adjacent to the root segment covered by cellular cementum, Dr. Garant asked

Drs. Melcher and Schroeder to comment on the possible significance of this anatomical relationship. Dr. Melcher noted that in his kinetic study of the contribution of cells from alveolar bone to the periodontal ligament (McCulloch, et al., Anat. Rec., 219:233-242, 1987), a significant correlation was observed between the position of protuberances of cellular cementum on the root surface and the openings of vascular channels from adjacent alveolar bone marrow spaces. However, Dr. Melcher was quick to caution making any direct connection at this time between the migration of paravascular cells from bone marrow into the periodontal ligament and the development of cellular cementum. Dr. Schroeder agreed that the idea was an attractive one which was supported by the anatomy of both tissues, and by the fact that cellular cementum was exclusively located on the apical part of the root.

Dr. Mackenzie pointed out that during tooth development cementum forms on the root surface after the epithelial root sheath undergoes fenestration, suggesting an inductive influence coming from the tooth side which switches the phenotype of fibroblasts in the tooth follicle into cementoblasts. He asked Dr. Melcher to comment if, in the fully formed root, there might not be some chemoattractant influence which drew cementoblast precursor cells from the bone side to the tooth side of the ligament. In responding, Dr. Melcher noted that extracellular substrates played an important role in regulating the expression of phenotype in connective tissue cells. He further noted that the results of recent experiments suggested that cell-substrate interactions, including chemoattractant influences, appeared to be significant in periodontal tissue function. (The reader should also note comments by Dr. Page elsewhere in this summary.)

Dr. Garant previewed recent work completed with his colleague, Dr. Moon-Il Cho, indicating that, in the formation of the initial layer of acellular extrinsic fiber cementum in mouse molar teeth, perifollicular fibroblasts migrated to the dentin surface followed by their differentiation into a typical cementoblast phenotype. The surprising finding, however, was that the cementoblast phenotype with polarized secretion toward the root surface was maintained for only one day, after which the cementoblasts appeared to return to a fibroblastic phenotype (Cho and Garant, Anat. Rec., in press). Thus, part of our difficulty in discussing the origin of acellular extrinsic fiber cementum was our incomplete knowledge of the onset and duration of cementoblastic activity.

Adult Growth

Dr. Mazeland, in her presentation, was concerned with

reviewing the evidence for increase in gingival width and face height with age. She noted that Ainamo (J. Perio. Res., 16: 595-599, 1976) reported an increase in gingival width to age sixty, possibly associated with an increase in face height. In her own work (Mazeland, J. Perio. Res., 15:429-433, 345-352, 1980), she found a slight increase in gingival width in the upper incisors only, which was associated with an increase in the maxillary alveolar process. On the basis of these results, she concluded that "continuous eruption of teeth in human adults takes place and is accompanied by an increase in height of the gingiva and the alveolar process." However, in her concluding paragraphs she states "when methodological errors in clinical and cephalometric measurements are taken into account, the changes in the vertical dimensions of the lower face, associated with continuous tooth eruption, are almost impossible to quantify." Noting an absence of calibrated examiners and generally a lack of duplicate measurements in previous clinical studies of tooth eruption, Dr. Mazeland suggested that "there is still no conclusive evidence for continuous tooth eruption and simultaneous increase in height of the gingiva and the alveolar process in man." Concern with the methodological aspects of these clinical studies was carried over into the discussion.

Dr. Ainamo asked if Dr. Mazeland had measured clinical attached gingiva in her studies. In response, Dr. Mazeland stated that she had measured visible gingiva from the muco-gingival borderline to the gingival margin, because she wanted to measure the gingiva anatomically present. Dr. Ainamo noted that in her own work she had taken recession into account by making measurements from the muco-gingival borderline to the cemento-enamel junction. Discussion followed on the merit of using the cemento-enamel junction to muco-gingival borderline measurement as opposed to the margin of the visible attached gingiva because of the unknown variable of gingival recession and edema associated with gingivitis. It would appear that if one wishes to determine growth of the alveolar process and/or the degree of tooth eruption, one must use the cemento-enamel junction to muco-gingival borderline measurement. On the other hand, determination of increases in facial height must be based on other facial skeletal landmarks. Whether or not the width of the anatomical attached gingiva measured from the gingival margin to the muco-gingival borderline has a positive correlation with either an increase in face height or the height of the alveolar process seems to remain problematic.

Dr. Picton offered the following observation: "On a conceptual basis it seems to me that we should introduce the idea of eruption and extrusion. The concept that we have is that remove the occlusal foeces and the tooth immediately starts to extrude and goes on quietly doing so in a somewhat logarithmic manner...restore the occlusal forces and of course there is the tendency for the tooth to be returned towards its previous position. So, eruption we conceive as being as it were the sum total of the balance of the forces over many hours, weeks even, and so it seems to me perfectly reasonable to think that over many years there could be a progressive extrusion leading to eruption of the tooth from its previous position."

Tooth Support

Dr. Picton reviewed what is known about the contribution of collagen fibers and the intervening molecules of the ground substance in tooth support. He noted that, as the periodontium is viscoelastic, time is an important factor in the response to force. The rate of loading and the history of previous loading also affects the magnitude of displacement. Although Dr. Picton noted that "unequivocal evidence on the mechanisms of tooth support is in short supply since, like eruption, most findings are subject to several interpretations --" he stated that the orientation of the periodontal ligament fibers appeared designed to resist force from any direction and that "tension is the mechanism which seems to have most structural evidence in its favor." He pointed out that indirect support for the tension hypothesis came from studies of lathyrogens which reduced the tensile strength of collagen molecules and increased the extrusive mobility of teeth. Alternative views of tooth support suggest that the extracellular matrix forms a compressive mattress. Picton noted that some experimental observations pointed to a simultaneous generation of tension and compression in the periodontal ligament. He concluded that "it is apparent that collagen may act as a three-dimensional tensional net but may also resist displacement of the tooth as a compressive mat."

Dr. Melcher asked Dr. Picton to comment on proteoglycans and their water-binding capacity as a factor in tooth support. Dr. Picton explained that, from an experimental point of view, if a tooth is isolated from any force acting on it for several hours, it extrudes and becomes progressively less mobile. If one analyzes the periodontal ligament of that tooth for proteoglycans and compares it with that from a normal tooth at time zero, one observes a marked increase in the size of the proteoglycans. Dr. Picton noted that the suggestion he wished to make from that data was "that the increase in size of the molecules might attract water to loose association with the molecule... Try though I have to think of changes in the collagen, crimping, angle, increase in blood volume, whatever it might be, I could think of no way of explaining the facts other than changes in the ground substance and it happens to fit with the changes which certainly occur. But I have not said the other way around so that the return of the loading in fact breaks down the molecular size. Though we have tried to do this by taking samples of the ligament at the end of the loading sequence... and several days later again collect the ligament. The results are by no means clear and straightforward."

Biology of Cementum

For many years, the biology of cementum has been overshadowed by interest in the development of the periodontal ligament and the biology of bone, dentin, and enamel. However, the recent publication of Hubert Schroeder's monograph and his presentation at this conference has generated a new level of interest in cementum which is likely to persist for some time.

Several conclusions presented by Schroeder challenge existing concepts and/or point to new opportunities for research. Chief among these was his proposal that acellular extrinsic fiber cementum was a product of periodontal ligament fibroblasts, and that "Acellular extrinsic fiber cementum is nothing more than calcified periodontal ligament fibers attached to the root surface." "All fibers are fibroblast products while the contribution of cementoblasts to acellular extrinsic fiber cementum is in doubt."

Cellular intrinsic fiber cementum is a purely cementoblast product while cellular mixed stratified cementum is a mixture consisting of layers of pure cellular intrinsic fiber cementum and acellular extrinsic fiber cementum. Resting lines seen in H+E light micrographs may at least in part be thin layers of acellular extrinsic fiber cementum.

A major part of Schroeder's paper was devoted to the demonstration that a positive correlation exists between the length of acellular extrinsic fiber cementum in single-rooted teeth and tooth survival during long-term treatment. Measurement of the average axial length of acellular extrinsic fiber cementum-covered root surfaces measured from the cemento-enamel junction to the level of the cellular mixed stratified cementum was made in a sample of forty-eight human teeth and correlated with the observed pattern of tooth loss during long-term treatment as reported by Hirschfeld and Wasserman (J. Periodontol., 49:225-237, 1978) and McFall (J. Periodontol., 53:539-549, 1982). Lateral incisors and canines, having a higher rate of acellular extrinsic fiber cementum to cellular mixed stratified cementum than central incisors and first premolars, showed greater survival times. It was suggested that the hardness and greater resistance of acellular extrinsic fiber cementum to root planing was a possible factor in the long-term prognosis of individual teeth subjected to long-term treatment. One other factor bearing consideration would be that acellular extrinsic fiber cementum is the attachment type of cementum.

Dr. Melcher questioned whether our concept that a periodontal ligament fibroblast can only do certain things (like make fibers) was still valid. "It was only fifteen years ago that we realized that they could phagocytize as well as make fibers. Perhaps like bone cells the periodontal ligament fibroblast can express different phenotypes which are regulated by different and yet-to-be discovered mechanisms. Thus, it may be possible that periodontal ligament fibroblasts make the extrinsic fiber and then regulate its mineralization."

Dr. Schroeder stressed the fact that extrinsic fibers were strictly parallel to each other and vertical to the tooth surface and in the other case (the intrinsic fibers) they were all parallel to the root surface. This suggested to him that "you have two different kinds of cells producing these fibers; however, both cells are structurally very similar and unless you catch the cementoblast trapped in its matrix (as a cementocyte) it is often difficult to identify features which distinguish it from a fibroblast."

Dr. Mackenzie cautioned the panel from becoming confused over semantics. "A fibroblast makes fibers and cementoblast makes cementum. Thus, the cell that makes acellular extrinsic fiber cementum, even though it structurally resembles a fibroblast, should be referred to as a cementoblast. We don't know enough about their biochemical properties to define them more precisely. We need to know more about their lineage. We need to know more about the plasticity of these cells. Experimental embryology has shown that there is nothing very much about the nucleus that is permanently shut off, and so in biological theory if we know enough about the mechanisms of control, any cell could potentially be switched into any other cell. During the development the phenotype of root sheath fibroblasts is switched to that of cementoblasts under an inducting influence from the tooth side at about the same time that the epithelial root sheath fenestrates."

Dr. Schroeder stressed that we should no longer speak of cementum as a single simplistic entity. "There are different types of cementum serving different purposes. Furthermore, they are different in origin and structure, there is a bone-like cementum (cellular intrinsic fiber cementum) and a ligament-type of cementum (acellular extrinsic fiber cementum) in which the only difference (morphologically) between it and periodontal ligament is that the collagen fibers are mineralized."

Dr. Page commented that for some time he and his colleagues have been convinced that root surfaces are important in what happens around them and that cementum may contain signals that may be sent to neighboring cells. He reported that he and his colleagues have prepared extracts from human cementum which have a potent mitogenic activity for fibroblast of gingival origin. These extracts also contain chemoattractant and attachment factors for fibroblasts which are potent down to one or two micrograms per milliliter concentrations. The remaining question which they have yet to answer is can these factors cause fibroblasts to differentiate into cells that make cementum. In response to questions, Dr. Page pointed out that these factors could not be isolated from bone. He further stated that, in view of Dr. Schroeder's results, it was important to see if these products were present in acellular extrinsic fiber cementum or cellular mixed stratified cementum, or both.

Dr. Mackenzie asked if any further progress had been made in Dr. Page's laboratory in identifying different fibroblast phenotypes, for in his opinion different fibroblasts might send different signals to the overlying epithelium. In response, Dr. Page reported that the C1Q-binding fibroblasts that he described some years ago appear to also have receptors for C3 which activate the cells. Thus, this fibroblast's phenotype may be activated during the inflammatory process. However, no other fibroblast phenotypes have been discovered.

Dr. Listgarten asked Dr. Schroeder to clarify how cementum was attached to dentin. In his reply, Dr. Schroeder referred to the work of Owens (Archs. Oral Biol., 18:889-897, 1973) which demonstrated the presence of a layer of unmineralized predentin on the root surface (between the surface and the layer of Tomes) which came into direct contact with newly deposited cementum matrix. Schroeder explained "the formation of a cementum matrix on top of a not yet mineralized dentin matrix and the mineralization of both simultaneously achieved the attachment." Dr. Listgarten stated that there was morphological evidence that collagen fibers could form perpendicular to mineralized dentin and eventually become mineralized and attached, thus he questioned the necessity of postulating that it was necessary to have an uncalcified surface prior to cementogenesis. Listgarten further cautioned about postulating that dentin had an inducing effect on cementoblasts, noting that there is probably "a functional aspect to cementogenesis which we don't understand."

Robert Frank pointed out that cells control the mineralization of extrinsic fibers and this may be a cementoblast function. Thus, even if the fibers are of periodontal ligament fibroblast origin, there is still a mineralization process that must be controlled.

Dr. Beerston commented on whether cementoblasts were needed for mineralization of the periodontal ligament. He described an experiment whereby previously frozen periodontal ligament became mineralized within two days, with a thick layer of new mineral deposited over the old layer of acellular extrinsic fiber cementum. This mineralization was formed in the absence of cells. Thus, Beertsen raised the hypothesis that mineralization is inhibited normally by periodontal ligament cells and that there is an intrinsic capacity in the periodontium to add mineral on top of the root surface.

Dr. Melcher observed that his studies had shown that periodontal ligament cells depress osteogenesis which could be viewed as consistent with inhibiting mineralization and somehow related to preserving periodontal ligament space from colonization by osteoblasts.

Stability of Gingival Epithelium

Dr. Ian Mackenzie reported the use of fluorescein labeled antibodies to a variety of keratins as a means of identifying different epithelial phenotypes in gingiva. Human oral gingival and oral sulcular epithelia express markers of stratifying epithelia and, in addition, oral gingival epithelium expresses the same keratins as palate and oral sulcular epithelium shares similar keratins as other lining epithelia. Junctional epithelium contains stratifying markers and keratin 19, a characteristic of simple epithelia, but is devoid of typical differentiation markers. Differences in keratins between basal and suprabasal cells in junctional epithelium suggest an unusual pattern of terminal differentiation in the junctional epithelium. Mackenzie also observed the expression of both simple and stratifying keratin markers in the outgrowths of epithelium from full thickness mucosal transplants. These epithelial outgrowths resembled junctional epithelium in that they failed to invade deep connective tissue, had a limited proliferative capacity, formed a basal lamina, and stratified without the normal pattern of terminal differentiation. Mackenzie suggested that the phenotypic similarities between junctional epithelium and outgrowths from mucosal epithelia onto deep connective tissue resulted from the non-permissiveness of the connective tissue. The cornerstone of Mackenzie's hypothesis lies in the production of instructive messages in lamina propria connective tissue which have a permissive effect on epithelial growth and differentiation. Thus, it is the absence of permissive factors in the periodontal ligament deep connective tissue which stabilizes the junctional epithelium, preventing its downgrowth along the root surface. It was further suggested that infiltration of the periodontal ligament by inflammatory cells changes the nature of the connective tissue, leading to the appearance of permissive factors which can lead to proliferation and growth of the junctional epithelium along the root surface during periodontal disease. Dr. Mackenzie noted that, although the molecular basis of epithelial-mesenchymal interactions had not yet been elucidated, the recent success in identifying the role of cytokines and growth factors in cell proliferation and differentiation led him to believe that it would be possible to discover the nature of the factors present in inflamed connective tissue which trigger the migration of the junctional epithelium.

Dr. Garant noted that Sharpey's fibers of the acellular extrinsic fiber cementum presented a barrier to epithelial migration and that perhaps it was their presence which set the apical limit of the junctional epithelium. Dr. Mackenzie responded that because of the results of his experiments it was not necessary to postulate the need for a barrier. In his view, it was an intrinsic property of junctional epithelium to be non-migratory; i.e., the "establishment of epithelium on a deep connective tissue automatically gives it this unusual, non-migratory phenotype." He further noted that there was plenty of evidence to support the idea that when epithelial cells are activated to migrate, they can go anywhere they please. For example, malignant epithelial cells can migrate through very dense connective tissue and in development epithelia wander a long way during budding to make glands. "We know from the work of Birkedal-Hansen that epithelia can produce collagenase and other proteolytic enzymes. So when epithelia are exposed to factors which are permissive it is clear that they can move through connective tissue barriers."

Several participants noted that inflammatory cells were always present near the sulcular and junctional epithelium. When asked if this was the case, why was it that permissive factors were not always produced, Dr. Mackenzie suggested that switching on epithelial downgrowth was a rare event. "Biology in its development is opportunistic. It takes what it can, what exists and moves it around to make what it wants to make. I think if the situation were that any old information at any old time produced the growth factor necessary for epithelial migration, then it wouldn't have used that method of stabilizing epithelium because it wouldn't work. My feeling is that it's a very rare set of circumstances that produce the permissive change required for that epithelium to grow down." Mackenzie noted that the non-migrating edge of an implant system was an acceptable model for looking at inflammation for the presence of permissive factors. Delayed hypersensitivity produced some outgrowth, but most of the time inflammation was insufficient. Mackenzie stated "that is my primary interest at the moment... to find out what it is that switches that epithelium on because I think that is essential to our understanding of why periodontal downgrowth occurs."

In responding to a question from Dr. P. Gjermo on whether bacterial products had any effect on epithelial downgrowth, Dr. Mackenzie observed that his model system was a mouse model and thus he had difficulty in deciding which bacteria were appropriate to test because, "we are not sure whether the human data [microbiological] is applicable to the mouse." He also noted that he did not know "of any bacterial products which have a direct stimulatory effect on the epithelium."

However, he expected that there might be some that would cause a depressant effect. Dr. Mackenzie reported that numerous recent studies indicated that epidermal cells had cell surface receptors for interleukins 1-7 (except 2), and that future research would lead to understanding how these substances effect epithelial metabolism. Dr. P. Baehni described that he had isolated bacterial products from cultures of *Bacteroides intermedius* and *B. gingivalis* which inhibited the *in vitro* growth of squamous carcinoma cells of human origin.

Philias R. Garant, Dean School of Dental Medicine,
Rockland Hall, State University of New York at Stony Brook
Stony Brook, New York 11794-8700, USA

Periodontology Today. Int. Congr., Zürich 1988, pp. 304–312 (Karger, Basel 1989)

Epidemiology of Periodontal Diseases

Firoze Manji

Kenya Medical Research Institute, Nairobi, Kenya

It was 22 years ago that the World Workshop in Periodontics was held in Ann Arbor, Michigan. As with the present conference, that workshop was held with the explicit intent of making a "scientific appraisal of current knowledge in the field" (RAMFJORD, KERR & ASH, 1966). Whereas at that meeting considerable confidence seemed to be expressed about the nature of the disease process, about the inevitability of the breakdown of the periodontal tissues in the absence of adequate oral hygiene, and about many of the determinants of the diseases, such confidence was notably absent in the presentations and discussions in this session. There is no doubt that at present we are in a period in which notions about periodontal diseases are in a state of flux, and the process of the recomposition of ideas, begun some 10 years ago, has yet to be completed. This may account for the divergences of opinion, ambiguities and sometimes lack of clarity over a number of issues discussed here, and may reflect that, despite the demise of many of the formerly accepted concepts about the epidemiology of periodontal diseases, we still have inadequate information about what constitutes the natural history of periodontal disease.

As well as reviewing those studies which have contributed to a re-evaluation of our understanding of the natural history of the periodontal diseases, the papers in this session reviewed the problems of defining the disease, of measuring the disease in epidemiological studies, of analyzing periodontal disease data (and thus of drawing valid conclusions from such data), and of using epidemiological data assessing treatment needs in populations. The following summary highlights some of the principle themes addressed during the session. In so doing, it may perhaps be useful to begin by summarizing those aspects of the epidemiology of periodontal diseases about which there appeared to have been a general consensus and which provide some measure of the extent to which concepts about periodontal diseases have changed over the last two decades.

Aspects of current concepts

A considerable amount of clinical, epidemiological and basic science research over the last decade has provided evidence which has forced us to re-evaluate previous concepts about the nature of periodontal diseases, what its features are, how it is distributed within the population, and which parameters are implicated in pathogenesis. It is generally accepted that the breakdown of periodontal tissues (as reflected clinically in the apical migration of the junctional epithelium and accompanying loss of bony support) is the outcome of complex interactions between plaque micro-organisms, host tissues, and the host's defence mechanism. Although a number of micro-organisms have been identified which have potentially pathogenic characteristics, their exact role (individually or in combination with other micro-organisms) in the initiation and progression of periodontal destruction is as yet unclear. Cross-sectional studies from a number of different countries have demonstrated, however, that a relatively small proportion of individuals in any given age cohort experiences severe periodontal destruction, the proportion so affected increasing with age. This is apparently as true for populations in industrialized countries as for many rural populations of the third world who exhibit considerable plaque and calculus accumulation, poor oral hygiene, and have minimal access to dental care. The association between age and periodontal breakdown observed in cross-sectional studies probably reflects the results of long-term plaque accumulation and an exhaustion of the tolerance of aging tissues. There appears to be considerable evidence that periodontal breakdown at a given site, or in a given individual, does not progress in a linear fashion, and evidence from clinical studies suggests that at many sites its progression may be characterized by periods of bursts and remissions; at present, however, we are not able to predict which sites are likely to undergo such bursts of activity or when remissions are likely to occur. The concept that all individuals are equally susceptible to periodontal disease, and that periodontal breakdown and loss of bony support are, in all individuals and at all sites, the inevitable consequences of plaque accumulation, is no longer tenable. Contrary to what was generally accepted a decade ago, there is considerable evidence today to demonstrate that periodontal disease is not the major cause of tooth loss in adults: this appears to be as true for populations in industrialized as for those in many third world countries.

What is periodontal disease?

In recent epidemiological studies the clinical features of the periodontium which have been taken as indicators of an experience of chronic disease have included inflammation of the marginal gingivae, level (or loss) of attachment of the junctional epithelium, and the depth of the periodontal pocket. (Parameters such as the extent and location of plaque and calculus are also sometimes measured, although principally as potential determinants of the disease rather than as a description of the diseased tissue itself). In any one individual, a number of these features may be present at different sites either singly or in combination, and to varying extent. In the discussions here, there appeared to be divergent views as to whether these features are clinical manifestations of a single disease entity or process, or of several different processes.

Dr Burt drew attention to the fact that since most gingivitis does not necessarily progress to breakdown of the periodontal tissues, we cannot be certain whether preventing gingivitis is a sufficient condition for preventing periodontal breakdown. Gingivitis and periodontitis have, he suggested, "separate though not unrelated bacterial etiologies". It was left unresolved, however, to what extent these signs of periodontal diseases may reflect distinct disease entities; to what extent the response of the gingivae to irritation in or around the margins reflect the processes which may be occurring deeper in the pocket; and to what extent inflammatory changes of the marginal tissues should be considered a "disease" as such, or merely an indicator of the activities of a healthy defence mechanism.

Dr Listgarten proposed that three criteria need to be concurrently present for a positive diagnosis of periodontitis: alveolar bone loss, increased probing depth and gingivitis (a definition reminiscent of that proposed in "Score 6" of Russell's PI (RUSSELL, 1956)). "In a situation where you only have gingivitis and alveolar bone loss, you don't have periodontitis," he insisted, "because you don't have pockets present." The central problem posed by such a definition, as pointed out by Dr Cutress and others, is that in many populations throughout the world - especially in those exhibiting poor oral hygiene and for whom there is minimal access to dental care - the major characteristic of periodontal breakdown is that of loss of attachment _without_ concurrent pocket formation. There is no doubt that in such cases there has been loss of bony support. Both Dr Listgarten and Dr Ainamo considered that such recession of the gingival margin should not be included in the definition of periodontitis in view of the fact that it may be caused, for example, by excessive brushing habits. Although perhaps true for populations in the industrialized world, it was suggested that this view ignores the fact that those populations manifesting recession as a major feature of periodontal disease _also_ manifest poor oral hygiene with considerable plaque and calculus accumulation around the marginal gingivae - indicative that trauma from brushing is unlikely to be an aetiological factor. Dr Cutress suggested that recession might perhaps be considered as being a form of "natural gingivectomy", while Dr Listgarten characterized such features as being primarily "gingivitis". The latter definition, Dr Marthaler suggested, was in conflict with the classic definition of gingivitis as being an inflammation confined to the marginal tissues, whereas periodontitis necessarily involved loss of bony support. Some suggested that recession may be taken an indicator of past disease activity whereas the presence of pockets might be considered as indicative of present disease. However, there does not yet seem to be evidence to indicate that a site with pocket formation is more likely to breakdown further than one without, and thus there are no grounds for postulating that the presence of pockets (with or without gingivitis) is an indicator of an "active" site. The view that the presence of a pocket constitutes a more serious pathological entity than gingival recession may perhaps reflect, it was suggested, an assumption that the one is amenable to "treatment", while the other is not. Dr Burt pointed out that increasingly the results of many clinical and epidemiological studies raised serious questions about how periodontal diseases ought to be treated, and at present we do not have sufficient information to do more than speculate on such issues. The difficulties about what constitutes the definition of periodontal diseases are, Dr Gjermo suggested, that in epidemiological studies we are usually measuring disease status, whereas the disease ought to be considered as a process.

Treatment needs and the need for treatment

The need for a definition of disease based on an assessment of the need for clinical intervention has been the underlying theme in the development of the CPITN, and was a subject addressed by both Dr Ainamo and Dr Cutress in their papers. Dr Cutress endeavoured to resolve the conflict faced by public health workers arising from on the one hand from current questioning of what might be considered as constituting effective periodontal therapy, and, on the other, of providing meaningful proposals for public health programmes. Dr Gjermo raised doubts whether there can be an objective definition of "need". Furthermore, the assumptions underlying the treatment categories of the CPITN could be taken as meaning that everyone should go to the grave with a perfect plaque-free periodontium, an assumption which, even if desirable, would in most societies be impractical from the point of view of the resources required. Dr Lang pointed out that the CPITN had a number of limitations in the parameters it measured, and provided little clarity as to what specific conditions were existing at any particular site. He pointed out that the CPITN was still rooted in the view that periodontal disease inevitably progressed in a linear fashion from gingival inflammation to pocket formation. Furthermore, it may be misleading to assume that the existence of any given condition necessarily requires the form of treatment proposed by the index. Dr Listgarten indicated that there is sufficient evidence to show that calculus does not have a major role in the pathogenesis of the disease, and thus to insist that calculus must be removed to achieve improvement of periodontal status may be misleading. Dr Cutress responded that assessment of population treatment needs provided a means for appraising what may be required, without presupposing what necessarily ought, in a given context, be done. Dr Ainamo's suggested that although there may be reasons to question the extent to which parameters such as calculus or gingival bleeding might be involved in the disease process, it was nevertheless the case that many patients considered it unsightly and unpleasant to have "smelly" mouths with much calculus. In that sense, they need to have some treatment. Thus the CPITN does in fact provide an assessment of treatment needs. It was pointed out, however, that such treatments were being provided primarily for subjective reasons, and as such the "need" for such treatment was entirely socially determined. In many rural populations, considerable calculus and plaque accumulation is common, and this is not necessarily viewed as unsightly. This does not, however, reflect that the amount of periodontal breakdown is any greater as a result, nor does it indicate that treatment would necessarily result in any alteration in the amount of periodontal breakdown in these populations.

Problems of Measurement

Although there were differences of opinion on a number of issues amongst the panelists, there was unanimity about the fact that we lack precision in the measurements that we make in epidemiological studies, especially measurements of loss of attachment. There are considerable difficulties in overcoming the problems posed by the relatively large size of measurement error when endeavouring to make an assessment of changes in attachment levels in longitudinal clinical and epidemiological studies. In part this may be due to the fact that at most sites (and in most individuals) the disease progresses rather slowly, and the actual changes in attachment levels tend to be rather small - especially when assessed in studies which are conducted over a relatively short periods of time. Although there may be a number of ways of reducing the effects of measurement error, including performing repeated measurements, there appears to be little room for improvement of current techniques of measurement. As Dr Burt expressed it, "periodontal measurement is rather like bicycling, where the rider is a far bigger performance variable than any aspect of the bike being ridden...(if) the rider is not very good, expensive refinements of the bike and its components will add only slight improvements to the bicycle's performance." While we may look forward to the days to come when sophisticated biological tests might be employed in the diagnosis of periodontal diseases, the availability of such tests may as yet be a long way away, especially, as Dr Page pointed out, in view of the present lack of clarity as to how we should define the disease. Dr Gjermo's paper emphasized that if it is accepted that periodontal disease is a process, then the difficulty faced is that the process itself is unobservable. This does not necessarily imply that the process is therefore unmeasurable, but that we may have to identify parameters which are indicators of the process. What such parameters might be remains, however, to be identified and Dr Gjermo, like many others, pinned his hopes on the development of potential biological markers.

There is no doubt that detailed recordings of periodontal parameters at four sites per tooth in every individual can be an arduous task. The necessity for so doing is, however, very much dependent upon the nature and purpose of the study. Partial mouth recordings may be useful for prevalence studies in which the purpose is to obtain estimates of disease levels in a population. Mr Sterne suggested that even taking four sites per tooth is still only a sample of all potential sites, and partial mouth recordings may be adequate for most studies provided it is accepted that some underestimation of the disease may occur as a result. Dr Listgarten suggested that since it is apparent that there are differences in the susceptibility of the different tooth-types in the same mouth, and differences in features of periodontal disease in different sites in the mouth, care may be needed in endeavouring to classify individuals by any one particular category; until much more is known about the nature and distribution of the diseases in different patients, we may need to look at as much data as we can from different sites of different tooth types. Dr Ainamo pointed out, moreover, that since periodontal disease is site specific, partial examinations may not be the best choice if one needs to know about the distribution of the individuals in a population with disease at one or more sites within the dentition.

Analysis and interpretation of epidemiological data

There is a widely held, though mistaken, view that epidemiology constitutes only the performing of surveys and presentation of purely descriptive results. Although such use of epidemiology is common, Dr Burt pointed out that, in addition, epidemiological research seeks to define determinants and risk factors, and ultimately to test hypotheses about the ethological factors in disease processes. Dr Listgarten's presentation set out to demonstrate that epidemiological data have no diagnostic value. In so doing he elegantly demonstrated that one of the central weaknesses of many epidemiological studies is the absence of adequate hypothesis testing, the result of which is that frequently erroneous conclusions about the aetiology and pathogenesis of diseases are produced. His conclusion that, because of such weaknesses, epidemiology cannot be of value beyond merely generating data was perhaps throwing the baby out with the bath water, especially since in proposing the use of diagnostic tests he recommended a basic tool frequently employed in the analysis of epidemiological data. Dr Listgarten pointed out a further weakness in many epidemiological studies: data presented in the form of averages provide little information about the distribution of the disease within a population, and this way of handling data often handicaps a clear understanding of the nature and extent to which various parameters are associated with disease. Such methods of presentation and analysis of data, he indicated, often did not adequately reveal the variations in response between individuals, and were unhelpful in assisting us to identify susceptible groups of individuals within a population. Dr Burt pointed out, however, that "there is nothing in the definition of epidemiology which says that data must be expressed in aggregate terms ... aggregated data is a method of data presentation not a research strategy."

Dr Burt pointed out that clinical studies may be distinguished from epidemiological studies not by the way in which data are analyzed or presented, but by the nature of the study design and questions being addresed. Whereas clinical research chooses its subjects on the basis of particular clinical characteristics related to the disease in question, epidemiological research requires people "who do and do not have the characteristics under study so that the relationship between exposure and disease can be better delineated". The common ground between clinical and epidemiological research comes with clinical trials: although the selection of the groups to be studied in clinical trials are predetermined by the nature of the hypotheses being tested, clinical trails then proceed using epidemiological principles.

Considerable problems can be posed by the way in which data are collected and subsequently analyzed, and inappropriate handling of data have led, in the past, to many misconceptions about the nature of periodontal diseases and associated determinants. Several examples could be highlighted, of which one is the relationship between calculus and periodontal diseases which Dr Listgarten describes in his paper. Another important example relates to present concepts about trends in periodontal diseases. It is believed that the prevalence of periodontal diseases has declined in industrialized countries over the last two decades (WHO, 1984). Dr Burt suggested that in view of the fact that methods of measuring of and reporting on periodontal disease data have changed considerably over the last two decades, it is difficult to be certain about trends. Although it is possible that oral hygiene may have improved, there appears to be little data to suggest that loss of bony support is any less prevalent today than previously. Our knowledge of periodontal diseases in the past has been based predominantly on surveys in which the PI has been used, but that index was based on a scoring system in which assumptions were made about the continuum between gingivitis and periodontal breakdown, and about the weights to be assigned to the different features of periodontal disease. Dr Burt stressed that in looking back at PI data from the past it is difficult to understand what the data actually mean.

Relatively little attention has been given in the past to the question of how periodontal disease data ought to be statistically handled. Mr Sterne highlighted in his paper that it is unacceptable for statistical tests to be performed on data from many diseased sites which have been grouped together without regard to the subject effect, since such ways of handling data are based on the mistaken assumption that the progression of disease at different sites in the same individual are independent. He proposed that variance components modelling may be an appropriate method of performing regression-like analyses of data which have a hierarchical structure (e.g. sites being nested under individuals). The method nevertheless provides results based on estimating the average response of the dependent variable to variations in one or more explanatory variables. There were inadequate discussions during the session as to how appropriate the proposed model might be for identifying, for example, "susceptible" groups of individuals within a population in whom the relationship between various parameters might be distinctly different from the average. As with many statistical techniques that are related to multiple regression, the results need to be carefully assessed before reasonable conclusions can be drawn: where explanatory variables are highly correlated, or worse, where important variables correlated to variables in the equation are omitted, many non-existing relationships may appear significant, positively correlated associations may appear as negatively associated ones, or *vice versa*. There is clearly a need to develop appropriate statistical techniques for use in periodontal research which may assist us to obtain answers to a variety of research questions and hypotheses which need to be addressed by epidemiologists and clinicians alike. It is doubtful, however, whether statistical methods *per se* can generate theories of periodontal diseases where the basic biological mechanisms of cause and effect are still poorly understood. Statistical methods are useful for determining associations. Much more than that is required, however, in order to postulate and substantiate cause-and-effect relationships.

Conclusion

There is no doubt that in many important ways our understanding of the nature of periodontal diseases have changed considerably since the World Workshop in 1966. The concluding remarks of Jens Waerhaug in the epidemiology session of that meeting nevertheless form a fitting epilogue for this one:

> "Epidemiology has already furnished the periodontal profession with valuable information, but it is still a science in rapid development. Therefore, associations which are

obscure today, may be clarified in the near future. Likewise, any type of therapy should be tested and evaluated in clinical trials before being introduced for general use. Even the effect of accepted, widely used and time-honored therapeutic methods and means should be questioned and re-evaluated in clinical trials. By an intelligent use of epidemiology and clinical trials it should be possible in the near future to base periodontal therapy mainly on facts and only to a very limited degree on opinion." (WAERHAUG, 1966)

References

RAMFJORD, S.P., KERR, D.A., and ASH, M.M. (Eds): World workshop in periodontics; (University of Michigan, Michigan 1966).

RUSSELL, A.L. A system of classification and scoring for prevalence surveys of periodontal disease. J. Dent. Res. 35: 350-359 (1956).

WAERHAUG, J.: Epidemiology of periodontal disease - review of literature. In: RAMFJORD, S.P., KERR, D.A., and ASH, M.M. (Eds): World workshop in periodontics; pp 181-211 (University of Michigan, Michigan 1966).

W.H.O.: Prevention, methods and programmes for oral diseases: Technical report series 713; (World Health Organization 1984).

Address

Dr Firoze Manji, Kenya Medical Research Institute, Medical Research Centre, Oral Health Programme, PO Box 20752, Nairobi, Kenya.

Periodontology Today. Int. Congr., Zürich 1988, pp. 313–323 (Karger, Basel 1989)

Periodontal Microbiology Today: Discourse on a Discordant Discussion

Richard P. Ellen

Faculty of Dentistry, University of Toronto, Toronto, Canada

Where is periodontal microbiology today? The exponential growth of information about bacteria colonizing periodontally is an expected by-product of the exponential proliferation of microbiologists now engaged in periodontology. Has there been a concomitant exponential growth in thought or creativity? Perhaps. If so, the open discussion at the conference did not reflect the true breadth of creative activity current in this field. Although many topics were mentioned, both panelists and audience alike - as if they had been cloned - seemed almost unanimously drawn to what can be categorized as clinical microbiology: the enumeration of microorganisms as related to disease status and the application of such findings to clinical use. While of great importance and of utmost interest to the majority of participants, the dominance of clinical microbiology in the discussion drew attention away from other "cutting edge" research on microbial ecology, physiology, host-parasite interactions at the molecular level, and molecular biology. But maybe that's where periodontal microbiology is today! The following is an interpretive summary highlighting major issues of the microbiology discussion.

Jan Carlsson's "What is a periodontal pathogen?" and Ann Tanner's "Is the specific plaque hypothesis still tenable?" should really be considered together. They deal with similar issues but certainly from different vantage points. Dr. Carlsson invoked knowledge of virulence and host-parasite interactions; Dr. Tanner dealt almost exclusively with numerical associations. Dr. Carlsson's main theme was that all bacteria in a periodontal pocket have the capacity to excite the host's inflammatory defenses. As defenses are not uniquely targeted against a few specific bacteria, a wide variety of microorganisms may induce host-mediated destructive mechanisms. Therefore, the term "periodontal pathogen" as applied to only a short list of bacteria should be dropped in deference to "pathogenic microflora." His view would also encompass a scenario that causative bacteria for periodontal diseases are most often present. Yet Dr. Carlsson did leave room for specificity by recognizing that some organisms specifically perturb the defense strategies of the host, thereby accelerating tissue destruction, but he weakened the statement with a strong reminder that such a "pathogen" would never function in isolation.

Dr. Tanner's conclusion that the specific plaque hypothesis - the term coined many years ago by Walter Loesche - is still tenable was based on experimental findings and observations that periodontal disease is not universal; that temporal phases of destructive activity coincide with the presence and elevated levels of certain species while inactivity can be associated with counts of other microorganisms; and that bacteria do invade periodontal tissues. She pointed to two reasons explaining why doubt still lingers about specificity. First, some investigators still consider gingivitis and periodontitis together as one entity, periodontal disease, whereas gingivitis includes sites inflamed but currently inactive in a destructive sense. Secondly, recognized periodontal pathogens can be detected in inactive sites and even spread from active to inactive sites, establishing a carrier state. During the discussion, both of these arguments were invoked in opposition to Dr. Carlsson's views. Experimental designs to test any hypothesis recognizing specificity must trudge through a quagmire of measuring disease "progression," "activity," "exacerbation," "burst," or whatever it is termed. This very risk spiced the discussion with a taste of irony, making Ann's seemingly more plausible arguments less 'tannerble'. Jan Carlsson's concepts (and strategy?) cleverly avoided this problem by tip-toeing around considerations of how to test his hypotheses in a clinical setting.

Abridged quotations which paced the discussion [moderator's interpretations]:

Dr. J. Slots: The carrier state is the problem in trying to define which bacteria are the pathogens. Many bacteria carried for a lifetime may cause mild diseases under experimental conditions or be associated with gingivitis, but they may not contribute directly to periodontitis. Others, perhaps more virulent, also in a lifelong carrier state, may emerge in the microflora, due to a host problem or even a local absence of inhibitory microorganisms, and these may contribute significantly to destructive disease, periodontitis. Regarding Dr. Carlsson's address, Koch did not address carrier states, and that's why his postulates cannot confirm causes for periodontitis.

Dr. J. Carlsson: That's correct. But he defined the pathogen and aimed treatment at it directly, precisely because he could show that it produced the disease [which we may not be able to do so clearly in periodontal diseases]. I introduced new terminology because it may be misleading to label all [or many] bacteria inhabiting a pocket "pathogen". [In response to Dr. J. Ebersole]: I did not say periodontitis was "multifactorial". But consider that a combination of virulence factors from many bacteria may be equivalent in biological activity to several factors from one bacterium.

Dr. G. Dahlèn: How does one define "specificity?" When we recognize certain bacteria and know their names, we call that infection "specific." When we don't know their names, we call that infection "non-specific." Perhaps we should call these infections of "unknown specificity." Are infections like pneumonias "nonspecific" because they can be caused by several different microorganisms? Periodontal infections might just as well be called "mixed anaerobic infections." Should we reserve "specific" for single-microorganism infections?

Dr. R. Attström: Most of this and Dr. Tanner's discussion of specificity revolve around the issue of disease activity; yet we do not have sensitive methods to determine activity. We cannot measure small changes, and our methods consider progression only in an apical direction. Lateral spread cannot be measured currently.

Dr. B. Guggenheim: By addressing "periodontal pathogen" we are going over old ground. Surely, following Rosebury, we should recognize those bacteria which are carried regardless of health or disease status. He used the term "amphibiotic," a valid term which should be used today. Also, bacteria resident in health can cause opportunistic infections. We might also use this term for periodontal infections. The trigger is the host response which affects microbial ecology.

Taking the liberty to discuss what was not discussed, I would like to ask Dr. Carlsson and Dr. Tanner the following:

To Jan Carlsson:

1. No one questioned your "keyhole" metaphor for researchers' compulsion to study virulence factors in isolation and then to enthusiastically push one view of pathogenesis. Is the measure of an organism's virulence proportional to the time spent studying it? Have we created a *B. gingivalis* and *Aa* cult? Or are these

readily cultivated bacteria really more virulent than some of the yet-to-be-cultivated spirochetes?

2. Experimentally, how can one determine the true pathogenesis of polymicrobial infections in a way more clever than done to this point? Is there a master key to all the keyholes?

To Ann Tanner:

1. Isn't all periodontal therapy, even targeted at Aa in LJP, nonspecific? Is it not merely the repopulation after nonspecific therapy which is specific?

2. Does the spread of periodontal pathogens from progressing to nonprogressing sites demonstrate that there really is a degree of dependence among sites within an individual?

3. Considering site carrier states and intersite transmision, how would one select appropriate sites to treat with locally administered antimicrobials?

Perhaps semantic arguments over what to call disease-associated bacteria are healthy. They focus on the middle ground, that microbial virulence is only one factor contributing to the host-parasite formula, rather than on the more pedantic arguments which create a clean but rather artificial division between "good guy" and "bad guy" bacteria. "Commensal", "amphibiotic", "opportunistic" are all variations of a theme recognizing that, in a given environment, like the gingival crevice, an otherwise virulent microorganism may have little, if any, irreversible or destructive effect on the host. Likewise, relatively avirulent bacteria, which might contribute little to attachment loss, even during active bursts, likely contribute to the inflammatory reaction. There is also a contrasting view that some periodontal infections are exogenous. The circumstances affording opportunists their opportunity are often host-environment driven, as emphasized in statements above made by both Dr. Slots and Dr. Guggenheim. Whether exclusively endogenous or occasionally exogenous, virtually all periodontal infections occur in a mixed flora milieu. How does one confirm which microorganisms in the mix are the "opportunists" or those which perturb host defenses the most? How does one experimentally confirm the relative relevance of Dr. Carlsson's various artificially generated "keyholes" of natural pathogenesis? An obvious approach is to take advantage of animal models in which hypotheses can be tested.

Roy Page's "Are there convincing models for periodontal diseases?" outlined the advantages and disadvantages of various systems used in the past. The major point was that, whereas the basics of tissue defenses were rather similar on a cellular and molecular level, the actual responses encountered were not precisely analogous to that seen in humans. Several anatomical and physiological features, including animal size and tooth eruption patterns, accounted for some differences. Dr. Page concluded that, yes, there are convincing models for testing well-targeted hypotheses but, no, there are no valid models directly applicable to human disease. To test a given microrganism superimposed on a mixed periodontal flora, Dr. Page considered the *Macaca* ligature-induced periodontitis model convincing enough, regarding recent experiments with *B. gingivalis*, that "it leads one to believe there is at least one clearly demonstrable periodontal pathogen and likely many more."

The ligature model was scrutinized from different standpoints. Dr. S. Holt, whose group recently published on *B. gingivalis* in this model, warned of the ligature model's complexity. He was not convinced that *B. gingivalis* would induce destruction in a situation where other bacteria were in low number. Moreover, the San Antonio colony evidently has some animals which carry no *B. gingivalis* but which experience progressive disease around ligated teeth colonized by other recognized pathogens. Dr. Guggenheim compared the ligature model to a foreign body reaction and thought it would be better to seek a model where periodontal disease occurred spontaneously. Dr. T. van Dyke pointed to the self-limiting nature of ligature-induced disease and suggested that spontaneous disease occurring around non-ligated teeth in ligated animals might be a relevant model. This was reminiscent of microbiological investigations by Kiel and co-workers, who suggested that periodontal pathogens spread from ligated to non-ligated sites. As moderator, I raised the question of whether the need to generate information confirming the pathogenicity of specific bacteria in periodontitis justified the use of monkeys for the ligature model. Several points, both logistical and philosophical, were made about animal care. Time did not allow a conclusive debate on this issue; it was left open, with the expressed hope of some that it should be considered more broadly in a forum composed of both scientists and philosophers.

The discussion also touched on the validity of rodent models. Verbal jousting between Dr. Page and Dr. B. Guggenheim recognized that, while conventional rats are useful for some hypothesis testing, the cellular response resembles a neutrophil-rich acute infection not seen often in human disease. Dr. P. Garant reminded the panel of his published work using a rat infection model which yielded long-term chronic responses with a plasma cell infiltrate. While offering the opportunity to test concepts of pathogenicity *in vivo*, the overall tone of the discussion supported Dr. Page's contention that, although convincing, the animal models all had weaknesses casting doubt on their validity.

If given the opportunity to question Dr. Page further, I would have raised these issues:

1. Is implantability of suspect pathogens still a great enough problem to invalidate rodent models? How does one implant and control an appropriate periodontal mixture?

2. You stated that a major problem is inadequate characterization of any animal diseases, even the oft-studied dog. What additional information is needed to use this model more intelligently?

3. Is the human the best animal model to study periodontal disease? How might this model be improved?

A natural progression from considering microbial specificity would be to debate the potential application of microbiology to monitoring and/or predicting disease activity. Jørgen Slots's "Does the analysis of the subgingival flora have value in predicting periodontal breakdown?" dealt with diagnostic efficiency of such tests and pointed to the effect of measurement error on the clinical side. Gunnar Dahlèn's "Sources of variations in the evaluation of the subgingival microbiota" dealt with sources of errors introduced by performing the microbiology.

Baye's Theorem, used by Dr. Slots to predict low probabilities for success of microbiology predictive tests, is nothing more or less than a mathematical modeling system in which concepts of predicting disease progression can be tested. The outcome depends on the values and validity of clinical measurements applied in the formula, as Dr. Slots did with data for prior probabilities taken from clinical studies by Dr. Listgarten. His major point was that progression of periodontitis occurs at too low an incidence for even a hypothetical supertest of very high nosologic specificity and sensitivity to be diagnostically accurate. It follows that the diagnostic efficiency would be raised by an increase in incidence as seen in high risk groups, like siblings of LJP patients. Clearly, the accuracy of measuring and analyzing disease activity would have an overriding impact on any predictive test. As mentioned over and over again, but perhaps most pointedly stated by Dr. T. van Dyke, "A 3-mm limit is not a very accurate measure of disease change."

Even if the clinical measurement problems could be sorted out, Dr. Dahlèn's address cast doubt on the accuracy of microbiology, especially in longitudinal monitoring, which might be applied in a clinical situation. He stressed that the principal source of error was reproducibility in obtaining an accurate and representative sample. From his address and a review published by Dr. Tanner (2), it is evident that little progress has been made to standardize sampling among various laboratories. On questioning, Dr. Dahlèn admitted there has been little published research directly comparing sampling methods.

Why do we need a test? What would we do with it if we had it? Why be so concerned to find a predictive test if we don't know what the etiologic agents are? These are the questions which were raised and in discussing these issues, the emphasis shifted away from activity prediction to the use of tests in general, in monitoring therapy for example:

Dr. J. Slots: When faced with a problem patient who is breaking down, a clinician wanting to use microbiology to help control the disease should be able to do so, even if our knowledge is not complete. That is why we established a testing center. Through this service, we can sample, determine the bacteria which are present and whether the microbiota contains a species we would rather get rid of, and determine the best way to suppress it. The clinical situation and the clinician identify a high-risk patient; then we sample. With present state of knowledge, we don't apply tests to predict or to screen all individuals. That would not be meaningful.

On questioning about a specific clinical situation, that of asymptomatic siblings of LJP patients, Dr. Slots stated that, as risk for future breakdown is 50%, a positive isolation of Aa in such siblings justifies therapeutic intervention aimed at eliminating Aa.

Even if predictive efficiency is not great, microbiologically oriented clinicians evidently still see efficacy in microbiological monitoring of selected patients. The discussion shifted to considerations of the microbiological methods used for laboratory identification and whether to monitor individually targeted or clusters of key species. Most of the debate focused on the comparative advantages of cultivation methods and oligonucleotide probes. Probes were favored because they can be synthesized to be ultraspecific and do not have to be limited to readily cultivable organisms. Multiple samples could be shipped without regard to viability, and be analyzed in one batch. Dr. Page and Dr. Tanner both supported testing of composite reagents consisting of two to several probes; Dr. Page gave examples of how combining probes raised the diagnostic specificity and selectivity to values approaching 1.0. Both Dr. Slots and Dr. U. Goebel supported the use of DNA probes in epidemiology research but adamantly questioned their value for clinical monitoring at this time. Dr. Slots spoke from the experience of administering a growing microbiology testing service; he estimated that one-third of the clinical problems of referral patients had little to do with bacteria for which probes are currently available. He warned that patients for whom samples are submitted are often suffering from systemic illness and taking a wide variety of medications, making the choice of an antibiotic for treating periodontitis critical. For example, many patients are infected with Candida and Pseudomonas. When dentists take samples, they are really asking what antibiotic to use. DNA probes cannot answer their needs and run the risk of overlooking opportunistic pathogens resistant to antibiotics.

Regardless of one's approach to sampling and method for identification, the discussion underscored the discomfort of several participants for concentrating attempts at microbiological monitoring and/or prediction on a narrow range of bacteria without knowing their relative importance in etiology. Compound this problem with Dr. Slots's contention that microbiological prediction is unlikely to be successful for diseases of low incidence, and what remains is that the most practical value of applied microbiology is in selecting antibiotics and in monitoring therapy for selected cases ... that is, classical hospital microbiology. Does this not return the debate to the beginning: what is a periodontal pathogen?

If I could question Drs. Slots and Dahlèn once again, I would ask:

To Jørgen Slots:

> You stated that, with increasing knowledge, other organisms will likely be useful prognosticators. Doesn't the Bayesian theory predict failure regardless of the microorganism chosen unless it is combined with knowledge of a high-risk group with a higher incidence of periodontitis?

To Gunnar Dahlèn:

1. You seemed to blame differences in microbial recoveries on sampling error rather than on true temporal shifts. Does your opinion mean that little can be gained from longitudinal monitoring until sampling variance can be controlled?

2. How would you react today to a statement of about 10 years ago attributed to Socransky: "Any way you sample is wrong"?

The innate virulence of some microorganisms is a clue that they may be involved in the pathogenesis of an infection. Afterall, species like B. gingivalis and Aa are not on most investigators' "hitlist" solely for their numerical association with advancing disease. The final two addresses,

Robert Frank's "Is microbial tissue invasion a reality during periodontal breakdown?" and Hans Preus's "The pathogenicity of Haemophilus actinomycetemcomitans, a new concept" focused not so much on individual virulence traits but on parasite into-actions with periodontal tissues.

Dr. Frank reviewed the microscopic evidence for the presence of bacteria within periodontal tissues and implied significance of this event in pathogenesis. There was general agreement that bacteria are found within the tissues during advanced periodontitis, but there was general disagreement on whether or not invasion enhanced the severity of disease. Since persons with gingival inflammation experience bacteremias, since bacteria have been shown between the junctional epithelium and tooth, and since almost all patients with periodontal disease manifest immune reactions to bacteria found in pockets, Dr. Page questioned the fuss made over whether whole bacteria or just antigen-bearing fragments entered the tissues. Dr. M. Listgarten raised the point that, since microcolonies were not seen as evidence of microbial proliferation within the tissues, the word "invasion" overstated what should be considered "penetration." Dr. Frank emphasized the depth to which "penetration" or "invasion" was seen and speculated whether bacteria in proximity to bone contributed to resorption, complementing the activity of various cytokines which would be released from host cells. Dr. B. Guggenheim suggested that, if bacteria invade, their presence deep within tissues might increase the radius of host exposure to bacterial antigens and other products. Moreover, he speculated that periodic invasion might contribute to bursts of disease activity. Dr. Preus introduced a concept, recently reported for Yersinia pseudotuberculosis (1), that virulence traits associated with invasion are linked to surface proteins (invasins) for which a specific gene has been identified. He presented results of some very preliminary experiments, which he is conducting, in which DNA extracted from Aa strains appeared to hybridize with a synthesized short oligonucleotide sequence thought to be homologous with a segment of the Yersinia "invasin" gene.

Comparing bacterial penetration into tissues to molecular events in chemotaxis of mammalian cells, several traits of potentially invasive periodontal bacteria were noted. Highly proteolytic bacteria (B. gingivalis, T. denticola), those able to degrade glycosminoglycans between epithelial cells (those above plus peptostreptococci) or those which produce volatile sulphur-containing compounds (bacteroides) may effectively promote passage of larger molecules. B. gingivalis can also degrade many proteins in the inflammatory defense systems. These bacteria can also bind to basement membrane components and collagen, which has been proposed to promote invasion. Periodontal bacteria also respond chemotactically to gradients of various stimuli. Dr. P. Adriaens introduced the concept that bacteria from the periodontal pocket also invade root surfaces and thus dentin might constitute a reservoir for bacterial recolonization of treated pockets.

Actinobacillus actinomycetemcomitans is known to invade tissues and to stimulate immune responses against its leukotoxin. Both Dr. L. Hänström and Dr. M. Wilton discussed new data demonstrating a high frequency of individuals, both diseased and healthy, with anti-_Aa_ or anti-_Aa_- leukotoxin antibodies in serum, even if they were not found to be positive for isolation of _Aa_ itself. Cross-reactions and other nonsampled body sites harboring these bacteria were considered possible explanations. Dr. Slots noted that these new findings conflict with previous work by Dr. Taichman, who reported that only 15% of healthy individuals have anti-leukotoxin antibodies. This demonstrates the difficulty of trying to correlate systemic immune responses with bacterial carrier states; elevated titres can last such a long time.

If I were able to question the panelists further:

To Robert Frank:

1. If PMN are important in preventing invasion, would invasion of certain bacteria, those with leukotoxins or those able to survive phagocytosis, be favored? Is invasion seen in LJP or ANUG primarily because these conditions are associated with PMN chemotactic defects?

2. How does immunosuppression by one bacterial species promote invasion by others?

To Hans Preus:

1. What is the evidence that, like some other bacterial toxins, _Aa_ leukotoxin is coded by a phage? Is there evidence that individuals with LJP respond with antiphage antibodies?

2. Obviously, hypotheses are there to test. You have proposed several. How would you design studies to support or refute the bacteriophage hypotheses which you have raised?

Ending this brief discussion of pathogenesis, it might be healthy to consider an overview of disease. Dr. Listgarten might have stated it best:

Dr. M.A. Listgarten: It is unlikely that what constitutes periodontal disease in one individual is common to all individuals who develop disease. It follows that disease is not just dependent on the presence of single organisms. Not only do host and bacteria interact, but there are interactions among bacteria themselves.

Conclusion:

Looking back at Periodontology Today, it seems as though creativity was reflected mostly in the questions posed in advance to the panelists and the ingenious ways in which they addressed their penetrating topics. As the panalists were sometimes at variance with one another, the discussion itself was lively, indeed. However, it drifted so many times into the bottomless depths of accurately measuring disease activity that one might wonder whether clinical periodontal microbiology is being stalled by circumstances beyond its control and, as a science, is not progressing (especially laterally) as rapidly as periodontitis itself. Periodontal microbiology today really encompasses a much broader field than that considered in Periodontology Today. The discipline has experienced several productive bursts of research activity during the 20 years of ERGOB history; few have been randomly directed and totally independent. Thus, some might conclude that microbiology has already made immeasurable progress. Yet in preparing this discourse on a discussion, I have tried to ask over and over: periodontal microbiology, where are you today? In return, a discordant answer. As in probing any issue, it is hard to identify exactly where we stand, and then again, who knows where we'll end up?

References

ISBERG, R.R.; VOORHIS, D.L., and FALKOW, S.: Identification of invasin: a protein that allows enteric bacteria to penetrate cultured mammalian cells. Cell. 50: 769-778 (1987).

TANNER, A.C.R. and GOODSON, J.M.: Sampling of microorganisms associated with periodontal disease. Oral Microbiol. Immunol. 1: 15-20 (1986).

Richard P. Ellen, Faculty of Dentistry, University of Toronto, 124 Edward Street, Toronto, Ontario M5G 1G6, Canada

Periodontology Today. Int. Congr., Zürich 1988, pp. 324–336 (Karger, Basel 1989)

Host Defenses

Mark Wilton

MRC Dental Research Unit, London, UK.

The host defense system has an obvious role in maintaining the integrity of periodontal tissues and the clinical evidence from general immunodeficency states supports a protective function for immunity,especially in relation to the polymorphonuclear leucocyte (PMN). It is generally agreed that our present knowledge of the microbial aetiology of the periodontal diseases, which indicates that some forms of disease have specific bacterial aetiologies, would indicate that it is changes in host defenses which determine whether disease starts, is chronic and protracted or, most especially, is acute and progressive. This breakdown of the defense system does not presume which plaque hypothesis (specific or the non-specific) is correct but can only use specific bacteria or their antigens to study associations between the clinical status of a patient and the immune response at the time of sampling.

The session on host defenses was designed to describe the current approaches to the study of the immune system utilising antibodies, lymphocytes, PMN and cytokines with periodontopathic bacteria and their antigens. It was hoped that the papers and their public discussion would lead to better understanding of host defense in periodontal diseases and indicate directions for future research. In the summary, the discussion is linked to each presentation and not in the sequence that the topics were raised.

An overview- the holistic approach to health and disease.

Dr Brandtzaeg urged us not to be narrow minded and to consider the whole system. Whilst accepting that the immune system was complex, and that all those elements which are known can be located (at least in theory) in the connective tissues and the crevice or pocket, the ultimate goal for the immune response was elimination of the foreign material. He had no doubt that there was an immune response to plaque bacteria but, since the plaque was never naturally eliminated completely, then in the periodontal context this could only mean the elimination of the tooth itself. Thus the persistence of plaque meant that the periodontium was an area of immunological conflict and frustration with an accompanying inflammatory response.

Whilst it is necessary that immunologists working with individual components of the immune system should recall that they are only studying a part of that system, economics and the amount of material for study precludes a totally integrated approach in any one laboratory. Thus the holistic approach will have to be either theoretical or consist of the exercise of putting the different data on each part together -just the purpose of this meeting!

The the failure to eliminate plaque was generally accepted but it was pointed out by several speakers that plaque was effectively outside the body (in the crevice or pocket) and that PMN, antibodies , complement and the cytokines have all been described in crevicular fluid. If they do not eliminate plaque they presumably could limit its growth,and as Dr Brandtzaeg reminded us, prevent invasion of the connective tissue by bacteria. In the connective tissue these mechanisms would then function as a second line of defense. If the ability to prevent invasion is one mechanism of defence, then the immune system is generally very effective since bacterial invasion is rare. It could, however, simply be that the bacteria are not invasive and that their pathogenicity is mediated by antigen penetration into the tissue. In that case the immune response would function primarily in the connective tissue and events in the crevice would be of secondary importance.

Thus the question of whether antigen penetration of the epithelium does actually occur is of some importance. Dr Ebersole felt that there was sufficient experimental evidence for the permeability of the epithelium to plaque antigens, whether intact and especially when damaged. Apart from rare demonstrations of intact bacteria in the connective tissues, there is no evidence that I am aware of which shows that any of the bacterial virulence factors are present in vivo. Whatever the route of the induction of immunity, the expression of the response (whether protective or damaging) must occur in the periodontal tissues. Dr Shenker felt that the failure to demonstrate antigens in the tissues was not important since the immune response was always present indicating that immune recognition had occurred irrespective of the route of sensitisation. Whatever the importance of the route by which the host becomes sensitised, sensitisation exists and thus the question is which antigens enter the tissues and how are they eliminated or, if phlogistic, neutralised. The point was repeatedly made by the panel and from the floor that we do not know which antigens are relevant in the pathogenesis of the diseases nor which bacteria these unknown antigens come from but we all assume that the defenses are mounted against them. When this is added to the difficulties with the meaning of changes in the loss of attachment, as measured by probing , expressed generally by the clinicians in the audience and particularly by Dr Birkedahl-Hansen's statement that probing changes were a product of loss of attachment and inflammation, then the possibility that immune status is frequently correlated with measurement error is a real one. This would lead to completely erroneous conclusions about the relationship of the immune response to a marker of destruction. It is an illustration of the extent to which immunologists are totally reliant upon other investigators to provide information on which to plan relevant laboratory studies.

Antibodies to periodontopathic bacteria are specifically induced.

Dr Ebersole presented studies utilising whole bacteria and outer membrane antigens and the immunoglobulin isotype and IgG subclass antibody responses to them. His investigations supported the concept that plaque bacteria induce specific antibodies and that the antibodies to plaque bacteria are not simply the product of a polyclonal response to agents such as lipopolysaccharide. In bringing a wide range of arguments to support his contention, he highlighted the importance of two areas that must engage immunologists in the future. Firstly, he has started to dissect the relevant,cell-surface antigens which will give more precision to the role of the immune response, whether diagnostic or in pointing to the aetiology of the diseases. Secondly, he has probed the relationships of isotype and sub-class profiles to these antigens and the clinical status of the patient. Although we know that the amounts of IgG antibodies to bacteria such as Bacteroides gingivalis or Actinobacillus actinomycetemcomitans are elevated in patients with disease, we now need better correlates with stages of disease (and with health). These will only come with the precise description of isotype and subclasses of antibodies to defined antigens which Dr Ebersole has discussed.

The meeting seemed to accept the evidence for specific induction but the concensus that emerged from the discussion was that already outlined above. Until we are told which are the relevant pathogens by the microbiologists then immunology cannot support or refute the concept of microbial specificity whether for diagnosis or to investigate the attenuation or elimination of virulence factors for pathogenesis. We can only add our own speculations to the other speculations about the mechanisms which might operate, whether to damage or protect, when the microbes interact with cells or their products generated by the immune responses.

One point, raised by Dr Mackenzie, was that dermatoligists have shown that depletion of Langerhans cells leads to specific immune tolerance. He asked whether this might be a mechanism in the pathogenesis of periodontal diseases. Replying, Dr Ebersole felt that there was presently no evidence for specific unresponsiveness in humans but that attempts to induce this in rats and young primates had not been successful. He admitted that all the present methods of investigation look for the presence of an immune response,not its absence. It was also pointed out by Dr Mangan that experimental tolerance-inducing systems succeeded only with soluble antigens but another speaker said that this did not rule out concurrent tolerance to a specific antigen within immune responses to other antigens on a bacterial surface even if that was induced by a mitogen or polyclonal B lymphocyte activator. In a brief discussion of the possible relationship of the secretory immune system to periodontal diseases, Dr Ebersole pointed out that there was no secretory tolerance in the presence of systemic tolerance induced by the feeding of antigens. There was evidence that pre-existing IgA antibodies would lead to a reduction of systemic antibody levels to the same antigen.

Dr Shenker questioned the validity of the term "high antibody titres" when the significance of the amounts of antibodies was presently unknown. The term might have precision in diseases caused by defined toxins such as diphtheria where low levels of antibody predisposed to re-infection. We needed to know much more about the meaning of the levels in relation to disease susceptibility or protection in patients with periodontal diseases. If the relevant antigens were uknown then we should not infer anything at present other than that the host had seen some antigens from some periodontopathic bacteria. Dr Mangan pointed out that the functional aspects of the immune responses were more likely to provide clues to the relationship of the responses to disease. He cited the need to test antibody functions, not just to estimate their levels. Although more difficult, cell-mediated immune responsiveness should not just consist of evidence for responsiveness such as thymidine incorporation (blastogenesis) assays but also measure the production of bioactive molecules such as the cytokines.

Dr Lang asked whether we should concentrate our studies on the host defenses in the periodontium if the panel felt that the systemic assays only provided evidence of sensitisation and told us nothing about the mechanisms operating at the site. He gave the example of the rat ligature model where the study of peripheral blood lymphocytes could be correlated with each stage of periodontal inflammation and the histological evidence of bone resorbtion. Responding,Dr Shenker agreed that a study of the site was important but felt that the questions to be asked in the investigation were critical. For instance, was there such an entity as the sensitive patient? If there was, what was the relationship of lymphocyte subsets in the tissues to disease and to the peripheral blood lymphocyte subsets. Regarding functional studies of cytokines, since there were no specific inhibitors of these molecules, their role in the cause of, or effect on, tissue events could only be inferred. Dr Reynolds agreed that there were no specific inhibitors of cytokines but all biological systems had at least one inhibitor so we must expect that they would eventually be identified.

In vitro lymphocyte studies and the pathogenesis of disease.

Dr Mangan discussed this important topic, prefacing his remarks with the observation that the immune response was at least as complicated as microbiology. Although *in vitro* studies showed that plaque bacteria both stimulate and suppress lymphocyte activation, they can do this both with specific antigens and non-specific mitogens. No measure of activation, whether blastogenic transformation, lymphokine production or the generation of cytotoxic cells correlated well with disease. He felt that the lack of correlation might be due to a number of factors such as failure of *in vitro* models to resemble the *in vivo* state or the need to study a number of different lymphocyte responses simultaneously. The best strategies for the future would be those utilising new techniques in cell and molecular biology. The continued use of the *in vitro* assays was necessary to dissect the immune response to plaque bacteria and to relate these where possible to the identification of cytokines with known function *in vivo*. Using strategies such as comparing health and disease, pre- and post therapy studies and human experimental gingivitis, we should come closer to identifying factors which relate to pathogenesis.

There was little discussion of this area which perhaps reflected the failure to confirm the early results of the positive correlations of lymphocyte blastogenesis and lymphokine production in response to plaque and specific bacterial antigens with gingivitis and periodontal destruction. As Figure 4 in Dr Brandtzaeg's paper shows, the trend for studies of cell-mediated immunity in periodontal diseases research has declined as studies of antibodies have become dominant using newer techniques such as ELISA. The data showing that the inflammatory infiltrate in the stable periodontal lesion is B lymphocyte and plasma cell dominated and that plaque contains mitogenic substances have reinforced the view that the antibody responses may be more relevant. The information on the regulatory networks in the immune system, especially the T lymphocyte control of B lymphocyte antibody production, was not available when the first *in vitro* lymphocyte assays were used in relation to periodontal diseases. As Dr Mangan asserted, and as Dr Shenker showed in his presentation, using the newer cellular technologies combined with studies of lymphocyte function such as immunosuppression may yet prove valuable.

Cytokines: mediators of osteoclast activation and bone resorption in perodontal diseases.

Dr Reynolds stated that in inflammatory diseases activated leucocytes produce many cytokines which not only affect the behaviour of other leucocytes but have profound effects on non-leucocyte populations. The cytokines such as the interleukins, tumour necrosis factors, interferons and transforming growth factors are critical factors in mediating host responses. Although many biological effects of the cytokines are beneficial to the host they also have the potential, especially in connective tissues, to cause damage. He proposed that production of cytokines by inflammatory cells in response to bacterial antigens in the periodontium is the major cause of periodontal tissue breakdown. In the specific context of bone, the osteoblast possessed receptors for all the factors implicated in both physiological and pathological bone resorption. This cell synthesises bone and controls the osteoclast to regulate bone removal.

In the wider context of connective tissue destruction, there is a need to study the mechanisms of action and the target sites for the cytokines on cells. At present there was much data on the biological effects of individual cytokines but we must study them in combination to resolve what appear to be mutually exclusive properties of each. The final need was to investigate the balances between enzymes causing tissue damage such as the metallo-proteinases released in response to cytokines and their inhibitors such as the tissue inhibitors of metallo-proteinases (TIMP) and the relationship of this balance to disease. He also claimed that cytokines were really the most complex despite the competing claims that had been made for the complexity of immunology, microbiology and epidemiology by other speakers.

Dr Meikle presented his studies of IL-1β production by peripheral blood monocytes from patients with adult periodontitis. As measured by radioimmunoassay, IL-1β production was high in many patients but there was no relationship to disease status suggesting that the patients might be in remission. Monocytes from the patients produced both IL-1β and biologically active Tumour Necrosis Factor (TNF) in response to LPS suggesting that the cells were pre-activated *in vivo*. There was no correlation between IL-1β and TNF production. Dr Shenker asked whether the fact that radioassays would also detect the biologically inactive IL-1β precursor might have compromised data interpretation. In reply, Dr Meikle stated that the IL-1 was active in two bioassays. Dr Reynolds also asserted that if one performed bioassays then the criticism was that they were not precise and if one only performed immunoassays, they were criticised in the terms that Dr Shenker had used. The obvious need was to do both but the bioassays lacked quantitation.

Again there was little discussion of this new, rapidly progressing area although it seemed to meet with general approval. This might be because the area is new and thus the amount of information is much less than that available for other aspects of host defences such as antibodies. Dr Wilton suggested we consider stopping the study of cells for the present and concentrate on assaying the cytokines. Dr Reynolds agreed and felt that this might produce new ideas provided that tissue breakdown was also measured. If multiple cytokines were assayed using radioassay and ELISA kits and comparisons made between disease and health then the data might provide pointers toward the types of cell are the most relevant to study. Dr Van Dyke described his own studies of gingival crevicular fluid (GCF) and said that IL-1β, TNF and PGE2 levels were correlated. Dr Shenker felt that this approach gave no insight into the relevant antigens and was also measuring an outcome of the immune response that was too distant from early events. Dr Birkedal-Hansen had an open mind but felt that it was important to dissociate the concept that inflammation and tissue breakdown were related. Since it was agreed that gingivitis was stable for many years we needed to know whether the inflammatory infiltrate actually caused the destruction of the ligament fibres and what triggers made a lesion unstable and progressive. Dr Van Dyke felt that all the cytokines were likely to be important and that their relationships to each other needed dissecting, particularly in longitudinal studies of individual sites.

Immunosuppression: an aetiopathogenic mechanism?

Dr Shenker stated his hypothesis for the immune response in periodontal diseases. There were two factors to consider in this context. Firstly that there were active responses, both cell-mediated and humoral, to periodontopathic pathogens. Secondly, that there was a persistent infection in the face of these immune responses. The responses were dynamic and would change according to the presence or absence of disease or whether disease was chronic or acute. The appropriate response was that which rapidly eliminated the pathogen and ended the disease.

If the disease became chronic, caused tissue injury and only then did the immune response develope, this delay would have three possible outcomes. First, and the most favourable, would be resolution of disease and this might be the basis for remission activity in the burst hypothesis. Second, there might be the induction of hypersensitivity with immune-mediated damage by both cellular (Type IV) and antibody (Types I, II and III) responses. Third, antigen overload at a site or an inappropriate immune response to irrelevant antigens would ensure that the disease continued. The reasons for delayed responses might be congenital, genetic or environmental,that is due to the pathogens themselves. Organisms especially powerful at this down-regulation of the immune response included A.actinomycetemcomitans which induced T suppressor lymphocytes, Treponema denticola which elicited suppressor activity in monocytes and Centipeda periodontii which kills B lymphocytes and monocytes. He concluded by stating that we know nothing of the events occurring before disease starts or in the earliest stages of disease. This information could only be obtained by studying subjects at risk for disease such as the siblings of patients with juvenile periodontitis to describe those immune events which accompanied the transition from health to disease.

There was little discussion of Dr Shenker's paper. This was unfortunate since his elegant work has shown not only that there are periodontal pathogens which are immunosuppressive but also delineated the subtleties of this effect by demonstrating that different bacteria affect different cell types. Down-regulation or elimination of specific immune responsiveness must have severe implications for host defense in the periodontium. The possibility that these immunosuppressive effects could be linked precisely with the onset of clinical disease is surely an exciting prospect. Dr Shenker told the meeting of an example from the prospective study of juvenile periodontitis in Philadelphia. One subject had developed clinical disease having had abnormal Helper/Suppressor T lymphocyte ratios and poor blastogenesis to two mitogens when first studied. These parameters normalised after three months and remained normal but the patient developed disease. Other investigations including microbiology, antibody levels, gingival crevicular fluid composition and cellular studies were still being carried out. It is only by performing prospective longitudinal studies in patients with known risk factors that we will obtain the information on the pathogenesis of periodontal diseases. Such an approach must include all the elements which have been implicated in causation-bacterial and immunological-and must also measure breakdown products of the tissues to provide clues to the mechanism(s) of damage.

Neutrophils and their interactions with subgingival bacteria.

Dr Van Dyke discussed the studies of his group using B.gingivalis and neutrophils (polymorphonuclear leucocytes-PMN). He prefaced his discussion by observing that PMN are the first line of defence against infectious agents including those of periodontal diseases. Interaction of PMN and subgingival bacteria takes place locally, usually in the crevice or pocket, but also in the connective tissues if the bacteria have invaded. They had examined the chemotactic, chemokinetic, phagocytic, bactericidal and superoxide generation response of PMN in response to B. gingivalis cells and LPS. The LPS was a powerful inhibitor of PMN function; both chemotaxis and chemokinesis were inhibited and the bactericidal property of PMN for Staphylococcus epidermidis was abolished. LPS did not affect the rate of superoxide production by normal PMN but when PMN from diseased patients were used low concentrations of LPS enhanced, and high concentrations depressed, superoxide generation. B.gingivalis were poorly phagocytosed by normal PMN in the presence of patients' serum containing high antibody levels. He concluded that LPS was a powerful virulence factor and that this, combined with poor uptake of the bacteria themselves, emphasised the extreme pathogenicity of this organism.

These experiments show the importance of studying virulence factors from suspected periodontal pathogens in relation to PMN. Clinical evidence clearly shows that the absence of the PMN or defective functions such as adherence or migration lead rapidly to infection of tissues generally which include the periodontium. Some forms of periodontal disease such as juvenile periodontitis are associated with defects of PMN function such as chemotaxis. It is reasonable to assume that the health of the periodontium is dependent on the complete range of PMN activity. Although as previously discussed, plaque is never eliminated totally, the ubiquity of the PMN in the crevice or pocket and their intimate relationship with the plaque surface would be likely to modulate plaque growth. Both the uptake and intracellular killing of plaque bacteria by crevicular PMN are known to occur and lysosomal enzymes eliminate bacterial attachment. All these functions are amplified by specific antibodies and complement at concentrations present in crevicular fluid. The specific opsonins are not just directed against the pathogenic bacteria but also against non-pathogens. There are other factors in the regulation of subgingival plaque growth such as bacteriocins and nutrient limitation but the interactions of PMN, antibodies and complement must surely help to regulate this flora.

The role of antibodies in defense was addressed by Dr Van Dyke during the subsequent discussion. He considered that the low level of B.gingivalis uptake by PMN could either be due to low avidity antibodies or the surface proteases of the bacteria destroying the opsonic capacity of bound antibody.

Since hyperimmune rabbit serum supported normal uptake, the high titres in the patient might be of low avidity antibody and would be unprotective. Individual bacteria have different avoidance mechanisms and the IgG-cleaving proteases might explain why disease persisted in the face of "high" antibody titres. Another plausible explanation might be the distortion of the IgG sub-class antibody response to produce non-opsonic sub-classes. Dr Ebersole reported that Dr Schenkein had recently shown that inhibition of protease activity by TPCK, but not zinc or mercury, restored phagocytic activity. Dr Soder presented the results of his studies showing that there were wide differences in uptake between strains of B.gingivalis; strain W83 was poorly phagocytosed but strain 381 was ingested well. Clinical isolates showed a range of uptake and the phagocytosis was serum dependent. Dr Van Dyke confirmed the greater uptake of his clinical isolates in serum and wondered whether strain W83 was capsulated. Dr Ebersole pointed out that growth conditions had an effect on capsule production and that human sera might lack a response to capsular antigens. Dr Charon asked whether bacteria needed to be killed in the crevice in contrast to the tissues. If bacteria adhered to the PMN, the loss of cells to the saliva would be sufficient protection for the crevice. In the tissues the PMN would not move and bacteria could be killed by mechanisms such as superoxide. Dr Van Dyke did not think that this was the case since it was host susceptibilty which was important, not just the type of bacteria present.

A clinical assessment of the burst hypothesis.

Dr Birkedal-Hansen introduced this final topic of the session. His approach had been to examine the clinical data of probing attachment levels, thought to support the burst hypothesis, from a statistical and biological perspective. He pointed out that both Swedish and American studies agreed that only a small percentage of sites, 3.2 to 3.9, lost attachment each year. By choosing a cutoff, usually 2-4 standard deviations from a mean of 2-3 mm so as to minimise the Type 1 error, it had been claimed that the fraction of losing sites exceeded that due to chance and could be held to support the burst hypothesis. Measurement error alone would not explain this disproportion. He pointed out that the statistical basis for the hypothesis had been challenged on statistical grounds and that modelling had shown that the autocorrelation of measurement error increased the Type 1 error which meant that there had in fact been no real change. At best the data could equally support the concept of continuing loss of attachment with varying rates. Probing measurements had disadvantages for assessing disease progression such as the large standard deviation due to measuring in 1mm increments meant that small changes cannot be measured. When statistical difficulties were added to biological problems such as probing force, site anatomy, probe position and inflammation (all leading to a large standard deviation), then "the noise overpowers the signal.".

He had two other areas of concern. The first was that selecting a cutoff meant that any site outside this would not be considered to have lost attachment and these might be the majority of sites. The cutoff might also have selected for an infrequent, unrepresentative disease occurring rapidly and thus miss all sites progressing slowly. Secondly, probing attachment gains of 1-2mm follow treatment and this "gain" may be due to resolution of inflammation and not to a functional connective tissue re-attachment. He concluded by saying that whilst probing attachment measurements may measure attachment, they may not also measure the progression of disease.What was needed was methods of functional attachment loss.

Dr Manji presented his stochastic model of disease activity which accounted for the problem of measurement error. The site of attachment responds with gain or loss to many small, independent, biological events and attachment level may be regarded as an example of Brownian motion. There will be periods of burst and remission even if disease is stationary and this will be constant with time. His computer simulation took a site measured 100 times a year for six years assuming a standard deviation of 0.5mm and a loss of 4mm. An accumulation of variable random events were entered assuming that disease was constant. He showed four outcomes. First, disease progressed linearly and changes were well within measurement error. Second, the site lost 4mm in the first year, repaired and then disease remitted in the 5th and sixth years. Third, there was steady loss for the first three years, sudden 4mm loss in the 5th year and then stability in the 6th year. Last,there was relative stability and considerable remission of attachment level for the six year period. Given these types of observations, he felt that it was inevitable that someone would propose a burst model. If the inputs were small, cumulative and multiple there was no reason to search for major biological reasons for events causing change but it could not, of course, preclude them. He concluded that activity and remission were due to an accumulation of random events which were essentially unpredictable, that it was not necessary to counterpose a burst model for a progressive loss model and that positive autocorelation between independent events would enhance episodes of disease activity/inactivity whilst negative autocorrelations would dampen them.

Dr Shenker felt that it did not matter whether disease was linear or burst in nature for aetiology. He said that the model had produced a lot of academic data with no information content. Dr Manji agreed that it did not address aetiology but said that to search for biological predictors of activity and remission was looking for a mirage. Dr Birkedal-Hansen felt that it was important to know which was the nature of progression, especially for study planning. Dr Tanner felt that the tolerance method was one approach. Since microbiology was cumbersome, to concentrate on sites that had changed minimised this. It had also provided information on new species, pathogenesis and the identity of bacteria associated with change. What was needed were better clinical methods such as computer assisted probes. Dr Shenker agreed models were important for planning clinical studies but still felt we were studying the wrong phase, too far from the beginning. He gave the example of diabetes where β cell destruction led to insulin therapy but said nothing about aetiology. It was found that the juvenile form of the disease was autoimmune, but this was only detectable at a very early stage. There was no evidence for autoimmunity at the time the patient presented. Mr Sterne said that the original papers on the burst hypothesis had been very vague about timing - "a few days to a few months" for the duration of activity - and had presented no convincing evidence. If the theory was accepted then study design became critical. If a burst was for a few days only then studies of aetiology would be practically impossible since observations of change must be made at the time they occur. He felt that the evidence was extremly weak for an acute burst hypothesis as opposed to changes in rates of progression over longer periods - a process which could be described neither as bursts nor as constant progression. His work on the Sri Lankan data of Dr Loe, looking at successive increments in attachment levels, allows the effect of measurement error to be distinguished from changes in the rate of disease progression. Dr Holt thought that the burst theory was interesting for two reasons. One was that it could show whether there were different types of disease and the other that variations in either the organisms present or in host responses could explain progression. Dr Guggenheim felt that clinicians knew that the disease was episodic even where the probing attachment level was apparently the same over a 5-10 year period.

Dr Graaf presented his study of ten patients where all sites in the mouth were probed each month for ten months. Sites with a 2mm loss and in remission were biopsied and sites which had progressed always had an increased inflammatory infiltrate at the tip of the papilla within one month of breakdown in contrast to non-progressive sites. Dr Birkedal-Hansen again questioned the validity of attachment loss where there was inflammation since 1.5 mm change would not necessarily be loss of attachment. If body height was measured in the population each year with a yardstick marked at one yard intervals, we would conclude correctly that a limited number of the population accounted for all the growth i.e. the children and adolescents. If we then just measured children, only those who passed a yard mark would be registered as having grown. The erroneous conclusions would be that only a small proportion of children grow and those who do grow awfully fast!

Moderator's conclusions.

I hope I have been accurate and fair to all participants and that the flavour comes over to those not present- discussion was always lively and good humoured. What did we learn?

My impression is that we know very little of defense before disease occurs or in early disease. We know a lot about established disease but we are no nearer to describing risk. Discussion concentrated on antibodies, perhaps because data is relatively easy to collect. The difficult task of probing subclasses within the IgG response and testing antibody functions has started. Study of the biological effects of virulence antigens is also starting. Proteases and their effects on antibodies or LPS down regulating phagocytic cell function were reported. Further back, in the afferent limb of immune responses, the effects of bacteria on lymphocytes and monocytes are known and we will learn which virulence factors cause this. This is knowledge of host defenses but we also learned how we are dependent on clinicians for the clinical status but also on how disease progresses in patients. Given the continuing difficulties with probing and the nature of disease progression, it is perhaps not surprising that immunologists have not come up with definitive answers.

Where are we going? Cytokines are certainly a coming area with much work to do. We should heed remarks about their complexity, however, and measure more than just one cytokine and then in relation to mechanisms of damage by enzymes. There are new technologies from molecular and cell biology but we must ask the right questions and design the right studies to answer them. Reference was made in the discussion to looking at local events, particularly cellular events, and new technologies are sensitive enough for this important step. What the session lacked was a speaker on the local host defences of the crevice and tissues. This is not to forget established techniques and the cells or antibodies measured but examination of carefully selected sites in selected patients will still yield much information about the functions of host defenses in the periodontium.

Address

Dr Mark Wilton, PhD, FRCPath, Medical Research Council Dental Research Unit, Periodontal Diseases Programme, 32 Newark Street, London E1 2AA (UK).

Periodontology Today. Int. Congr., Zürich 1988, pp. 337–345 (Karger, Basel 1989)

Treatment of Periodontal Diseases

Niklaus P. Lang

University of Berne, School of Dental Medicine, Berne, Switzerland

After having discussed the biology, the structure and function of the periodontal tissues, the epidemiology and the host-parasite interactions in periodontal diseases, the relevance of this knowledge for the treatment of these diseases in daily practice has to be discussed and emphasized.

The session on treatment considered the diagnostic criteria and their reliability in distinguishing between active and inactive lesions and in predicting future progression of the disease. Furthermore, an attempt was made to specify treatment goals.

In reviewing treatment modalities, two types were pointed out:
- Debridement therapies (mechanical or chemical)
- Regenerative therapy.

Definition of Treatment Goals

Most clinical efforts are directed at the elimination of disease and the maintenance of health. While it is accepted that periodontal diseases are caused by microorganisms and involve all the defense mechanisms of the host, it is not clear when anti-infectious therapy will lead to the "cure" of these infectious diseases. Dr. U. VAN DER VELDEN pointed to the fact that the definition of "cure of a disease" may have several interpretations. While "cure" in the true sense of the word is defined as "restoring health, soundness and normality", this goal may not be achievable in all situations. A relevant strategy for "curing" a disease, therefore, may be aimed at the reduction or remission of symptoms, which necessitates reliable diagnostic criteria. Since periodontal diseases are microbial diseases, the complete elimination of the infectious agents would have to be achieved. "Cure" in the true sense of the definition would then be impossible.

Conclusive evidence as to the nature of the infection in individual cases is still lacking. Whether periodontal diseases are classical, mixed or opportunistic infections, are important considerations in determining treatment goals. Dr. VAN DER VELDEN clearly stated that adequate microbiological tests are not yet available to document cure and hence, the only practical periodontal treatment goal remains the response to treatment of the patient, i.e. the remission of symptoms.

Reliability of Diagnostic Criteria

Dr. J. EGELBERG took a pragmatic and very provocative approach to answer the questions of

When are we done with therapy?

What is enough treatment?

The decision of whether or not therapy is effective is obviously still based on clinical parameters. However, the standards to be achieved appear to be based on clinical experience rather than on sound scientific evidence. For most clinical conditions in the oral cavity, there are simply no hard and fast criteria for diagnosis. Because of this difficulty, it is frequently not possible to find information on how well clinical diagnostic parameters compare to a trustworthy standard. Therefore, another clinical parameter, such as changing attachment levels, which admittedly is imperfect, but is considered the best available, has to be chosen for a standard. The clinicians, therefore, quickly learn that establishing diagnoses is an imperfect process, resulting in a probability rather than a certainty of being right. The clinician must become familiar with the mathematical relationship between the properties of diagnostic tests and the information they yield. A simple way of looking at the relationship between a test's results and a true diagnosis is the presentation of a two-by-two table (figure 1). The test is considered to be either positive (abnormal) or negative (normal), and disease progression is either present or absent. There are then four possible interpretations of test results, two of which are correct and two wrong. Assessment of the test's accuracy rests on a sound assessment of the truth, i.e. to know whether or not the disease progression is truly present. Since such a "gold standard" is hard to determine in the case of periodontal disease (usually a loss of probing attachment of 2 mm or more is used), evaluations of clinical tests have to be interpreted with care.

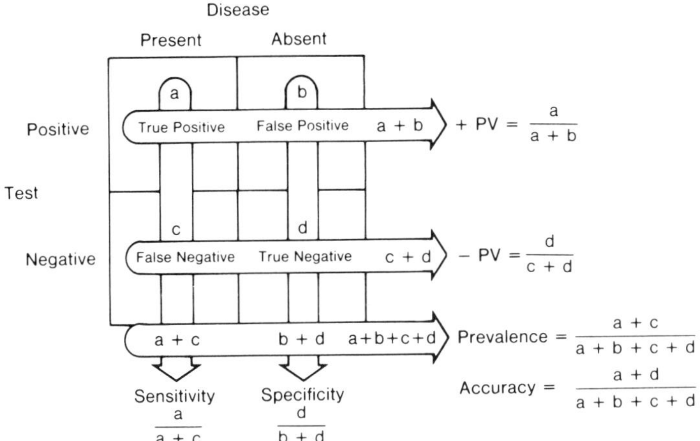

Figure 1. Diagnostic Test Characteristics and Definitions. (Design Courtesy of the Department of Clinical Epidemiology and Biostatistics, McMaster Health Sciences Centre) (+ PV: positive predictive value; - PV: negative predictive value).

Sensitivity and specificity of diagnostic tests are usually determined. Sensitivity is defined as the proportion of subjects with disease progression who have a positive test (defined by clinical parameters). Specificity is the proportion of subjects without the disease who have a negative test (defined by clinical parameters). For the clinician, the predictive value of a test may be of more significance than sensitivity and specificity. The predictive value of a test indicates the probability for disease progression in a subject/site with a positive or negative test result. It is determined by sensitivity and specificity of the test as well as the prevalence of disease in a population. The more specific a test is, the better will be the predictive value of a negative test and conversely, the more sensitive a test is, the better will be the predictive value of a positive test. As the prevalence decreases, the predictive value also decreases because there is a greater chance of obtaining false test results. Since the prevalence for progressing periodontitis may be smaller than previously thought (NIH 1987), it is not surprising to find that clinical parameters have little predictive value.

As pointed out by Dr. J. EGELBERG, the predictive value of clinical parameters rarely exceeds 25 % if bleeding on probing, suppuration or initial probing depth are used as single tests or in combination to predict future attachment loss. Using data from two clinical trials (BADERSTEN ET AL. 1988, CLAFFEY ET AL. 1988), Dr. J. EGELBERG documented that improved predictive values could be achieved, if the data were obtained from a reevaluation 2-3 years following the completion of active periodontal treatment. In this context, increasing probing depth appeared to be the most predictable parameter for future disease progression. Increasing probing depth after 2 years seems to be a much better predictor than residual probing depth. Although Dr. J. EGELBERG pointed out several times that the "gut-feeling" of the clinician or the "smell and look" of a clinical condition would be just as good predictors than a single clinical parameter assessed at a single observation, the outcome of these two studies offered some hope for better prognostic tests in the future. However, it should be realized that only repeated evaluations of probing depth and bleeding on probing are necessary to improve the predictability of these clinical diagnostic criteria.

In searching for additional diagnostic criteria to assess the presence of actively progressing lesions, the analysis of the components of crevicular fluid may be very helpful. However, Dr. G. CIMASONI alluded to the difficulties of obtaining representative and reproducible samples. The successful efforts at standardization have led to several observations which will be important in the development of biochemical tests based on gingival fluid samples obtained at chairside.

The depth of penetration of the filter strip papers does not seem to affect the dynamics of fluid production (at least not in shallow pockets). In discontinuous sampling, the intervals between samplings have to be shorter than 30 sec. in order to obtain a constant flow rate. There does not appear to be a pool of fluid in a given sulcus. The amount of lysosomal proteases in the gingival fluid seems to reflect the number of polymorphonuclear leucocytes in a given sample. This is also the reason why a biochemical analysis of gingival fluid should not only include the volume of fluid, but also the number of PMNs. In Dr. G. CIMASONI's opinion, the number of biochemical markers to be used as predictors for disease progression is small (Elastase, Cathepsin G, α_2, α_1 antitrypsin) and depends on carefully standardized procedures. Longitudinal enzymatic analyses have to be performed before biochemical parameters are ready for chairside use by the practitioner.

The panel as well as most of the discussants agreed that single clinical parameters alone are not satisfactory in predicting future loss of periodontal attachment. However, it is evident that scientific analyses of longitudinal clinical trials have offered enough evidence to demonstrate trends to evaluate the efficacy of therapy in a more objective way. Clearly, initial therapy with oral hygiene instruction, scaling and root planing should be followed by a long period of evaluation (2 years) and then, increasing probing depth compared to baseline seems to be the best predictor of the need for further therapy. Furthermore, absence of inflammatory parameters such as bleeding on probing in repeated examinations is a good predictor of health (LANG ET AL. 1986). Therefore, clinical parameters, although not completely satisfactory, are still the best way to assess the effect of therapy.

Dr. R. ATTSTROEM pointed out that our assessment of treatment will in all instances evaluate the effect of "sub-optimal cleaning", at least in the subgingival area, since it has been demonstrated that these areas are never free of microorganisms.

Finally, the discussion focused on the significance of clinical parameters in sorting out patients at higher risk for the disease. Like microbiological parameters, clinical parameters play an important role in this process. Certainly, even better predictors not only for disease progression, but also for maintenance of health have to be developed in well-controlled clinical studies.

Anti-infectious Therapy

Since it is well established that perfect supragingival plaque control plays a key role in the prevention of gingivitis, the discussion emphasized its general importance to periodontal therapy. Both mechanical and chemical plaque control were discussed.

Debridement Therapy

Dr. R. ATTSTROEM addressed the question: Under what conditions would supragingival plaque control not be successful? Optimal supragingival plaque control measures should keep the subgingival environment free of microorganisms. However, it is agreed that such a goal is practically impossible to achieve if residual periodontal pockets are present. This fact was elegantly summarized by Dr. T. IMFELD: Supragingival plaque control is efficient in preventing periodontal disease and dental caries when a periodontal pocket has not yet developed. In the latter case, supragingival plaque control is only helpful in preventing caries; professional cleaning of the subgingival environment has to supplement the efforts in the supragingival region.

Supported by his own studies and some in the literature (SIEGRIST & KORNMAN 1982), Dr. R. ATTSTROEM presented evidence that the relative proportions of presumptive periodontopathic microorganisms such as Bacteroides gingivalis correlate well with the presence of supragingival plaque and hence, the degree of supragingival plaque control would influence the subgingival microbiota. However, this opinion was not shared by everybody. Dr. P. BAEHNI commented on his dark-field microscopic data (LAVANCHY ET AL. 1987) and claimed that there was no influence of supragingival plaque control on either the existing subgingival microbiota or on its recolonization following debridement. Controversy still exists as to what subgingival cleaning really means. While it is accepted that sterilization of an existing pocket is not feasible, a significant reduction of the bacteria below the threshold level for disease can be achieved with debridement therapy, which is reason enough to be optimistic. Therefore, the pessimism that most periodontal treatments may result in incomplete subgingival cleaning and hence, be inadequate may not be justified. The discussion reemphasized the need for microbiological parameters to monitor treatment efficacy. Dr. J. EGELBERG indicated that there is enough evidence to use relative proportions of either spirochetes or periodontopathic microorganisms as indicators of adequate subgingival cleaning. Furthermore, hope was expressed that chairside tests will be available to monitor a pathogenic environment by determining the presence of proteases originating from certain periodontopathic bacteria (GUSBERTI ET AL. 1986). It is obvious that all these tests, be they specific for certain bacteria or less specific, will have to be evaluated in well-controlled longitudinal clinical trials before they can be recommended for general clinical use.

Some emphasis was also placed on the role of the host response. Evidently, supragingival plaque control would be ineffective in a compromized host as demonstrated by Dr. R. ATTSTROEMS's "Experimental neutropenia" model. Likewise, it was agreed that the host response's role in maintaining a subgingival environment free from disease is very difficult to evaluate. Dr. B. GUGGENHEIM used the analogy of "a time bomb which may explode anytime". Because bacteria are always present in a residual pocket following subgingival cleaning, the host response may be responsible for the activation of the disease process resulting in loss of attachment.

Chemotherapy in Periodontal Treatment

The problems about the efficacy and completeness or adequacy of therapeutic approaches with antiseptics and/or antibiotics also were addressed. While it was clear from Dr. M. ADDY's statement that the use of antiseptics, such as chlorhexidine, is highly effective in controlling supragingival plaque, the discussion focused on the rationale for using antibiotics in the treatment of advanced periodontitis. Obviously, mechanical debridement may not reach an optimal level in all cases and hence, the question of adjunctive antibiotic therapy is intriguing. However, it has to be realized that there is very little scientific evidence, and there are no longitudinal studies available which would support such an approach. Dr. M. ADDY clearly pointed out that in today's practice too many guesses dominate and too few guidelines are available. The side-effects, including development of resistant strains, superinfections by other microorganisms, development of hypersensitivity reactions and the toxicity encountered especially with combinations of drugs preclude the use of antibiotics as a routine procedure. The transmission of plasmid-dependent drug resistance is potentially a serious problem (tetracyclines).

It was agreed that mechanical debridement has to be performed prior to or at least simultaneously with chemotherapy. Even the use of tetracyclines in Juvenile Periodontitis was questioned after Dr. J. WENNSTROEM pointed to the results of a 7-year controlled clinical trial, which showed no additional benefits above those obtained with routine mechanical debridement. Nevertheless, antibiotics offer an additional approach to the treatment of certain periodontal diseases, if very important principles are observed. These were clearly specified by Dr. A.J. VAN WINKELHOFF and agreed upon by all discussants:

1. It is possible to affect periodontal tissues by the systemic route using antibiotics.
2. The potential side-effects from the use of antibiotics has to be balanced against the severity of the disease. A microbiological diagnosis should be made prior to their use.
3. In carefully selected cases, chemotherapeutic drugs may be indicated, if the purpose of their use is to eliminate certain indicator microorganisms also suspected to be periodontal pathogens.

Everybody agreed that mechanical debridement is always the first choice of therapy and that chemotherapy should be used for selected cases as a second choice. This includes the group of "refractory" or "reinfected" cases, where multiple sites show disease progression despite good maintenance care.

Regenerative Therapy

One of the goals of periodontal therapy is to restore the tissues which have been lost as a result of periodontal disease. Of course, a complete regeneration, which would restore the original structure, architecture and function of periodontal tissues, is still an unrealized objective long wished for by the practitioner. Recent studies have clearly documented that complete regeneration of periodontal tissues hardly ever occurs with conventional therapies. These tissues heal by repair rather than by regeneration. A long junctional epithelium most often is the result of successful therapy. Studies have also shown that the reestablishment of a connective tissue fiber attachment to the root surface is not always accompanied by regrowth of alveolar bone and yet, long junctional epithelia or connective tissue fiber attachments without complete "bone-fill" appear to be just as resistant or susceptible to periodontal disease as attachments of normal length and original bone levels. Obviously, loss of periodontal attachment is unrelated to the presence or absence of the bone component of the periodontium (NYMAN ET AL. 1984). There is, therefore, no scientific rationale for placing bone or bone substitutes into periodontal defects in order to obtain regeneration, unless the remaining bone is inadequate for stabilizing the tooth in function.

Dr. T. KARRING deplored the use of bone grafting procedures and reviewed a new principle for regenerating periodontal tissues. Dr. S. NYMAN and Dr. T. KARRING have demonstrated that the cells of the periodontal ligament are capable of regenerating a functional periodontium. This is achieved by the placement of membranes under mucoperiosteal flaps in an attempt to "guide" cells from the remaining periodontal ligament along the root surface in a coronal direction. As a result, new cellular cementum is deposited. This cementum functions well, despite the frequently observed artifactual split between the new cementum and the dentinal surface in histologic sections. Before the procedure of "guided tissue regeneration" can be advocated with sufficient predictability, additional longitudinal studies are needed.

The panel recognized the potential danger of early commercialization of this principle, which could jeopardize a potentially valuable treatment of periodontal defects.

References

BADERSTEN, A.; NILVÉUS, R., and EGELBERG, J.: Scores of plaque, suppuration and probing depth to predict probing attachment loss. 5 years of observation following nonsurgical periodontal therapy. Submitted for publication in J. Clin. Periodontol. (1988).

CLAFFEY, N.; NYLUND, K.; KIGER, R.; GARRETT, S., and EGELBERG, J.: Diagnostic predictability of scores of plaque, bleeding, suppuration and probing depth for probing attachment loss. 3 1/2 years of observation following initial periodontal therapy. Submitted for publication in J. Clin. Periodontol. (1988).

GUSBERTI, F.A.; SYED, S.A.; HOFMANN, T., and LANG, N.P.: Diagnostic methods for the assessment of potential periodontal disease activity: enzymatic activities of bacterial plaque and their relationship to clinical parameters. In LEHNER, T. and CIMASONI, G., The borderland between caries and periodontal disease III., pp. 165-174 (Médecine et Hygiène, Genève 1986).

LANG, N.P.; JOSS, A.; ORSANIC, T.; GUSBERTI, F.A., and SIEGRIST, B.E.: Bleeding on probing. A predictor for the progression of periodontal disease? J. Clin. Periodontol. 13: 590-603 (1986).

LAVANCHY, D.L.; BICKEL, M., and BAEHNI, P.C.: The effect of plaque control after scaling and root planing on the subgingival microflora in human periodontitis. J. Clin. Periodontol. 14: 295-299 (1987).

NATIONAL INSTITUTES OF HEALTH: Oral health of United States Adults. National Findings from the national survey of oral health in U.S. employed adults and seniors: 1985-1986 (U.S. Department of Health and Human Services).

NYMAN, S.; ERICSSON, I.; RUNSTAD, L., and KARRING, T.: The significance of alveolar bone in periodontal disease. An experimental study in the dog. J. Periodont.Res. 19: 502-525 (1984).

SIEGRIST, B., and KORNMAN, K.S.: The effect of supragingival plaque control on the composition of the subgingival microbial flora in ligature-induced periodontitis in the monkey. J. Dent. Res. 61: 936-941 (1982).

Niklaus P. Lang, University of Berne School of Dental Medicine, Freiburgstrasse 7, 3010 Berne, Switzerland

Author Index